F
A

Pharmacotherapy of Diabetes: New Developments

Improving Life and Prognosis for Diabetic Patients

Pharmacotherapy of Diabetes: New Developments

Improving Life and Prognosis for Diabetic Patients

edited by

Carl Erik Mogensen

Medical Department M
Diabetes and Endocrinology
Aarhus University Hospital
Denmark

Springer

Carl Erik Mogensen, MD
Professor of Medicine
Medical Department M
Diabetes and Endocrinology
Aarhus University Hospital
DK-8000 Aarhus C
Denmark

Library of Congress Control Number: 2006939509

ISBN- 978-0-387-69736-9 e-ISBN- 978-0-387-69737-6

Printed on acid-free paper.

9 8 7 6 5 4 3 2 1

springer.com

Dedication

This book is dedicated to my teacher and mentor and my very good friend, Knud Lundbæk (1912–1995). He was a dedicated physician taking care of diabetic patients as well a researcher and teacher for many young physicians. After his retirement, he explored new areas, namely the interrelationship between different cultures. He was really a foresighted man.

Carl Erik Mogensen, Aarhus, March 2007

Introduction

In 1991, I wrote with Eberhard Standl in a book on pharmacology of diabetes: "Treatment of diabetes has become an increasing challenge to the clinicians in recent years. A rapid development has taken place within a number of pharmalogical areas, both with respect to insulin-dependent and non-insulin-dependent diabetes, and also within the prevention and treatment of complications of both types of diabetes."

This is even more true today. Since then we have observed a rapid development in the area with new drugs for treatment of hyperglycemia – both oral agents and new insulin preparations. Indeed, within the area of complications, there are also many new perspectives in the treatment strategy. Combination treatment with agents that treat hyperglycemia is more and more important, also in combination with several agents controlling the complications has become more and more common. It is not unusual that patients receive four or five or six or even more drugs.

Problems within diabetes treatment can usually be divided into two phases, namely (i) acute and short-term treatment of patients and related to well-being and near-perfect physical abilities for professional and leisure activities, most often related to good metabolic control. (ii) On the other hand, the long-term perspective is preventive treatment of complications, both microvascular and vascular complications. Under special situations such as pregnancy, treatment is critical. A number of co-morbid situations are important: heart disease (although not always specifically related to diabetes), obesity (an increasingly important problem), and lipid management (very common). Since 1991, we have seen a rapid development in the treatment of one important issue, namely treatment of erectile dysfunction, which is even more important in diabetic than in nondiabetic individuals.

The so-called metabolic syndrome is also becoming more and more pertinent and an increasing number of patients fulfill that criterion (although it may not be a true syndrome); therefore, multifactorial intervention is important. Indeed, this book is meant as a working guide and a source for more basic knowledge regarding pharmacological treatment, for the practising diabetologist, the internist, and the general physician.

It has been a great pleasure for me to work with many colleagues, most of them personal and/or professional friends that I have known for many years. They represent, I believe, the clinical excellence in diabetes treatment, and it has been possible to collect all the chapters within a few months, which is quite remarkable when you have some experience in editing books.

Finally, I would like to thank the publishers – Springer, who are very much involved in diabetes treatment in general. It has been a pleasure to work with them throughout the whole process – from creating the idea to seeing the book on the street.

References

1. Pharmacology of diabetes. Present practice and future perspectives. Eds C.E. Mogensen and E. Standl. Walter de Gruyter, Berlin/New York, 1991.

Editorial assistant: Birgitte Josefine Henriksen

Aperitif

Edwin Gale, Bristol, UK

Why should anyone bother to put a textbook together? I have often wondered about this, even while doing the job myself. All those who have engaged in this activity will tell you that the work will be harder than you can imagine, that chasing reluctant authors is a depressing business, and that there are easier ways of making money. Worse still, the book you produce will typically have many competitors, and is destined to suffer from built-in obsolescence. All these are questions for those who create a textbook. For you, the reader, the question is: should you consider looking further into this one?

I think you should. The reason, I suggest, is that physicians treat patients, and that this is a book about treatment. Therapy for diabetes is life-long, monotonous, demanding, and has benefits that are mostly deferred into a distant future. Pleasing though it is for patients to learn that their cholesterol, blood pressure, or glycated haemoglobin have fallen within the target range, the fact is that they often feel no better in consequence, and may sometimes actually feel worse. The main argument we can offer them in defence of a demanding diabetes regimen is that—as Maurice Chevalier said of old age – it is so very preferable to the alternative.

A celebrated physician once remarked that it is not the disease that has the patient, but the patient that has the disease, that matters. Nowhere is this more true than for diabetes, for which no treatment will work unless the patient is committed to its success. Insulin is often its own argument, since patients feel so much better for it that they are often reluctant to stop. This is not the case when it comes to pills: people like to ask for them, but are less enthusiastic when it comes to swallowing them on a regular basis—and no medication will work if the patient is not taking it.

Doctors are, or should be, passionate advocates for the benefits of the treatment they offer. Their passion and their advocacy provide the core element in therapy. However, how do we know which treatment is best? Guidelines are necessary and useful, but choosing the right set of treatments, with the help of the person who will have to take them, is the essence of good medicine. And here the choices become ever more complex. Since diabetes is so intimately involved with lifestyle, especially in the overweight, behaviour change is the necessary prelude to any other intervention. Beyond this point, the options proliferate. There are currently nine classes of glucose lowering medication in development or on the pharmacist's shelf, each with its advantages and disadvantages. Further choices as to lipid-lowering and antihypertensive agents will have to be made, with the possible addition of anti-obesity medication. And behind these routine elements of therapy come all the special situations, pregnancy, foot ulcers, erectile dysfunction, and so forth. The diabetes physician must be equipped to deal with all of these, and this is a book which covers them all, which is refreshingly up to date, and currently seems to have no competitors.

It might seem that there is no lack of good advice about medication for diabetes. Specialist associations issue an unending stream of guidelines, and government agencies are increasingly guided by advisory bodies such as the National Institute for Clinical Excellence (NICE) in the UK, bodies which review the evidence and advice as to how money for health care should be spent. Meanwhile, big Pharma continues to generate new therapies, at ever-increasing cost to the consumer. According to one analysis, global drug costs of US$3.8 billion dollars for diabetes in 1995 expanded to an estimated US$17.8 billion in 2005, and are projected to hit US$27.9 billion by 2010 [1]. As these estimates reveal, we have entered a realm of unsustainable costs and diminishing returns. And it is here, at the cutting edge of pharmacological intervention, that evidence-based medicine lets us down, for the sources of information are controlled by those who wish us to invest in their therapy.

How then do we make the best choice for the patient sitting in front of us? At the end of the day, the wisest advice will usually come from experienced, impartial, and critical clinicians, which is what this book has to offer.

Reference

Hauber A, Gale EAM. The market in diabetes. Diabetologia 2006;49:247–252.

Contents

Contributors

Henning Beck-Nielsen
Department of Endocrinology, Odense University Hospital, Kloevervaenget 6, 4, 5000 Odense C, Denmark, henning.beck-nielsen@ouh.regionsyddanmark.dk

Toke Bek
Department of Ophthalmology, Århus University Hospital, DK-8000 Århus C, Denmark, toke.bek@mail.tele.dk

D. John Betteridge
Department of Medicine, University College London Medical School, 5 University Street, WC1 6JJ London, UK, rmhajbe@ucl.ac.uk

Andrew J.M. Boulton
Universities of Manchester, UK, Miami, FL, USA Consultant Physician, Manchester Royal Infirmary, Manchester, UK, ABoulton@med.miami.edu

Knut Borch-Johnsen
Director Steno Diabetes Center, Niels Steensensvej 2, DK 2820 Gentofte, Denmark, kbjo@steno.dk

Mark Cooper
Baker Heart Research Institute, P.O. Box 6492 St Kilda Road Central, Melbourne VIC 8008, Australia, mark.cooper@baker.edu.au

Anders Dejgaard
Novo Nordisk A/S, Bagsvaerd, Denmark, ade@novonordisk.com

Niels Ejskjaer
Department of Medicine M (Endocrinology and Diabetes), Aarhus University Hospital, DK 8000 Aarhus C, Denmark, niels.ejskjaer@as.aaa.dk

Markolf Hanefeld
Science and Technology Transfer\NGWT TU Dresden, Centre for Clinical Studies, Fiedler Str. 34 Dresden 01307, Germany, hanefeld@gwtonline-zks.de

Jan Erik Henriksen
Odense University Hospital, Kloevervaenget 6, 4, 5000 Odense C, Denmark, jan.erik.henriksen@ouh.regionsyddanmark.dk

Kjeld Hermansen
Department of Endocrinology and Metabolism C, Aarhus University Hospital, Tage-Hansens Gade 2, DK-8000 Aarhus, Denmark, kjeld.hermansen@as.aaa.dk

Jannik Hilsted
Rigshospitalet, University of Copenhagen, Copenhagen, Denmark, jhilsted@rh.dk

Serge Jabbour
211 South Ninth Street, Ste 600, Philadelphia, PA 19107, Serge.jabbour@jefferson.edu

Sten Madsbad
Department of Endocrinology, Hvidovre Hospital, University of Copenhagen, Copenhagen, Denmark, sten.madsbad@hh.hosp.dk

Elisabeth R Mathiesen
Department of Endocrinology 2132, Rigshospitalet, University of Copenhagen, Blegdamsvej 9, DK 2100, Copenhagen Ø, Denmark, em@rh.dk

Carl Erik Mogensen
Medical Department M, Aarhus University Hospital, Nørrebrogade 44, DK-8000 Aarhus C, Denmark. carl.erik.mogensen@ki.au.dk

Niels Møller
Medical Research Laboratories, Aarhus University Hospital, Nørrebrogade 44, Dk-8000 Aarhus C, Denmark, nielsem@dadlnet.dk

Michael Nauck
Diabeteszentrum Bad Lauterberg, Kirchberg 21, D-37431 Bad Lauterberg im Harz Germany, M.Nauck@diabeteszentrum.de

Torsten Toftegård Nielsen
Aarhus University Hospital, Skejby, Brendstrupgaardsvej, DK-8200 Aarhus N, Denmark, *toftegaard@ki.au.dk*

Oluf Pedersen
Steno Diabetes Center, Niels Steensens Vej 2, 2820 Gentofte, Denmark, oluf@steno.dk

Johan V. Poulsen
Department of Renal Medicine C, Skejley Sygehus, Aarhus University Hospital, DK-8200 Aarhus N, Denmark. vpj@sks.aaa.dk

Per Løgstrup Poulsen
Medical Department M, Aarhus University Hospital, Nørrebrogade 44, Dk-8000 Aarhus C, Denmark, logstrup@dadlnet.dk

Gerald M. Reaven
Division of Cardiovascular Medicine, Stanford University School of Medicine, Falk Cardiovascular Research Center, Stanford, CA 94305, USA, greven@cvmed.stanford.edu

Lars Rejnmark
Medical Department M, Aarhus University Hospital, Aarhus Sygehus, Nørrebrogade 44, DK-8000 Aarhus C, Denmark, rejnmark@post6.tele.dk

Bjørn Richelsen
Department of Medicine and Endocrinology C, Århus Sygehus, THG, bjoern.richelsen@as.aaa.dk

Jørgen Rungby
Department of Endocrinology C, Aarhus University Hospital, Tage-Hansensgade 2, DK-8000 Aarhus C, Denmark, jr@farm.au.dk

Gerit Holger Schernthaner
Medical University Vienna, University Clinic, Waehringer Guertel 18–20, 1090, Vienna, Austria, gerit.schernthaner@meduniwien.ac.at

Guntram Schernthaner
Rudolfstiftung Hospital-Vienna, Juchgasse 25, A - 1030 Vienna, Austria, guntram.schernthaner@wienkav.at

Monika Shirodkar
Division of Endocrinology, Diabetes & Metabolic Diseases Department of Medicine, Thomas Jefferson University Hospital, Philadelphia, Pennsylvania, USA

Aino Soro-Paavonen
Baker Heart Research Institute, Diabetes and Metabolism Division, 75 Commercial Road, 3004, Melbourne, Victoria, Australia, aino.soro-paavonen@baker.edu.au

Harald Stingl
Rudolfstitung Hospital, Department of Medicine 1, Juchgasse 25, Vienna, Austria, harald.stingl@wienkav.at

Krogsgaard Thomsen
CSO of Novo Nordisk, Novo Allé 1, DK-2880 Bagsværd, Denmark, MKT@novonordisk.com

Alberto Zanchetti, MD
Centro Interuniversitario di Fisiologia Clinica e Ipertensione, Università di Milano and Istituto Auxologico Italiano, Ospedale Maggiore, Via F. Sforza 35, 20122 Milan, Italy, alberto.zanchetti@unimi.it

Section: Overview

1
Pharmacoepidemiology of Diabetes

Jørgen Rungby and Andrew J. Krentz

Keywords: Pharmacoepidemiology, Pharmacoeconomics, Pharmacosurveillance.

The Epidemiology of Antidiabetic Drugs

Type 1 Diabetes

Type 1 diabetes requires insulin treatment soon after diagnosis and thereafter insulin must be continued life-long without interruption. By some definitions type 1 diabetes may have shorter or longer periods early in the disease during which insulin is not yet needed. Insulin secretagogues are often used in such cases before the diagnosis becomes clear, but they will eventually fail to control hyperglycaemia as marked insulin deficiency becomes established. Furthermore, as the obesity epidemic also strikes in patients with type 1 diabetes, combinations of classical insulin treatment regimens with insulin sensitizers, metformin, and in some countries, thiazolidinediones, are becoming more common. Nonetheless, for the 5–10% of the world's diagnosed diabetics who have type 1 diabetes, insulin monotherapy remains lifesaving therapy. The prevalence of type 1 diabetes varies enormously with population genetics, a subject that has been thoroughly discussed elsewhere. Within the seven major insulin markets (USA, Japan, France, Germany, Italy, Spain, UK – total sales) the prevalence of type 1 diabetes ranges from 0.2% (Japan) to 0.7% (Germany). In these countries alone, more than 3.1 million (with an expected increase to 3.4 million in 2011) people are affected. Even though insulin treatment is mandatory, a number of issues cause continued concern from a pharmacoepidemiological viewpoint.

Availability of Insulin

Unfortunately insulin, even in standard formulations (porcine, bovine or human insulin in vials for subcutaneous injections), is not necessarily accessible to all patients with type 1 diabetes. In a survey by the International Diabetes Federation (IDF) Task Force on Insulin performed in 2003 [1], only 44 and 40 out of 74 responding countries reported uninterrupted access to insulin for people with type 1 or type 2 diabetes, respectively. Thus, in 30 countries, people with type 1 diabetes were without continuous access to insulin. Cost remains a major cause of lack of access. However, availability, transportation problems and poor quality of insulin were also reported as major issues. There are considerable regional differences with African countries reporting the worst situation. An unfortunate consequence of low access to insulin is pressure on health personnel and authorities to give preference to people with type 1 diabetes over people with type 2 diabetes. However, as highlighted recently by Beran and Yudkin [2] the life expectancy of patients with type 1 diabetes in parts of sub-Saharan Africa remains extremely short. This situation has changed little in some countries over the last decade. On a global basis, the commonest cause of death in a child with diabetes eight decades since the discovery of insulin is lack of access to the drug. The recent decision by

NovoNordisk to make insulin available to 50 of the world's poorest counties at no more than 20% of the average price in Europe, North America and Japan has been applauded [3]. However, the impact of this initiative has so far been limited.

New Insulin Formulations

In many countries, animal insulin in vials remains the cheapest and most accessible form of insulin, although in North America human insulin is now the cheaper option. The paradigms for insulin treatment have changed within the last two decades with the introduction of insulin analogues and, to a certain extent, increasing use of insulin pumps as an alternative to subcutaneous injections. Currently a new change is emerging, namely the use of non-injection insulins, with inhaled insulins becoming available in some countries [4]. In contrast to the situation in type 2 diabetes, there is as yet no convincing evidence for insulin treatment during the pre-diabetes phase of type 1 diabetes. The market therefore reflects the prevalence and availability of insulin and, unfortunately, health economy politics including reimbursement policies.

The Global Insulin Market

Sales of rapid-acting analogues of insulin now exceed those for human sequence insulin. Humalog and Novolog (Novorapid) had combined sales totalling US$1555.2 million in 2005 compared with US$870.2 million for all other rapid-acting insulins, Humalog being the market leader. The intermediate-acting insulins, Humulin and Novolin (Insulatard) being the dominant examples, sold US$1050.8 million in 2005, which was a small decrease compared with 2004. The market (US$1576.8 million in 2005) for prolonged-duration analogues is dominated by Lantus, with Levemir gaining some ground since its introduction. All insulins, including premixed formulations with a sale of US$2256.1 million in 2005 and dominated by Novolog Mix, Novolin Mix and Humalog Mix, are used for both type 1 and type 2 diabetes (all data from [5]). As a consequence there has been a general increase in the use of insulin. Data from recent years in Denmark (with an estimated 25,000 patients with type 1 diabetes and more than 200,000 patients with type 2 diabetes) are shown in Fig. 1. Data from France [6] showed a tripling of the use of insulin from 1976 to 1989 most likely driven by the increasing burden of type 2 diabetes. In addition, the adjuvant use of novel amylinomimetics has gained some ground in the USA.

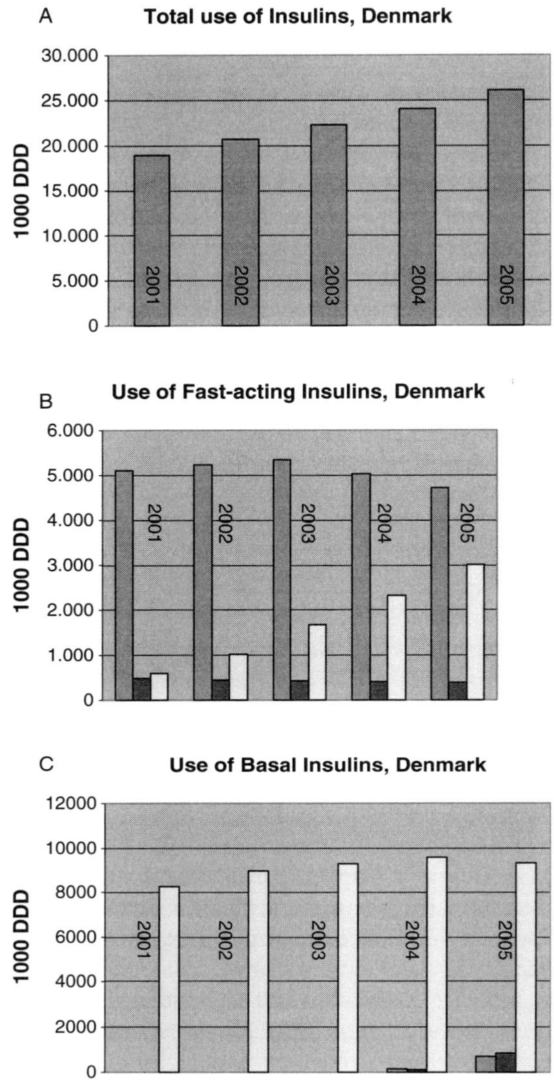

FIG. 1. Trends in the use of insulin in Denmark in the new millennium, all insulins (defined daily doses, DDD) (A), fast-acting insulins (left human insulin, middle lispro, right aspart) (B), basal insulins (left glargine, middle detemir, right human insulin) (C). (From The Danish Medicines Agency at www.dkma.dk.) The numbers reflect the use of insulin in 44,467 patients in 2001, increasing to 56,501 in 2005. Total use of analogues is increasing.

Prescribing of Insulin in Type 1 Diabetes

Internationally, guidelines for the treatment of type 1 diabetes vary little between countries. In essence, the goal remains near-normal glucose levels without inducing severe hypoglycaemia. The options available are legion although the intrinsic limitations of subcutaneous insulin delivery continue to act as a barrier to attainment of this goal in the majority of patients. Although some regimens appear to offer certain advantages over others [7], the choice of treatment remains dependent on the availability of insulin preparations (and delivery systems), local professional expertise and provision of support, and individual preferences of both patients and the diabetes healthcare team. As stated above, while paradigms of care may change, the choice of therapy often reflects the impact of factors other than evidence for treatment efficacy (and safety). For example, in otherwise comparable markets (Denmark and Sweden), the use of continuous subcutaneous infusion systems varies significantly [8] according to reimbursement policies.

Type 2 Diabetes

In the majority of subjects type 2 diabetes is usually not well controlled by lifestyle modifications and so presents major challenges to pharmacotherapy. The increasing number of ways to attack the cardinal metabolic defects of type 2 diabetes – insulin resistance and beta-cell failure – leaves patients and doctors with numerous possibilities for pharmacological interventions. The forecast of increased prevalence of diabetes in the coming years raises enormous ethical and practical questions, which must be resolved to supply patients with the necessary drugs. Data from the IDF suggest that overweight and obesity will affect major proportions of the population in the USA and large European countries, with France at 36% and the USA at 51.9% [1] by 2011, the latter increasing from 45.5% in 2005. Unless this trend is reversed, which at the moment appears unlikely, type 2 diabetes will affect significant proportions of the population. In 2005, Italy registered 6.2% of its population as having type 2 diabetes (increasing from 6.0% in 2004); corresponding figures from the USA were 6.1% and 5.9%. In the USA, diabetes mortality increased form approximately 68,000 deaths in 1999 to 74,000 deaths in 2003. Diabetes is the sixth leading recorded cause of death in the USA [5].

Availability

Varying with socioeconomics and health policies, the availability of oral or injectable antidiabetic agents varies. However, basic drugs for beta-cell stimulation, the sulphonylureas, and for treating insulin resistance and increased hepatic glucose output (the biguanides) remain cheap, effective and widely accessible. Alpha-glucose inhibitors and, in particular, thiazolidinediones, retarding the rates of intestinal glucose absorption and tissue insulin resistance, respectively, are alternatives that have been increasing in use and availability.

The Market for Antidiabetic Agents for Type 2 Diabetes

Including insulin, half of the global diabetes market is accounted for by the USA. Other major markets are Germany (7%), the UK (4%) and France (3%). Highly populated countries with substantial numbers of people with diabetes such as Russia and Brazil each account for approximately 1% of the market. The market is dominated by (54%) original branded drugs; however, generics account for some of the market and unknown numbers of patients are treated with "generics" in countries such as China and India where licensing regulations are less strict [5]. Oral antidiabetic drugs account for 58% of the total market worth US$18.6 billion in 2005, an increase of 11.5% compared with 2004. The market is led by the thiazolidinediones with a pioglitazone turn-over worth US$ 2.544 billion in 2005 (rosiglitazone US$ 2.258 billion, rosiglitazone/metformin combination US$ 382.7 million, metformin US$ 518.7 million, glimepiride US$ 857.9 million, vogiblose US$ 547.1 million). There are few descriptions of regional differences in prescription patterns. It can only be assumed that, as for insulin, availability varies and expectedly even more so since several oral antidiabetics can be used to achieve the same treatment goals in the individual patient. When drugs for associated conditions are included, it is likely that for some high-prevalence countries, Germany, for example [9], diabetes may account for more than 20% of total pharmacy costs; cardiovascular drugs are the most important cost factor, reflecting the rates of atherosclerotic complications.

Prescribing of Antidiabetic Drugs for Type 2 Diabetes

Although hard end-point studies are somewhat sparse in diabetology, little doubt exists that near-normal blood glucose levels are beneficial, relieving symptoms and preventing long-term vascular complications. Guidelines are legion, and treatment goals are becoming increasingly ambitious. For example, the latest IDF guidelines for the treatment of type 2 diabetes [10] aim for HbA_{1c} levels lower than 6.5%. Since this goal is rarely achieved through lifestyle measures alone, oral antidiabetic agents are usually required. Initially, monotherapy is commenced with the most appropriate drug, based on the clinical and biochemical profile of the patient, and in the light of safety considerations. For most patients, drugs from different classes are required in varying combinations, insulin being ultimately necessary in many patients. Current guidelines recommend metformin and sulphonylureas as first-line therapy. Other regimens may be equally effective or even more so. However, comparative studies are sparse. With very prevalent diseases such as type 2 diabetes, pharmacoeconomics become extremely important. Thus, both the economy of society at large and the economy of the individual patient must be taken into account when choosing drug therapy. Safety issues remain important since treatment will often be continued for many years or even life-long, during which time complications, for example, nephropathy or cardiovascular disease, that may alter the safety profile of certain drugs may develop.

Trends in the Use of Antidiabetic Drugs

A recent survey [11] of antihyperglycaemic drugs in ten European countries showed that their use increased in all countries but with very different treatment patterns. The use of insulin doubled from 1994 to 2003 in some countries (England and Germany) but remained stable in others (Belgium, Portugal, Italy). The use of biguanides increased substantially, whereas the use of sulphonylureas increased more moderately in most countries. Insulin accounted for more than 50% of the daily antidiabetic doses in Sweden, the corresponding number in Portugal was <20% (Fig. 2). In an

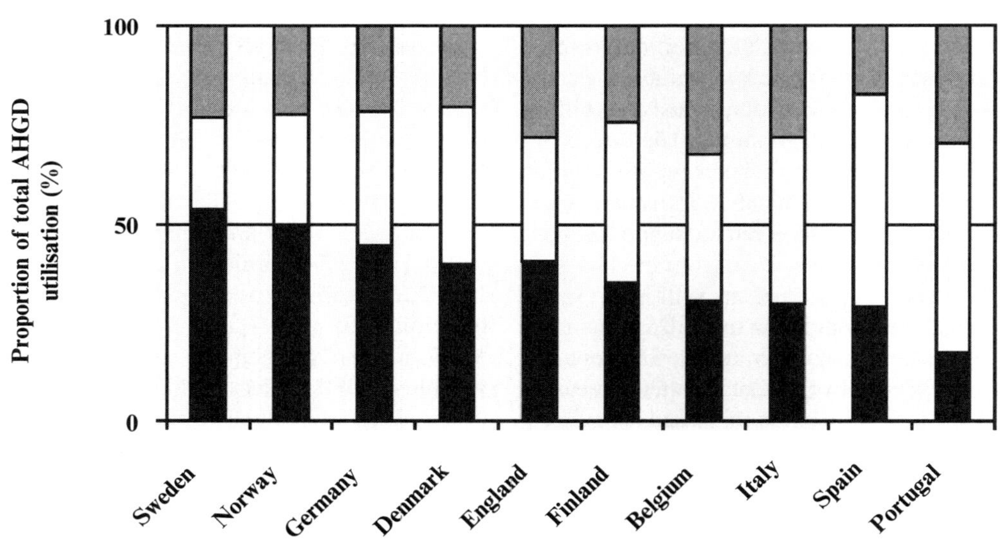

FIG. 2. Use of insulins (black), sulphonylureas (white) and biguanides (grey) as proportions of the total use of antidiabetics drugs in ten European countries (2003). Regional variation is substantial. Reproduced with permission from [11].

interesting comparison between Finland and Denmark (with the expected prevalence of diabetes being 7.2% and 6.9% in 2003, respectively) it was found that in 2000, 3.15% of the population in Finland (insulin 1.76%, oral agents 2.40%) was treated with antidiabetic drugs, the corresponding numbers for Denmark was 1.96% for any antidiabetic treatment (insulin 0.78%, oral agents 1.31%) [11]. It is unlikely that differences in detection levels of diabetes or different diabetic phenotypes, let alone drug availability, can explain such a difference. Local therapeutic convention is a plausible explanation. As described in a comparison of two neighbouring communities in Sweden [12] tradition (specialized diabetes clinician compared with non-specialist clinicians) may have major influences on both drug type and dose. Along with progressively more aggressive treatment of glycaemia, the use of cardiovascular and lipid-lowering drugs also increases with time in patients with diabetes [13]. Although the result is improvements in a number of biochemical risk factors, the relation between prescriptions and improved survival remains somewhat elusive since time-related changes are severely confounded by improved diagnostic awareness and, particularly in the case of diabetes, of recent changes in diagnostic levels of blood glucose [14].

The impact of recommendations or guidelines (more similar between countries for cardiovascular diseases) has been studied in the Euroaspire programme [15]. Among patients with coronary heart disease there appears to be room for improvement in aspects of cardiovascular prescribing if international guidelines were to be rigorously applied. For antidiabetic drugs, however, it has been shown that changes in recommendations coincide with substantial changes in drug prescription [16].

Use of drugs to prevent diabetes or to treat related diagnoses (e.g. polycystic ovary syndrome) may result in changes in prescription patterns in the future. Such changes may confound the interpretation of data on drug use. At present there is some evidence for the efficacy of metformin, troglitazone (now withdrawn), orlistat, rosiglitazone and rimonabant [17–19] on delaying the development from impaired glucose tolerance to diabetes. However, use of these drugs to prevent diabetes is not currently recommended.

Pharmacoepidemiology of Diabetes: Safety Considerations

While phase 1 and 2 trials are necessary for the demonstration of early safety in humans, phase 3 trials (randomized controlled trials) are unsurpassed in design for the demonstration of the effects of a drug on the disease course (efficacy). Post-marketing phase 4 trials vary in design; however, they are often not suited to evaluate therapeutic effects (effectiveness) in the population as a whole and long-term safety in non-selected groups of patients. Pharmacoepidemiology offers methods, retrospective but often including prospective follow-up designs, that allow for the surveillance of larger populations for longer periods. In many cases, as has recently been described for glargine, a long-acting insulin analogue, efficacy and effectiveness measurements are comparable in type and magnitude [20]. Unfortunately, safety issues have in some cases been undetected, and to some extent overlooked, as was the case for troglitazone in the late 1990s [21,22]. It should be borne in mind that well-established antidiabetic drugs such as metformin, sulphonylureas and insulin, even when used appropriately, are associated with appreciable rates of morbidity and, less frequently, mortality [23].

Diabetes-related pharmacoepidemiological research, applying state-of- the-art methodologies, may prove to be a helpful tool in choosing which drugs to prescribe. Recently we [24, 25] and others [26] have evaluated the safety of sulphonylureas by epidemiological methods. Based on preclinical evidence it was suspected that some sulphonylureas were preferable to others with respect to the main cause of mortality in type 2 diabetes, myocardial infarction. In population-based studies from Italy and Denmark similar results have shown a significantly reduced risk of myocardial infarction and mortality (relative risks being approximately 0.8) for gliclazide and glimiperide when compared with other sulphonylureas. This applies for monotherapy as well as for combination therapy when sulphonylureas are used together with antidiabetic agents from other classes. The results were unchanged by corrections for a large number of potential confounding factors, a key issue in epidemiological research that can now be met with an increasing use of detailed databases that allow simultaneous registrations of treatment, disease and mortality data and a large number of socioeconomic parameters. The estimated number of participants in a prospective controlled trial designed to test this hypothesis would be >60,000 for a 5-year period making the performance of such a study less than likely on economic and practical grounds.

Thus, structured epidemiological surveillance of established diabetes treatments can powerfully complement more established methods used during the development of new drugs.

References

1. The IDF E-atlas. Issued at www.eatlas.idf.org by International Diabetes Federation (IDF), Avenue Emile De Mot 19, B-1000 Brussels, Belgium.
2. Beran D, Yudkin JS. Diabetes care in sub-Saharan Africa. Lancet 2006;368:1689–1695.
3. Gale EA. Dying of diabetes. Lancet 2006; 368:1626–1628.
4. Rungby J, Brock B, Schmitz O. New strategies in insulin treatment: analogues and noninvasive routes of administration. Fundam. Clin. Pharmacol. 2005; 19(2):127–132.
5. Riley S. The Diabetes Market Outlook to 2011. Business Insights Reports, 2006.
6. Papoz L. Utilization of drug sales data for the epidemiology of chronic diseases: the example of diabetes. The EURODIAB Subarea C Study Group. Epidemiology 1993;4(5):421–427.
7. Hermansen K, Fontaine P, Kukolja KK et al. Insulin analogues (insulin detemir and insulin aspart) versus traditional human insulins (NPH insulin and regular human insulin) in basal-bolus therapy for patients with type 1 diabetes. Diabetologia. 2004;47(4):622–629.
8. Hermansen K, Bendtson I, Borch-Johnsen K et al. [Insulin pump treatment in Denmark] Ugeskr Laeger 2004;166(42):3685–3689.
9. Rathmann W, Haastert B, Roseman JM et al. Prescription drug use and costs among diabetic patients in primary health care practices in Germany. Diabetes Care. 1998;21(3):389–397.
10. IDF Clinical Guidelines Task Force. Global guideline for Type 2 diabetes. Brussels: International Diabetes Federation, 2005.
11. Melander A, Folino-Gallo P, Walley T et al. Utilisation of antihyperglycaemic drugs in ten European countries: different developments and different levels. Diabetologia 2006;49(9):2024–2029.
12. Olsson J, Lindberg G, Gottsater M et al. Differences in pharmacotherapy and in glucose control of type 2 diabetes patients in two neighbouring towns: a longitudinal population-based study. Diabetes Obes Metab. 2001;3(4):249–253.
13. Wandell PE, Brorsson B, Aberg H. Drug prescription in diabetic patients in Stockholm in 1992 and 1995 – change over time. Eur J Clin Pharmacol. 1997; 52(4):249–254.
14. Wandell PE, Gafvels C. Drug prescription in men and women with type 2 diabetes in Stockholm in 1995 and 2001: change over time. Eur J Clin Pharmacol. 2002;58(8):547–553.
15. Euroaspire II study group. Lifestyle and risk factor management and use of drug therapies in coronary patients from 15 countries. Eur Heart J. 2001;22 554–572.
16. Stalhammar J, Berne C, Svardsudd K. Do guidelines matter? A population-based study of diabetes drug use during 20 years. Scand J Prim Health Care. 2001; 19(3):163–169.
17. Padwal R, Majumdar SR, Johnson JA et al. A systematic review of drug therapy to delay or prevent type 2 diabetes. Diabetes Care. 2005;28(3):736–744.
18. Kahn SE, Haffner SM, Heise MA et al. Glycemic durability of rosiglitazone, metformin, or glyburide monotherapy. N Engl J Med. 2006;355(23):2427–2443.
19. Scheen AJ, Finer N, Hollander P et al. Efficacy and tolerability of rimonabant in overweight or obese patients with type 2 diabetes: a randomised controlled study. Lancet 2006;368(9548):1660–1672.
20. Thisted H, Johnsen SP, Rungby J. An update on the long-acting insulin analogue glargine. Basic Clin Pharmacol Toxicol. 2006;99(1):1–11.
21. Gale EA. Troglitazone: the lesson that nobody learned? Diabetologia 2006;49:1–6.
22. Gale EA. Lessons from the glitazones: a story of drug development. Lancet 2001;357(9271):1870–1875.
23. Krentz AJ. Comparative safety of oral antidiabetic drugs. Expert Opinion in Drug Safety 2006; 5:827–834.
24. Thisted H, Jacobsen J, Thomsen RW et al. Use of sulphonylureas and mortality after myocardial infarction in diabetic patients: a Danish nationwide population-based study. Diabetologia 2006;490(091 Suppl. 1):57–58.
25. Johnsen SP, Monster TB, Olsen ML, Thisted H, McLaughlin JK, Sorensen HT, Lervang HH, Rungby J. Risk and short-term prognosis of myocardial infarction among users of antidiabetic drugs. Am J Ther. 2006;13(2):134–40.
26. Monami M, Luzzi C, Lamanna C et al. Three-year mortality in diabetic patients treated with different combinations of insulin secretagogues and metformin. Diabetes Metab Res Rev. 2006; 22(6): 477–82.

2
New Definitions of Diabetes: Consequences

Knut Borch-Johnsen

Keywords: Diagnosis, IFG, IGT, classification, definitions.

In 1980, the World Health Organisation (WHO) ended a long phase of confusion by providing international standards for diagnosis and classification of diabetes [1]. Before this, confusion existed with respect to the glucose threshold for diagnosis of diabetes and other categories of glucose intolerance as well as the glucose load used for the oral glucose tolerance test. As always, however, new scientific data and insight combined with health political issues have led to several revisions of the diagnostic criteria and classification of patients with diabetes as well as with other categories of glucose intolerance. The first revision was made in 1985 [2], the second in 1999 [3] and most recently the third revision came out in 2006 [4] based on a collaborative effort between WHO and the International Diabetes Federation (IDF). In addition to these global definitions, national agencies like the American Diabetes Association (ADA) [5,6] as well as international organizations such as the IDF [7] have provided definitions that are not fully in accordance with the WHO definitions of diabetes, glucose intolerance and the metabolic syndrome (Table 1). This lack of concordance has not only created confusion among researchers but also among clinicians. As a consequence of the use of different diagnostic criteria, studies and trials may no longer be directly comparable as "diabetes" "IGT" or "IFG" no longer represents the same population in different studies. Finally, the fact that leading personalities within the field of diabetes have identified themselves with some definitions and not with others as the "fathers and mothers" of the different definitions has split observers and users into groups of "believers" rather than into scientific orientation.

This chapter focuses on the following questions related to definition and classification of diabetes:

- What are the criteria used to identify diagnostic thresholds for DM and impaired glucose regulation (IFG and IGT together)?
- Redefining diabetes – what are the consequences for prognosis and diagnostic tests?
- Reclassifying diabetes – how to differentiate between type 1 and type 2 diabetes?
- Establishing a third category – IFG – why and what is IFG?
- Lowering the threshold for IFG – what are the consequences?
- Open questions by 2007

What are the Criteria Used to Identify Diagnostic Thresholds for DM and Impaired Glucose Regulation (IFG and IGT Together)?

Diabetes is a disease characterised by abnormal glucose metabolism, a risk of developing microvascular complications specific to diabetes and a markedly increased risk of developing macrovascular complications. Consequently, all three elements have been used in trying to define diagnostic thresholds or cut points for diabetes.

Defining diabetes by glucose distribution: In some populations [8,9] but certainly not in all [10] the glucose distribution is bimodal, suggesting that there are distinctly different glucose distributions

TABLE 1. Changes in diagnostic criteria for diabetes and glucose intolerance (all values are plasma glucose in mmol/L).

Category		WHO 1985	WHO 1999	WHO 2006	ADA 1997	ADA 2003
Diabetes	Fasting	7.8	7.0	7.0	7.0	7.0
	2 h	11.1	11.1	11.1	11.1	11.1
Impaired Glucose Tolerance (IGT)	Fasting	<7.8	<7.0	<7.0	<7.0	<7.0
	2 h	7.8–11.0	7.8–11.0	7.8–11.0	7.8–11.0	7.8–11.0
Impaired Fasting Glycaemia (IFG)	Fasting	Not defined	6.1–6.9	6.1–6.9	6.1–6.9	5.5–6.9
	2 h	Not defined	<7.8	<7.8	Not recommended	<Not recommended
Normal (NGT)	Fasting	<7.8	<6.1	<6.1	<6.1	<5.5
	2 h	<7.8	<7.8	<7.8	<7.8	<7.8

ADA (American Diabetes Association) does not recommend the use of an oral glucose tolerance test. Consequently the use of ADA-criteria will normally not allow for identification of individuals with IGT or diabetic individuals where only the post-challenge value is abnormal.

in individuals with and without diabetes. This bimodality was an essential element in deciding on the 2-h post-OGTT cut-point for diabetes in 1980 and 1985 [1,2] with the final cut-point of 11.1 mmol/l largely based on data from the Pima Indian population in the USA. A recent analysis based on global, epidemiological data shows that bimodality is not a universal phenomenon, but furthermore in population where this is found, the actual cut-point in the bimodal distribution varies between populations. In other words, defining diagnostic threshold values for diabetes based on distributions of glucose values at the population level is not particularly helpful.

Defining diabetes by microvascular complications: The microvascular complications in the retina and the kidney are to a large extent specific to diabetes. Based on this observation the ADA expert committee in 1997 [5] was able to define thresholds for fasting and 2-h post-OGTT glucose values based on data from Egypt and the USA. This analysis led to the lowering of the fasting plasma glucose threshold from 7.8 to 7.0 mmol/L. Low numbers in the populations included, however, left this analysis with considerable uncertainty with respect to the optimal cut-point.

Defining diabetes by macrovascular complications: Although microvascular complications are only specific to diabetes, macrovascular complications remain the leading cause of death in diabetic individuals. Consequently, it has been suggested that abnormal glucose values should be defined as the glucose values in fasting and following an OGTT, which are associated with an increased risk of developing or dying from CVD (cardiovascular disease). Several publications from the DECODE-study have tried to follow this track. For fasting glucose values this analysis would support a threshold of 7.0 mmol/L while for the 2-h value there is no threshold but a continuous increase in mortality with increasing glucose value from the normal range, through the IGT range to diabetes as defined at present [11].

In conclusion none of the three approaches described here have proven to be superior in defining diabetes. Nevertheless, the use of microvascular complications still appears to be the most rational way as this is the only approach based on a feature specific to diabetes. This view was also adopted by WHO in the 2006 version of diagnostic criteria for diabetes. Thus, the focus should be on providing additional scientific data that could be helpful by conducting epidemiological surveys in individuals without previously diagnosed diabetes, where standardised screening for retinopathy using methods that can detect the very early stages of retinopathy are included as part of the study.

Redefining Diabetes – What are the Consequences for Prognosis and Diagnostic Tests?

Following the change in diagnostic threshold for diabetes by ADA in 1997, a large range of studies analysed the potential consequences of changing the diagnostic criteria for diabetes. The largest and most systematic effort was done through the DECODE-study initiated under the European Diabetes Epidemiology Study Group [12]. This collaborative effort used population-based epidemiological studies of diabetes based on the use of a standard 75-g oral glucose tolerance test from a large number of centres in Europe to analyse the effect of revising the diagnostic criteria. Most of the publications are based on data from between 25,000 and up to 50,000 individuals.

The first DECODE-publication [12] clearly showed that there is only a partial overlap between individuals diagnosed based on the revised fasting glucose criteria and those diagnosed on the basis of the 2-h post-challenge value. Approximately 1/3 are diagnosed by the fasting value only, 1/3 by the 2-h value only and the remaining 1/3 are diabetic based on both the fasting and the 2-h value. The same study demonstrated some phenotypic differences between those diagnosed based on the fasting and those diagnosed based on the 2-h value. Those with diabetic fasting values only tended to be younger and more obese than those diagnosed based on the 2-h value.

As the two groups were different in phenotype, the emerging question was whether this had an impact on prognosis [13]. As demonstrated in Table 2 the 2-h post-OGTT glucose value was more strongly associated with prognosis (all cause mortality and death from CVD) than fasting plasma glucose, and individuals with diabetic fasting, but normal post-OGTT values, did not have any excess mortality at all.

These studies were the first to challenge the concept that the more convenient diagnosis based on fasting glucose values equalises the more complicated diagnosis based on the oral glucose tolerance test. The observations were, however, confirmed by others, and this was the rationale for WHO in modifying the diagnostic criteria in 1999, where WHO in contrast to the ADA recommended the use of the oral glucose tolerance test in epidemiological surveys as well as in the diagnosis of diabetes in individuals at high risk based on the fasting plasma glucose.

In conclusion, the revised diagnostic criteria for diabetes, suggested by ADA in 1997 and subsequently confirmed with minor modification by WHO in 1999, increased the number of individuals with diabetes to a moderate extent. They identified a fasting plasma glucose level that statistically (but not necessarily clinically) corresponded better to the diagnostic 2-h value, but initiated studies that clearly demonstrated that the prognostic impact of fasting versus 2-h post-challenge glucose is not identical.

Reclassifying Diabetes – How to Differentiate Between Type 1 and Type 2 Diabetes

So far the focus on the 1997 ADA and 1999 WHO revision of the diagnostic criteria has been on the impact of the revised diagnostic thresholds. Another often neglected but equally (or even more) important revision relates to the classification of patients. In 1985, patients were classified as having insulin-dependent (IDDM) and non-insulin-dependent (NIDDM) diabetes based on the underlying disease, that is, whether beta-cell dysfunction was reduced to a level where insulin was needed to survive without entering ketoacidosis (insulin-dependent diabetes) or whether the patient had diabetes based on insulin resistance (with or without associated beta-cell dysfunction) where the patient would survive without insulin, but where insulin could be necessary to maintain acceptable metabolic

TABLE 2. All cause excess mortality by fasting and 2 hour glucose in the DECODE study (Adopted from ref 11).

		Fasting plasma glucos (mmol/L)			
		≤6.1	6.1–6.9	7.0–7.7	≥7.0
2-h plasma glucose (mmol/L)	≤7.7	1	1.1	1.4	1.4
	7.8–11.0	1.6	1.3	1.7	1.7
	≥11.1	2.1	1.9	2.2	2.3

control. From 1985 and onwards several clinical studies [14] as well as practical clinical experience demonstrated that a large proportion of patients characterised as non-insulin dependent would subsequently need insulin to maintain acceptable metabolic control. This often led to confusion with respect to classification of the individual patient, and increasingly patients were re-classified from NIDDM to IDDM. This clinical observation combined with a wish to establish a classification based on a combination of clinical stages and aetiological types [15] led WHO to abandon the terms IDDM and NIDDM and to reintroduce the terms Type 1 and Type 2 diabetes. This development was helped by the identification of several markers of autoimmunity linked to the destruction of beta cells such as islet cell antibodies (ICA), insulin auto- antibodies (IAA) and auto-antibodies to glutamic acid decarboxylase (anti-GAD). Consequently, the revised classification included as the two main groups

- Type 1 diabetes (beta-cell destruction, usually leading to absolute insulin deficiency). In this group 85–90% are antibody positive for at least one of the antibodies ICA, IAA or GAD, while a smaller group (10–15%) have total beta-cell destruction without any signs of autoimmunity. Within the group of patients with type 1 diabetes there is a smaller group that have antibodies, but are not insulin-requiring for survival at least for several years. These patients are characterised by a slower disease process and very slow loss of beta-cell function and this group is often referred to as latent autoimmune diabetes in adults (LADA).
- Type 2 diabetes (predominantly insulin resistant with relative insulin deficiency or predominantly an insulin-secretory defect with/without insulin resistance). These individuals consequently have a relative not an absolute insulin deficiency. At the same time this group of individuals have no other known specific aetiology. At present this group comprises 70–80% of all cases of diabetes (even more in some parts of the world), but given the fact that molecular biology combined with other scientific disciplines continuously identifies an increasing number of "specific types" this group will gradually diminish. Apart from this the specific types will not be discussed further in this chapter.

One problem related to the change in classification to an aetiological definition is that the diagnosis of a so-called type 1 process is based on measurement of autoimmune markers, which is not a part of routine clinical practice, and markers that currently have none or very limited impact on the treatment regiment for the individual patient. As a consequence of this, a patient with diabetes with considerable residual beta-cell mass and obviously not insulin requiring from a clinical point of view, but with an ongoing autoimmune process, will be diagnosed as having type 2 diabetes unless admitted to a centre where measurement of auto-antibodies for some reason (typical research) is a part of routine clinical practice. In this case, in real life, the classification of the patient would therefore reflect the centre at which the patient is treated, not the underlying disease process. This would clinically be a minor problem, but with 5–15% of patients with type 2 diabetes being antibody positive, and given that treatment guidelines differ and type 1 diabetes patients are treated centrally while type 2 diabetic patients are treated in general practice, this would have tremendous impact on the organisation of the health care system if all patients had antibodies measured and subsequently were remitted accordingly.

Another problem that has not been solved is that even in the general population with normal glucose tolerance following an OGTT 2–5% are antibody positive [16,17]. This would suggest that some antibody positive individuals with clinical T2DM are truly type 2 diabetic where antibody positivity reflects a "by chance finding" and not necessarily an ongoing autoimmune disease process.

Establishing a Third Category – IFG – Why and What is IFG?

The new category – Impaired Fasting Glycaemia – was introduced by the ADA expert committee in 1997. This was in many ways the logical consequence of their recommendation to stop using the OGTT, as this would make the diagnosis of IGT impossible. The hope was that through establishing the new category IFG it would be possible to identify a group comparable to the IGT with respect to risk of progression to diabetes and risk of developing CVD.

As already discussed, the DECODE-study showed that while IGT is associated with an increased risk of developing CVD this is only the case in IFG-individuals if they also have abnormal 2-h glucose values [11,13]. In other words, isolated IFG is not associated with increased risk of CVD or increased all cause mortality. It has also been shown that while IGT is often associated with other abnormalities associated with the metabolic syndrome as dyslipidemia and hypertension, this is not the case for isolated IFG (at least not to the same extent) [18].

The different phenotypes of individuals with IFG and IGT have led to the question whether these two conditions reflect the same underlying pathogenic mechanisms. An answer to this question is important, as several trials have shown that progression from IGT to diabetes can be prevented by life style intervention (diet and physical activity) [19–22]. These interventions are likely to exhibit their effects through increased insulin sensitivity and modifications in body composition. Consequently, the interventions are only likely to be effective in the case of insulin resistance as the underlying mechanism. If, however, IFG is more linked to beta-cell dysfunction than to insulin resistance (which would be in compliance with the relative absence of metabolic abnormalities in IFG-individuals), then life style intervention would be less likely to have an effect on this group of individuals. It should also be noted that IFG only identifies approximately 25–30% of all individuals with IGT in a given population. In conclusion it should therefore be noted that IFG and IGT are not the same conditions; they are not characterised by the same phenotypic abnormalities; and they are not associated with the same risk of progression to diabetes or risk of developing CVD. Therefore, the clinical relevance of IFG as a clinical category or risk group remains questionable.

Lowering the Threshold for IFG – What are the Consequences?

The most recent revision of the diagnostic criteria for IFG by ADA [6] lowered the diagnostic threshold for IFG 6.1–5.6, so now the diagnostic interval for IFG according to ADA is 5.6–6.9. The major reason for redefining IFG was an attempt to improve the alignment of IFG and the corresponding intermediate category based on the oral glucose tolerance test [impaired glucose tolerance (IGT)] in predicting the future development of type 2 diabetes. The proposed new diagnostic threshold is derived from receiver–operator characteristic curves of the different levels of fasting plasma glucose that predict the development of diabetes. The optimal cut-point (optimising the sum of sensitivity and specificity) was between 5.2 and 5.7 mmol/L [6]. A secondary, but equally important consideration was to increase the proportion of individuals with IGT identified as having IFG. With the previous definition (6.1–6.9) [18] only 29% of individuals with IGT also have IFG. Lowering the diagnostic threshold to 5.5 mmol/L would increase this proportion to 69%. Identification of patients with IGT is important from the perspective of preventive medicine, as this is the group where intervention studies have proven effective in preventing progression to diabetes as discussed above [19–22].

We used the DETECT-2 database [23] to analyse the consequences of change in diagnostic criteria on concordance between IFG and IGT, on the CVD-risk profile in individuals with IFG and on the public-health impact of modifying the diagnostic criteria [24]. We analysed the impact on concordance based on populations from Denmark, France, USA, India and China. In these countries the prevalence of IGT was 12.0, 8.2, 20.3, 11.2 and 10.3%, respectively, and based on the old criteria for IFG only 3.5, 3.5, 4.4, 3.0 and 2.8% were IGT and IFG positive. As indicated above, one aim was to increase the fraction of IGT individuals identified through IFG, and this was a success as the prevalence of combined IGT and IFG positivity based on the new criteria increased to 7.2, 6.1, 9.4, 7.2 and 5.2%, respectively, in the five countries. However, everything comes with a price. The increased probability of identifying individuals with IFG was only possible because the prevalence of IFG increased dramatically from 11% to 16% with the old criteria to 29–46% with the new criteria. Consequently, the probability of an individual with IFG also having IGT decreased from approximately 27% to 20%. As expected, the cardiovascular risk profile is even less atherogenic in individuals classified as IFG based on the new diagnostic criteria from ADA, as illustrated in Table 3 based on data from the Inter99 study from Denmark [24,25].

TABLE 3. The cardiovascular risk profile according to the diagnostic criteria in the Inter99 population [24] (from ref [24]).

	IFG_old (6.1–6.9 mmol/L)	IFG new (5.6–6.0 mmol/L)	p-value
N	1,645	788	
% Women	29.6	38.4	<0.0001
Age	49.4(6.8)	47.4(7.4)	<0.0001
SBP (mmHg)	139.5(17.4)	133.1(15.8)	<0.0001
DBP (mmHg)	88.0(11.4)	84.4(10.6)	<0.0001
Total-cholesterol (mmol/L)	5.9(1.2)	5.7(1.1)	<0.0001
HDL-cholesterol (mmol/L)	1.3(0.4)	1.4(0.4)	0.002
Triglyceride[a] (mmol/L)	1.5(0.6)	1.2(0.5)	<0.0001
Fasting insulin (pmol/L)	47.0(0.6)	37.8(0.5)	<0.0001
2-h insulin (pmol/L)	211.2(0.9)	160.1(0.9)	<0.0001
BMI (kg/m^2)	28.4(4.8)	27.0(4.4)	<0.0001
Waist (cm)	94.6(12.3)	90.0(12.1)	<0.0001
% daily smoker	64.4	64.5	N.S

Values are mean (SD), where stated percentage are given.
[a]Values are geometric means and coefficient of variation.

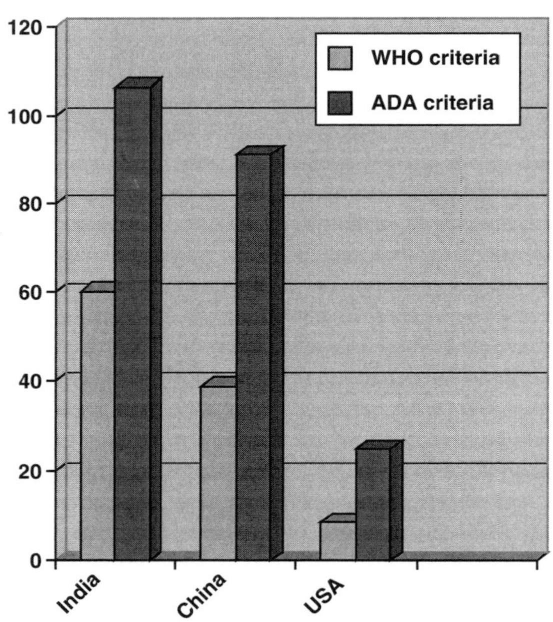

FIG. 1. Number of individuals with IFG in India, China and USA in the age group 45–64 years based on the WHO and ADA diagnostic criteria for IFG by 2005 (based on the DETECT-s study (modified from [24])).

The public health impact of the ADA-revision of the diagnostic criteria is illustrated in Fig. 1. We used population-based studies from India, China and USA and the demographic data from WHO for these three countries to illustrate the effect by calculating the number of individuals in the age group of 45–64 years that would have IFG based on the WHO and ADA criteria, respectively. The effect was dramatic in all three countries leaving the number of individuals characterised as having IFG so high that any possibility of individual-based prevention programme would seem impossible to even think of.

In conclusion, from this part of the chapter the revised diagnostic criteria for IFG seem to have limited relevance. The additional individuals identified by the revised criteria seem to be at low risk of developing CVD; they have lower probability of also having IGT and meanwhile the overall number of individuals diagnosed as having IFG will be double to triple. All together this explains why WHO did not follow ADA in their 2006 version of diagnostic criteria for diabetes and impaired glucose regulation [4].

Open Questions by 2007

With the recent publication from WHO and IDF on definition and diagnosis of diabetes mellitus and intermediate hyperglycaemia [4], a natural question could be – have we now reached the end of the road? Unfortunately, the only possible answer is a no. Science is progressing, and as part of this, our understanding of the underlying aetiology and pathogenic mechanisms behind abnormalities in glucose metabolism will improve. Definition and classification of diseases must (or at least should) always be following progress in our understanding of the disease aetiology. When it comes to definition and classification of diabetes there are a number of open questions.

1. Could the diagnosis of diabetes be simplified? This was the intention of the ADA-recommendation in 1997, where they recommended discontinuation of the logistically complicated and time-consuming oral glucose tolerance test and recommended that all diagnostic tests should be based on fasting glucose. Unfortunately, this strategy did not fulfil its aim, and consequently the WHO retained the OGTT. An alternative would be to replace the diagnosis based on fasting plasma glucose or the OGTT with a diagnosis based on HbA_{1c} as it reflects the average plasma glucose over a period of 2–3 months and as it does not require any special preparation such as fasting. HbA_{1c} is associated with the risk of retinopathy in the same manner as fasting or 2-h glucose [5] and is associated with the risk of developing CVD even in the non-diabetic range [26]. There is, however, still a considerable variability dependent on the laboratory method used although standardisation is ongoing [27], and the association between HbA_{1c} and the category of normal or impaired glucose metabolism is not clear-cut [28]. If the diagnosis was to be made on HbA_{1c} and not on glucose, this would clearly lead to the reclassification of individuals and it would require global standardisation of the method. Consequently, this change will not happen in the near future, but it may happen in the more distant future.
2. Should intermediate hyperglycaemia (IFG and IGT) be redefined? As outlined above, the rationale for maintaining IFG as a separate category is somewhat weak. On the other hand, there is a need for identifying individuals at high risk of developing diabetes with the aim of initiating targeted intervention in these. At present little is known with respect to the underlying mechanisms behind IFG and IGT, but several studies are ongoing. These studies will tell us whether we will need this category also in the future.
3. How should patients with auto-antibodies (anti-GAD in particular) be classified? According to the 1999 WHO classification, all these individuals are expected to have an ongoing type 1 process classifying them as having type 1 diabetes independent of the actual glucose levels. From a scientific point of view this seems rational, but in practice this creates confusion. If the principle was followed rigorously then up to 10–15% of all current type 2 diabetic patients should probably be reclassified, almost doubling the pool of patients classified as having type 1 diabetes. Generally, patients with type 1 diabetes are treated in specialised centres but would that be relevant for all patients now classified as having type 1 diabetes and what would be the correct treatment for these patients to preserve their residual beta-cell function. All these answers are presently unanswered and call for further studies leading to clarification and ultimately to new classification guidelines.

References

1. WHO Expert Committee on Diabetes Mellitus. Second Report. Technical Report Series 646. Geneva: WHO, 1980.
2. World Health Organization Study Group. Diabetes Mellitus. WHO Technical Report Series 727. Geneva: WHO, 1985.
3. World Health Organization. Definition, diagnosis and classification of diabetes mellitus and its complications. Report of a WHO consultation. Part 1: Diagnosis and classification of diabetes mellitus. Geneva: WHO, 1999.
4. World Health Organization. Definition and diagnosis of diabetes mellitus an intermediate hyperglycaemia. Report of a WHO/IDF Consultation. Geneva: WHO, 2006.
5. The Expert Committee on the diagnosis and classification of diabetes mellitus. Report of the expert committee on the diagnosis and classification of diabetes mellitus. *Diabetes Care* 1997;20:1183–1197.
6. The Expert Committee on the diagnosis and classification of diabetes mellitus. Follow-up report on the diagnosis of diabetes mellitus. *Diabetes Care* 2003; 26:3160–3167.
7. Alberti KG, Zimmet P, Shaw J. The metabolic syndrome-a new worldwide definition. *Lancet* 2005; 366:1059–1062.
8. Rusforth NB, Bennett PH, Steinberg AG, nBurch TA, Miller M. Diabetes in the Pima Indians: evidence of bimodality in glucose tolerance distributions. *Diabetes* 1971;20:756–65.

9. Lim T-O, Bakri R, Morad Z, Hamid MA. Bimodality in blood glucose distribution. Is it universal? *Diabetes Care* 2002;25:2212–2217.
10. Borch-Johnsen K, Colagiuri S, Vistisen D on behalf of the DETECT-2 collaboration. Is there a bimodal distribution of plasma glucose. American Diabetes Association Annual Scientific Meeting, 2006, *Diabetes* 2006;55(Suppl. 1):A19, Abstract 77.
11. The DECODE Study Group. Glucose tolerance and cardiovascular mortality: comparison of fasting and 2-hour diagnostic criteria. *Archives of Internal Medicine* 2001;161:397–405.
12. DECODE Study Group on behalf of the European Diabetes Epidemiology Study Group. Will new diagnostic criteria for diabetes mellitus change the phenotype of patients with diabetes? British Medical Journal 1998;317:371–375.
13. DECODE-Study Group. Glucose tolerance and mortality. Comparison of the WHO and ADA diagnostic criteria. *Lancet* 1999;354(9179):617–621.
14. Turner RC, Cull CA, Frighi V, Holman RR. Glycemic control with diet, sulfonylurea, metformin, or insulin in patients with type 2 diabetes mellitus: progressive requirement for multiple therapies (UKPDS 49). UK Prospective Diabetes Study (UKPDS) Group. *JAMA* 1999;281:2005–2012.
15. Kuzuya T, Matsuda A. Classification of diabetes on the basis of etiologies versus the degree of insulin deficiency. *Diabetes Care* 1997;20:219–220.
16. Bosi EP, Garancini MP, Poggiali F, Bonifacio E, Gallus G: Low prevalence of islet autoimmunity in adult diabetes and low predictive value of islet auto antibodies in the general adult population of northern Italy. *Diabetologia* 1999;42:840–844.
17. Ruige JB, Batstra MR, Aanstoot HJ, Bouter LM, Bruining GJ, De Neeling JN, Heine RJ: Low prevalence of antibodies to GAD65 in a 50- to 74-year-old general Dutch population. The Hoorn Study. *Diabetes Care*, 1997;20:1108–1110.
18. DECODE Study Group. Is fasting glucose sufficient to define diabetes? Epidemiological data from 20 European studies. *Diabetologia* 1999;42:647–654.
19. Pan X, Li G, Hu Y-H, Wang J, Yang W, An Z et al. Effects of diet and exercise in preventing NIDDM in people with Impaired Glukose Tolerance. The Da Qing IGT and Diabetes Study. *Diabetes Care* 1997;20:537–544.
20. Tuomilehto J, Lindstrom J, Eriksson JG, Valle TT, Hamalainen H, Ilanne-Parikka P et al. Prevention of type 2 diabetes mellitus by changes in lifestyle among subjects with impaired glucose tolerance. *New English Journal of Medicine* 2001;344:1343–1350.
21. Knowler WC, Barrett-Connor E, Fowler SE, Hamman RF, Lachin JM, Walker EA et al. Reduction of the incidence of type 2 diabetes with lifestyle intervention or metformin. *New English Journal of Medicine* 2002;346;393–403.
22. Chiasson JL, Josse RG, Gomis R, Hanefeld M, Karasik A, Laakso M. Acarbose for prevention of type 2 diabetes mellitus: the STOP-NIDDM randomized trial. *Lancet* 2002;359:2072–2077.
23. Glümer C, Vistisen D, Borch-Johnsen K, Colagiuri S; DETECT-2 Collaboration. Risk scores for type 2 diabetes can be applied in some populations but not all. *Diabetes Care* 2006(Feb);29(2):410–414.
24. Borch-Johnsen K, Colagiuri S, Balkau B, Glümer C, Carstensen B, Ramachandran A, Dong Y, Gao W. Creating a pandemic of prediabetes: the proposed new diagnostic criteria for impaired fasting glycaemia. *Diabetologia* 2004;47:1396–1402.
25. Glümer C, Jørgensen T, Borch-Johnsen K. Prevalence of diabetes and impaired glucose regulation in a Danish population – The Inter99 study. *Diabetes Care* 2003;26(8):2335–2340.
26. Khaw KT, Wareham N, Luben R, Bingham S, Oakes S, Welch A, Day N. Glycated haemoglobin, diabetes and mortality in men in Norfolk cohort of European Prospective Investigation of Cancer and Nutrition (EPIC-Norfolk). British Medical Journal 2001;322:15–18.
27. Jeppsson JO, Kobold U, Barr J, Finke A, Hoelzel W, Hoshino T, Miedema K, Mosca A, Mauri P, Paroni R, Thienpont L, Umemoto M, Weykamp C. Approved IFCC reference method for the measurement of HbA1c in human blood. Clinical Chemistry and Laboratory Medicine, 2002;40:78–89.
28. Davidson MB, Schriger DL, Peters AL, Lorber B. Relationship between fasting plasma glucose and glycosylated haemoglobin: Potential for false-positive diagnoses of type 2 diabetes using new diagnostic criteria. *JAMA*, 1999;281:1203–1210.

Section: Pharmacotherapy of Diabetes

3
The Insulin Resistance Syndrome: Concept and Therapeutic Approaches

Gerald M. Reaven

Keywords: Insulin resistance syndrome, insulin resistance, hyperinsulinemia, obesity, weight loss

Introduction

Approximately 70 years ago Himsworth and colleagues completed a series of elegant experiments demonstrating for the first time the importance of insulin resistance in human disease [1–5]. The results of their experiments challenged the prevailing dogma that "all cases of human diabetes could be explained by a deficiency of insulin," and suggested, "a state of diabetes might result from inefficient action of insulin as well as from a lack of insulin." Furthermore, they proposed that diabetes could be subdivided into two categories "according to which of these disorders predominates into insulin sensitive and insulin insensitive types."

As prescient as Himsworth's findings were, the view that diabetes was one disease, secondary to an absolute deficiency of insulin, remained conventional wisdom until 1960 when Yalow and Berson introduced the insulin immunoassay [6]. Using this specific measurement of plasma insulin concentration to compare normal subjects to patients with type 2 diabetes, they concluded "that the tissues of the maturity-onset diabetic do not respond to his insulin as well as the tissue of the nondiabetic responded to his insulin." To use Himsworth's terminology, Yalow and Berson provided evidence that patients with maturity onset (type 2) diabetes were insulin insensitive.

Despite the findings of Yalow and Berson, the notion that a defect in insulin action could play a role in human disease continued to be debated until the introduction in the following decade of specific methods with which to quantify insulin-mediated glucose disposal [7, 8]. Once these methods were available it was demonstrated over the next several years that the vast majority of patients with either impaired glucose tolerance (IGT) or type 2 diabetes were insulin resistant [7–11], and that the presence of insulin resistance in normoglycemic individuals predicted the developoment of type 2 diabetes [12,13]. Thus, approxmately 40 years later, there was general agreement that "insulin insensitivity," as defined by Himsworth, is a characteristic defect in patients with type 2 diabetes.

The importance of insulin resistance in the pathophysiology of type 2 diabetes is no longer an issue. However, it has become apparent in the past two decades that the clinical implication of this defect in insulin action extends far beyond its role in the etiology of states of glucose intolerance. Values of insulin-mediated glucose disposal vary six- to eight-fold in apparently healthy individuals [14,15], and a significant number of patients with normal glucose tolerance are as insulin resistant as patients with type 2 diabetes [16]. Insulin-resistant, nondiabetic individuals secrete the amount of insulin needed to maintain normal or near-normal glucose tolerance. However, the combination of insulin resistance and compensatory hyperinsulinemia is hardly benign. For example, the more insulin resistant and hyperinsulinemic an individual is, the greater the simulation of hepatic triglyceride (TG) synthesis, and the higher the plasma TG concentration [17–19]. Plasma high-density lipoprotein cholesterol (HDL-C) concentrations are significantly lower in insulin-resistant/hyperinsulinemic individuals, and both a high TG and a low HDL-C concentration are independently related to insulin resistance/hyperinsulinemia [20]. There is also evidence that the prevalence of insulin resistance/hyperinsulinemia is increased in patients with essential hypertension [21,22]. Since cardiovascular disease (CVD) risk is increased in association with all three of the abnormalities associated with insulin resistance [23–25] – high TG, low HDL-C, and hypertension – it seemed apparent that type 2 diabetes was not the only clinical syndrome likely to develop in insulin-resistant individuals. In 1988, the findings listed in Table 1 were subsumed under rubric of Syndrome X [26], with the suggestion that this cluster of related abnormalities significantly increased the risk of CVD.

TABLE 1. Syndrome X – increased risk of cardiovascular disease.

- Insulin Resistance
- Compensatory Hyperinsulinemia
- Varying Degrees of Glucose Tolerance
- ↑ Plasma TG Concentration
- ↓ Plasma HDL Cholesterol Concentration

The concept of Syndrome X was introduced to emphasize the fact that type 2 diabetes was not the only clinical syndrome related to insulin resistance, and was focused on risk of CVD. We now know that the insulin-resistant individuals are more likely to develop many more abnormalities than those listed in Table 1 (see Table 2), and the number of clinical syndromes that occur more commonly in insulin resistant individuals is not limited to type 2 diabetes and CVD as seen in Table 3. Based upon these findings, the notion of Syndrome X has outlived its usefulness, and as the number of abnormalities and clinical syndromes more likely to occur in insulin-resistant individuals continues to grow, the concept of an Insulin Resistance Syndrome (IRS) now seems to be a more appropriate term to designate the protean manifestations associated with insulin resistance [27,28]. At the same time the list of clinical syndromes more likely to occur in insulin-resistant individuals was growing, the World Health Organization (WHO), the Adult Treatment Panel III (ATP III) of the National Cholesterol Education Program, and the International Diabetes Federation (IDF) proposed the establishment of a new diagnostic category; the metabolic syndrome [29–31]. Although the details of how to diagnose the meta-

TABLE 2. Abnormalities associated with insulin resistance/compensatory hyperinsulinemia.

- Some Degree of Glucose Intolerance
  - Impaired Fasting Glucose
  - Impaired Glucose Tolerance
- Dyslipidemia
  - ↑ Triglycerides
  - ↓ HDL-C
  - ↓ LDL-Particle Diameter (small, dense LDL-particles)
  - ↑ Postprandial Accumulation of TG-rich lipoproteins
- Endothelial Dysfunction
  - ↑ Mononuclear Cell Adhesion
  - ↑ Plasma Concentration of Cellular Adhesion Molecules
  - ↑ Plasma Concentration of Asymmetric Dimethylarginine
  - ↓ Endothelial-Dependent Vasodilatation
- Procoagulant Factors
  - ↑ Plasminogen Activator Inhibitor-1
  - ↑ Fibrinogen
- Hemodynamic Changes
  - ↑ Sympathetic Nervous System Activity
  - ↑ Renal Sodium Retention
- Markers of Inflammation
  - ↑ C-reactive Protein, WBC, etc.
- Abnormal Uric Acid Metabolism
  - ↑ Plasma Uric Acid Concentration
- Increased Testosterone Secretion (ovary)
- Sleep Disordered Breathing

TABLE 3. Clinical syndromes associated with insulin resistance.

- Type 2 Diabetes
- Cardiovascular Disease
- Essential Hypertension
- Polycystic Ovary Syndrome
- Nonalcoholic Fatty Liver Disease
- Certain Forms of Cancer
- Sleep Apnea
- Congestive Heart Failure

bolic syndrome vary with the definitions of the three organizations, they all share the goal of trying to identify individuals at increased CVD risk. The utility of the overall concept, let alone the relative advantages and disadvantages of the three different definitions of the metabolic syndrome, can be debated [32–35], but that critique is outside the purview of this chapter. Instead, the effort will be to focus on the broader concept of the IRS, and what interventions might be useful to prevent and/or attenuate the adverse clinical outcomes associated with insulin resistance.

Insulin Resistance, Hyperinsulinemia, and the IRS

Insulin resistance is not a disease, but a physiological abnormality that increases the likelihood that one or more of the abnormalities listed in Table 2 will be present. Furthermore, because the abnormalities seen in Table 2 occur more commonly in insulin-resistant individuals, they are at increased risk to develop one or more of the clinical syndromes listed in Table 3. However, the relationship between insulin resistance and the changes seen in Tables 2 and 3 is complicated, and the abnormalities and clinical syndromes listed in these tables can occur in the absence of insulin resistance. It must also be emphasized that insulin-resistant individuals do not *necessarily* develop any of the clinical syndromes listed in Table 3.

The focus of this chapter does not permit an extensive discussion of the complex relationship between insulin resistance, compensatory hyperinsulinemia, and the abnormalities and clinical syndromes that makeup the IRS, and reviews of these issues are available [27,28]. However, it is important to briefly discuss the relationship between insulin resistance, compensatory hyperinsulinemia, and differential tissue insulin sensitivity in the pathogenesis of the abnormalities and clinical syndromes that make up the IRS. To begin with, type 2 diabetes is the only clinical syndrome listed in Table 3 that is not associated with a significant degree of hyperinsulinemia. Obviously, in this instance, it is the failure of the pancreatic β-cell to adequately compensate for the insulin resistance that is responsible for the development of the clinical syndrome [16]. In the case of the other abnormalities and clinical syndromes listed in Tables 2 and 3, it is the relationship between insulin resistance, compensatory hyperinsulinemia, and the individual tissue response to the chronically elevated plasma insulin concentrations that is responsible for the observed pathophysiology. In this context, it is necessary to address the question of differential tissue insulin sensitivity, for if this phenomenon did not exist, there would be no IRS. For example, the ability of insulin to stimulate muscle glucose uptake and inhibit free fatty acid (FFA) release from the adipose tissue is highly correlated [36]. In insulin-resistant individuals, daylong increases in plasma insulin (muscle insulin resistance) and FFA (adipose tissue insulin resistance) concentrations act upon a liver that is insulin sensitive to stimulate hepatic TG synthesis [17,18]. One consequence of these events will be an increase in hepatic very low-density lipoprotein (VLDL)-TG synthesis and secretion, leading to hypertriglyceridemia, while at the same time there will be a tendency for the fat content of the liver to increase and nonalcoholic fatty liver disease to develop. The kidney is another example of an organ that retains normal insulin sensitivity in the presence of muscle and adipose tissue insulin resistance, and the compensatory hyperinsulinemia increases renal sodium retention and decreases uric acid clearance, thus contributing to the increased prevalence of essential hypertension and higher plasma uric acid concentrations in individuals with the IRS [37]. A third example is polycystic ovary syndrome (PCOS), where insulin increases testosterone secretion by ovaries that are likely to be hypersensitive to the stimulatory effects of insulin [38].

Thus, although insulin resistance at the level of the muscle and the adipose tissue may be the fundamental abnormality that underlies the IRS, it is the compensatory hyperinsulinemia, preventing the development of type 2 diabetes in insulin-resistant individuals, which is responsible for most, if not all, of the abnormalities and clinical syndromes that constitute the IRS. In other words, if differential tissue sensitivity to insulin did not exist, and if all tissues were equally resistant to the action of insulin, there would be no IRS.

Interventions Aimed at Improving Insulin Sensitivity

It is not possible within the confines of this chapter to discuss all possible therapeutic approaches to the abnormalities and clinical syndromes that comprise the IRS. For example, although type 2 diabetes is one of the clinical syndromes that occur more commonly in insulin-resistant individuals, guidelines outlining appropriate treatment are readily available, and need not be reviewed here. Instead an attempt will be made to selectively address issues considered to be of particular clinical relevance; decisions for inclusion and exclusion that will clearly reflect the biases of the author.

If insulin resistance/compensatory hyperinsulinemia play a primary role in the pathogenesis of the IRS, it seems obvious that increasing insulin sensitivity, and thereby also lowering circulating plasma insulin concentrations, should be the treatment of choice. Unfortunately, as should soon become apparent, the situation is not quite that simple. In this next section, an attempt will be made to clarify the preceding, somewhat opaque, sentence.

Weight Loss

It has been clear for more than 30 years that overweight/obese individuals are more likely to be insulin-resistant/hyperinsulinemic, and that weight loss in these individuals will improve insulin sensitivity, associated with lower plasma insulin concentrations and an improved lipoprotein phenotype [39]. It is now well-recognized that a variety of metabolic abnormalities improve when overweight/obese individuals lose weight, and that this intervention can lead to substantial clinical benefit. For example, it has been shown that weight loss leads to clinical improvement in patients with essential hypertension [40], PCOS [41], and nonalcoholic fatty liver disease [42]. Of greater relevance to this book is the finding that weight loss, in association with an increase in physical activity, can delay the progression of IGT to frank 2 diabetes [43,44]. However, rather than discuss these findings in detail, since they have been addressed in many other presentations, the emphasis in the remainder of this section will be on some issues that are less commonly considered and are perhaps less well-appreciated.

Although the gravity of the obesity epidemic is well appreciated, efforts to deal with it effectively are compromised by widespread pessimism concerning the ability to achieve sustained weight loss in overweight/obese individuals. The problem is further confounded by continuing controversies concerning the relative superiority of weight-loss diets that vary widely in their macronutrient content. In the absence of compelling evidence that compliance is greater with any specific macronutrient combination, other than the necessity that individuals are willing and able to follow a diet containing less energy than they use, it does not seem possible to propose the "best" diet to help overweight/obese individuals with the IRS lose weight.

In this context, it must be emphasized that not all overweight/obese individuals are insulin resistant and at increased risk to develop the adverse consequences associated with the defect in insulin action. Prospective studies from our research group have indicated that the upper-third of an apparently healthy population is sufficiently insulin resistant to develop the adverse clinical syndromes of the IRS, whereas those in the lower-third are at much less risk [45,46]. Although approximately 75% of individuals in the most insulin-resistant tertile are overweight/obese, 30% of those in the most insulin sensitive tertile are also overweight/obese, and at low risk of the IRS [47]. Thus, it seems sensible that the most intensive efforts at weight loss be initiated in those overweight/obese individuals that will benefit the most if the intervention is successful. Obviously, the first step in achieving that goal would be to identify those overweight/obese persons that are also insulin resistant, and it appears that there is a relatively simple way to accomplish that task [48].

How to Identify Overweight/Obese Individuals Who Will Benefit the Most From Weight Loss

Since there is no simple clinical way to quantify insulin resistance, the alternative is to either initiate similar efforts at weight loss in all overweight/obese persons, or use surrogate estimates of insulin resistance to identify those that will benefit the most from weight loss. Health care professionals electing the second course usually rely on measurements of fasting plasma insulin (FPI) concentrations, or various formulae involving the use of both fasting plasma glucose (FPG) and insulin concentrations (HOMA-IR, QUICKI, FPG × FPI, etc.) to identify insulin-resistant persons. FPI concentrations are reasonably predictive of direct measures of insulin resistance in nondiabetic individuals, but the relationship (r-value ~0.6) only accounts for ~36% of the variability in insulin action, and the use of the more complicated surrogate estimates of insulin action does not substantially increase the magnitude of the relationship [15,49]. More importantly, plasma insulin measurements are not standardized, and it is not possible to interpret the clinical significance of values from one laboratory to another. We have shown in overweight/obese individuals that the plasma TG/HDL-C concentration ratio is as good a surrogate marker of insulin resistance as is FPI concentration, and has the added ability to identify individuals who have the atherogenic profile that characterizes the IRS, and are thereby at increased risk of CVD [48]. Based upon the results of these studies, we have suggested that an overweight/obese person with a TG/HDL-C concentration ratio (mg/dL) ≥3.0 is highly likely to be both insulin resistant and at increased CVD risk; the higher the value, the less sensitive and the more specific the ratio, while values <3.0 increase sensitivity and lose specificity. This approach is certainly not perfect, but it does provide a way to decrease the number of overweight/obese individuals that deserve intensive weight loss efforts, and identify those that will benefit the most if weight loss can be accomplished.

Insulin-Resistant Individuals Can Lose Weight

Although there appears to a perception that insulin-resistant/hyperinsulinemic individuals cannot lose weight, several studies, performed in different ethnic groups, have indicated that insulin-resistant individuals, using either insulin concentrations as a surrogate measure of insulin resistance, or direct measures of insulin-mediated glucose disposal, either gain the same, or less weight, over time [50–54]. Furthermore, the ability to lose weight in response to calorie-restricted diets does not vary as a function of differences in either insulin resistance or daylong circulating insulin concentrations [55,56]. Consequently, although it is very difficult to carry out successful weight loss programs, the impediment is not because the individual may be insulin resistant/hyperinsulinemic.

Benefits of Weight Loss in Insulin-Resistant, Overweight/Obese Individuals

As indicated at the beginning of this section, it was shown many years ago that insulin sensitivity improved when insulin-resistant, nondiabetic, overweight/obese individuals lost weight, associated with a decrease in the plasma insulin response to oral glucose and lower plasma TG concentrations [39]. Similar improvements in insulin sensitivity have been demonstrated in several subsequent studies, and we have also shown following moderate weight loss that the slightly elevated daylong plasma glucose and FFA concentrations seen in nondiabetic, insulin-resistant, overweight individuals return to the values of equally overweight, insulin-sensitive person [55–57]. Although the daylong hyperinsulinemia that characterizes nondiabetic, overweight, insulin-resistant individuals also declines with weight loss, it usually does not fall to the level seen in insulin sensitive, equally obese individuals [55–58]. Concentrations of C-reactive protein (CRP) and asymmetric dimethylarginine are also higher in insulin-resistant than in insulin-sensitive individuals matched for adiposity [57,58], and fall in association with weight loss in insulin-resistant persons. Thus, a moderate amount of weight loss in insulin-resistant, overweight/obese individuals improves insulin sensitivity, resulting in changes in carbohydrate and lipid metabolism, and markers of vascular inflammation and endothelial dysfunction that would decrease risk of type 2 diabetes, CVD, and other clinical syndromes associated with the IRS.

Pharmacological Interventions

There are three pharmacological agents often referred to as "insulin sensitizers"; two thiazolidenedione (TZD) compounds (rosiglitazone and pioglitazone) and metformin. Despite the frequency with which this term is applied to metformin, in the absence of weight loss, insulin-stimulated glucose disposal does not increase in metformin-treated individuals [59–61]. It is outside the province of this chapter to discuss the mechanism of action of metformin, nor its use as an effective treatment of type 2 diabetes or PCOS, but the clinical utility of metformin does not seem to reside in its ability to enhance insulin-stimulated glucose uptake.

In contrast, there is no question that TZD compounds will enhance insulin-stimulated glucose uptake in insulin-resistant, nondiabetic individuals, associated with a decrease in daylong plasma insulin and FFA concentrations [62,63]. In addition, there is evidence that TZD compounds have potentially clinically beneficial effects, independent of their ability to enhance insulin sensitivity, for example, decreasing circulating inflammatory markers and increases in plasma adiponectin concentrations [62,64].

In addition to their clinically useful metabolic benefits, TZD compounds are approved for treatment of type 2 diabetes, and have been shown to decrease hepatic steatosis in patients with nonalcoholic fatty liver disease [65] and result in pregnancy when given to women with PCOS [66]. In light of this appealing clinical profile, the possibility that these compounds might be particularly effective in reducing CVD, and preventing the development of type 2 diabetes in particularly susceptible individuals, that is, insulin resistant, but without known disease. At the present time there are no data indicating that the development of CVD can be decreased when a TZD compound is given to insulin-resistant, nondiabetic individuals, with no evidence of CVD. On the other hand, there is information concerning the use of "insulin sensitizers" in delaying the progression to type 2 diabetes of individuals classified as having prediabetes.

Diabetes Prevention Program

The study [44] was initiated with two pharmacological treatment arms (metformin and troglitazone); however, the hepatic toxicity of troglitazone resulted in a premature closure of that portion of the study. As discussed above, although metformin is unlikely to act by increasing insulin-stimulated glucose disposal, it is often considered to be an "insulin sensitizer." Be that as it may, the report of the diabetes prevention program (DPP; [44]) found that the administration of metformin, 850 mg, twice/day, resulted in a 31% decrease in the incidence of type 2 diabetes during the average follow-up period of 2.8 years. Parenthetically, the life-style intervention of weight loss and increased physical activity led to a 58% decrease in the incidence of diabetes, and this intervention was statistically more effective than metformin.

The results of metformin treatment arm are often viewed as evidence that "diabetes was prevented." However, it is essential to distinguish between preventing type 2 diabetes, as compared with simply lowering plasma glucose concentration by administering an effective anti-hyperglycemic agent. In the case of metformin, 668 individuals were willing to stop the drug for 1–2 weeks, and within this period ~8% of these apparently nondiabetic subjects met the diagnostic criteria for diabetes [67]. Based on these data, the authors concluded that 26% of the initial impact of metformin to delay the appearance of type 2 diabetes in the initial study was related to the anti-hyperglycemic effect of metformin. On the other hand, since the period of withdrawal was relatively short, an average of 11 days, it could be argued that this estimate may well be an underestimate.

The DREAM Trial

The second large trial [68] attempting "to prevent" type 2 diabetes involved the administration of rosiglitazone RSG), 8 mg/day for 2 years, to more than 5,000 volunteers with either IGT or impaired fasting glucose (IFG). At the end of the study period, significantly fewer RSG-treated subjects had type 2 diabetes than the placebo-treated group (10.6% vs. 25.0%, $p < 0.001$). Not unexpectedly, the mean decrease in both FPG (0.5 mmol/l) and plasma glucose concentration 2 h after oral glucose (1.6 mmol/l) were lower in those receiving RSG. There was also a significant decrease in both systolic (1.7 mmHg) and diastolic (1.4 mmHg) blood pressure in the RSG-treated group. The improvement in glycemia in those receiving RSG was seen despite an average increase in body weight of 2.2 kg. Several measures of CVD were also evaluated, without any evidence that RSG-treated individuals were faring better. Indeed, there was a significant increase in the number of subjects with "confirmed heart failure" in RSG-treated subjects ($p = 0.01$), and the composite evidence of CVD was actually somewhat lower in placebo-treated subjects ($p = 0.08$).

Although the authors state that a withdrawal period is planned, there are currently no data available similar to the DPP study regarding how often the RSG was "treating" type 2 diabetes, rather than delaying its progression.

Pharmacological Interventions Aimed at Decreasing CVD Risk

Theoretically, if insulin sensitivity is enhanced in insulin-resistant persons, the associated improvement in CVD risk factors should lead to a decrease in CVD. Although there is substantive evidence that weight loss and treatment with TZD compounds will improve insulin sensitivity in insulin-resistant individuals, associated with an improved CVD *risk* profile, there are no clinical trials that provide experimental evidence that either approach will decrease CVD *events*. In the absence of such information, it is necessary to consider the potential clinical utility of addressing specific CVD risk factors, associated with the IRS, in an effort to decrease CVD. In the next section, therapeutic approaches to two such factors – dyslipidemia and hypertension – will be considered.

Dyslipidemia

Although a high plasma TG was the first abnormality in lipoprotein metabolism shown to be associated with insulin resistance and compensatory hyperinsulinemia [17,18], it is now apparent (see Table 2) that the dyslipidemia in the IRS consists of high TG and low HDL-C concentrations, smaller and denser LDL-particles, and the postprandial accumulation of TG-rich remnant lipoproteins [69]. Since all of these changes increase risk of CVD [24,25,70,71], it seems reasonable to suggest that clinical interventions aimed at improving this highly atherogenic lipoprotein profile would be highly desirable. Furthermore, since a low HDL-C concentration, a shift to smaller and denser LDL-particles, and an increase in postprandial lipemia are highly related to an increase in the plasma TG-pool size [69], treating hypertriglyceridemia offers a rational target to decrease the adverse effect of the dyslipidemia of the IRS on CVD risk. Given this theoretical context, it should not be surprising that evidence from both the Helsinki Heart Study and the Veterans Affairs HDL Intervention Trial (VA-HIT) study showed that CVD was decreased with administration of gemfibrozil [72,73], a drug that lowers plasma TG concentration. It is of particular interest that the data from the VA-HIT study also indicated that the greatest decrease in CVD associated with gemfibrozil treatment was seen in those individuals classified as being insulin resistant on the basis of their FPI concentration [74].

Based upon these data, it seems reasonable to conclude that insulin resistance/compensatory hyperinsulinemia is highly likely to be present in apparently healthy individuals displaying the atherogenic lipoprotein profile characteristic of the IRS, and such persons will benefit from treatment with gemfibrozil.

Essential Hypertension

Approximately 50% of patients with essential hypertension are insulin resistant/hyperinsulinemic [75], and it is this subset of patients with essential hypertension that have the atherogenic lipoprotein phenotype characteristic of individuals with the IRS: high TG and low HDL-C concentrations, smaller and denser LDL-particles, and an exaggerated degree of postprandial lipemia [69]. Furthermore, there is evidence that it is these patients in whom essential hypertension is present as a component of the IRS that are at the greatest CVD risk [76–79]. The importance of the link between the dyslipidemia present in insulin-resistant/hyperinsulinemic patients with essential hypertension and CVD has received considerable support from results of the Copenhagen Male Study. In one publication [78], Jeppesen and colleagues demonstrated that blood pressure, per se, was less predictive of CVD in individuals with the characteristic dyslipidemia of the IRS – a high TG and a low HDL-C concentration – than in those without these changes in lipid metabolism. These findings support the view that the development of CVD in individuals with a high TG and low HDL-C concentration was independent of differences in baseline systolic or diastolic blood pressure. In contrast, the higher either systolic ($p < 0.001$) or diastolic ($p < 0.03$) blood pressure was at the beginning of the study, the greater the incidence of CVD in those without the dyslipidemia of the IRS.

In a second study [79], participants in the prospective Copenhagen Male Study were divided into three groups on the basis of their fasting plasma TG and HDL-C concentrations. Individuals, whose plasma TG and HDL-C concentrations were in the upper third or lower third, respectively, of the whole population, were assigned to the high TG-low HDL-C group. At the other extreme, a low TG-high HDL-C group was composed of those individuals whose plasma TG and HDL-C concentrations were in the lower third and upper third, respectively, of the study population for these two lipid measurements. The intermediate group consisted of those participants whose lipid values did not qualify them for either of the two extreme groups. The results of their analysis indicated that the development of CVD in patients with hypertension in the lowest TG and highest HDL-C category was no different than in normotensive individuals with a similar lipoprotein profile, and the greatest incidence of CVD was seen in patients with hypertension who also were in the highest TG and HDL-C group.

Based upon these findings, it seems reasonable to suggest that lowering blood pressure is a necessary, but not sufficient, approach to reducing CVD in patients in whom essential hypertension is present as one of the manifestations of the IRS. Thus, at the simplest, the choice of drugs used to lower blood pressure should be selected with awareness of their possible deleterious effect on the adverse CVD risk factors often present in patients high blood pressure. For example, it is probably not the best approach to treat a patient, who has a high TG and a low HDL-C concentration, with more than 12.5 mg of hydrochlorothiazide, and in the absence of a previous myocardial infarct, to use a beta-blocker. More importantly, aggressive treatment of the dyslipidemia, if present, seems to be highly justified. It must be emphasized that there is no evidence that this approach will decrease CVD risk in hypertriglyceridemic patients with essential hypertension. On the other hand, given the evidence that the atherogenic lipoprotein profile of the IRS greatly increases CVD risk [24,25,70,71], and the results of the VA-HIT and Helsinki Heart studies [72–74], it would seem prudent to aggressively treat hypertriglyceridemia when present in patients with essential hypertension.

Conclusion

Insulin-mediated glucose disposal varies widely in the population at large, with approximately 50% of the variability in insulin action resulting from differences in lifestyle variables; with degree of adiposity and physical fitness each accounting for approximately (25%). The remaining 50% is familial, likely to be of genetic origin, with powerful ethnic differences. Type 2 diabetes develops when insulin-resistant individuals cannot secrete the increased amounts of insulin needed to overcome the insulin resistance. However, the majority of insulin-resistant individuals are able to maintain the degree of hyperinsulinemia required to prevent manifest decompensation of glucose homeostasis. Although compensatory hyperinsulinemia prevents the development of frank hyperglycemia in insulin-resistant persons, insulin-resistant/hyperinsulinemic individuals are at greatly increased risk of being somewhat glucose intolerant, with a dyslipidemia characterized by a high plasma TG and low HDL-C concentration, and an increase in blood pressure. These changes increase CVD risk, and because the importance as CVD risk factors of insulin resistance/compensatory hyperinsulinemia and its associated cluster of abnormalities was not widely appreciated at the time, the term Syndrome X was introduced in 1988 to focus attention on these relationships.

An enormous amount of new information relevant to the role of insulin resistance in human disease had appeared since the introduction of the concept of Syndrome X, and the abnormalities related to insulin resistance have broadened considerably. At the same time, it has become clear that the adverse clinical outcomes associated with insulin resistance extend far beyond type 2 diabetes and CVD. For example, in addition to type 2 diabetes and CVD, insulin-resistant individuals are at increased risk to develop essential hypertension, PCOS, nonalcoholic fatty liver disease, congestive heart failure, sleep disordered breathing, cognitive dysfunction, and certain forms of cancer. In addition, insulin resistance and its consequences have been shown to complicate protease inhibitor treatment of HIV/AIDS, as well as the use of atypical antipsychotic drugs in patients with schizophrenia. Consequently, it is suggested that the various abnormalities and clinical syndromes more likely to occur in insulin-resistant individuals be subsumed under the rubric of the IRS.

To discuss the treatment of *all* of the manifestations of the IRS is beyond the competence of this individual, and would seem to require the creation of a multiauthored monograph. It did seem possible that some clinical utility might result from a consideration of lifestyle and pharmacological approaches to enhancing insulin sensitivity in apparently healthy, nondiabetic, insulin-resistant individuals, and this has been the main focus of the chapter. In the case of the dyslipidemia and essential hypertension associated with the IRS, an additional attempt was made to consider potential interventions, above and beyond improving insulin sensitivity, which might be useful in an effort to reduce risk of CVD. It is clear that we have learned a great deal since the original observation of Himsworth that a defect in insulin action could lead to a disease: type 2 diabetes. The clinical problems associated with insulin resistance will only increase as the world grows more obese and less physically active, and the need to develop therapeutic approaches much more effective than the relatively primitive ones discussed in this chapter will become paramount.

References

1. Himsworth HP. The mechanism of diabetes mellitus. I. Lancet 1939;II:1–6.
2. Himsworth HP. The mechanism of diabetes mellitus. II. The control of blood sugar level. Lancet 1939;II: 65–68.
3. Himsworth HP. The mechanism of diabetes mellitus. II. The control of blood sugar level (cont). Lancet 1939;II:118–132.
4. Himsworth HP. The mechanism of diabetes. III. Human diabetes mellitus. Lancet 1939;II:171–175.
5. Himsworth HP. The syndrome of diabetes and its causes. Lancet 1949;2:465–473.
6. Yalow RS, Berson SA. Immunoassay of endogenous plasma insulin in man. J Clin Invest 1960; 39:1157–1175.
7. Shen S-W, Reaven GM, Farquhar JW. Comparison of impedance to insulin mediated glucose uptake in normal and diabetic subjects. J Clin Invest 1970; 49:21518.
8. DeFronzo RA, Tobin JD, Andres R. Glucose clamp technique: a method for quantifying insulin secretion and resistance. Am J Physiol 1979;237:E214–E223.
9. Ginsberg H, Olefsky JM, Reaven GM. Further evidence that insulin resistance exists in patients with chemical diabetes. Diabetes 1974;23:674–678.
10. Ginsberg H, Kimmerling G, Olefsky JM, et al. Demonstration of insulin resistance in untreated adult onset diabetic subjects with fasting hyperglycemia. J Clin Invest 1975;55:454–461.
11. Reaven GM. Insulin resistance in noninsulin-dependent diabetes mellitus. Does it exist and can it be measured? Am J Med 1983;74 (Suppl. 1A):3–17.
12. Warram JH, Martin BC, Krowlewski As, et al. Slow glucose removal rate and hyperinsulinemia precede the development of type II diabetes in the off-spring of the diabetic parents. Ann Intern Med 1990;113: 909–915.
13. Lillioja S, Mott DM, Spraul M, et al. Insulin resistance and insulin secretory dysfunction as precursors of non-insulin dependent diabetes mellitus N Engl J Med 1993;329:1988–1992.
14. Hollenbeck CB, Reaven GM. Variations in insulin-stimulated glucose uptake in healthy individuals with normal glucose tolerance. J Clin Endocrinol Metab 1987;64:1169–1173.
15. Yeni-Komshian H, Carantoni M, Abbasi F, et al. Relationship between several surrogate estimates of insulin resistance and quantification of insulin-mediated glucose disposal in 490 healthy, nondiabetic volunteers. Diabetes Care 2000;23:171–175.
16. Reaven GM, Hollenbeck CB, Chen Y-DI. Relationship between glucose tolerance, insulin secretion, and insulin action in non-obese individuals with varying degrees of glucose tolerance. Diabetologia 1989;32:52–55.
17. Reaven GM, Lerner RL, Stern MP, et al Role of insulin in endogenous hypertriglyceridemia. J Clin Invest 1967;46:1756–1767.
18. Olefsky JM, Farquhar JW, Reaven GM. Reappraisal of the role of insulin in hypertriglyceridemia. Am J Med 1974;57:551–560.
19. Tobey TA, Greenfield M, Kraemer F, et al. Relationship between insulin resistance, insulin secretion, very low density lipoprotein kinetics, and plasma triglyceride levels in normotriglyceridemic man. Metabolism 1981;30:165–171.

20. Laws A, Reaven GM. Evidence for an independent relationship between insulin resistance and fasting plasma HDL-cholesterol, triglyceride and insulin concentrations. J Int Med 1992;231:25–30.
21. Ferrannini E, Buzzigoli G, Bonadona R. Insulin resistance in essential hypertension. N Engl J Med 1987;317:350–357.
22. Shen D-C, Shieh S-M, Fuh M, et al. Resistance to insulin-stimulated glucose uptake in patients with hypertension. J Clin Endocrinol Metab 1988;66:580–583.
23. Kannel WB. Blood pressure as a cardiovascular risk factor: prevention and treatment. JAMA 1996;275: 1571–1576.
24. Castelli WP, Garrison RJ, Wilson PWF, et al. Incidence of coronary heart disease and lipoprotein cholesterol levels: the Framingham Study. JAMA 1986;256:2385–2387.
25. Austin MA, Hokanson JE, Edwards KI. Hypertriglycridemia as a cardiovascular risk factor. Am J Cardiol 1998;81(4A):7B–12B.
26. Reaven GM. Role of insulin resistance in human disease. Diabetes 1988;37:1595–1607.
27. Reaven GM. The insulin resistance syndrome. Curr Atheroscler Rep 2003;5:364–371.
28. Einhorn D, Reaven GM, Cobin RH, et al. American College of Endocrinology position statement: the insulin resistance syndrome. Endocrine Practice 2003;9:237–252.
29. Alberti KG, Zimmet PZ. Definition, diagnosis and classification of diabetes mellitus and its complications. Part 1: diagnosis and classification of diabetes mellitus provisional report of a WHO consultation. Diabet Med 1998;15:539–553.
30. Executive Summary of Third Report of The National Cholesterol Education Program (NCEP) Expert Panel on Detection, Evaluation, And Treatment of High Blood Cholesterol In Adults (Adult Treatment Panel III). JAMA 2001;285:2486–2497.
31. Alberti KGMM, Zimmet P, Shaw J and for the IDF Epidemiology Task Force Consensus Group. The metabolic syndrome – a new worldwide definition. Lancet 2005;366:1059–1062.
32. Reaven GM. The metabolic syndrome: Requiescat in pace. Clin Chem 2005;51:931–938.
33. Kahn R, Buse J, Ferrannini E, et al. The metabolic syndrome: time for a critical appraisal. Joint statement from the American Diabetes Association and the European Association for the Study of Diabetes. Diabetes Care 2005;28:2289–2304.
34. Gale EA. The myth of the metabolic syndrome. Diabetologia 2005;48:1679–1683.
35. Reaven GM. The metabolic syndrome: is this diagnosis necessary. Am J Clin Nutr 2006;83:1237–1247.
36. Abbasi F, McLaughlin T, Lamendola C, et al. The relationship between glucose disposal in response to physiological hyperinsulinemia and basal glucose and free fatty acid concentrations in healthy volunteers. J Clin Endocrinol Metab 2000;85:1251–1254.
37. Reaven GM. The kidney: an unwilling accomplice in syndrome X. Am J Kidney Diseases. 1997;30: 928–931.
38. Baillargeon JP, Nestler JE. Commentary: polycystic ovary syndrome: a syndrome of ovarian hypersensitivity to insulin. J Clin Endocrinol Metab 2006;91; 22–24.
39. Olefsky JM. Reaven GM, Farquhar JW. Effects of weight reduction on obesity: studies of carbohydrate and lipid metabolism. J Clin Invest 1974;53:64–76.
40. Su H-Y, Sheu WH-H, Chin H-ML, et al. Effect of weight loss on blood pressure and insulin resistance in normotensive and hypertensive obese individuals. Am J Hypertens 1995;8:1067–1071.
41. Moran LJ, Noakes M, Clifton PM, et al. Dietary composition in restoring reproductive and metabolic physiology in overweight women with polycystic ovary syndrome. J Clin Endocrinol Metab 2003;88: 812–819.
42. Dixon JB, Bhathal PS, Hughes NR, et al. Nonalcoholic fatty liver disease. Improvement in liver histological analysis with weight loss. Hepatology 2004;39:1647–1654.
43. Tuomilehto J, Lindstrom J, Eriksson JG, et al. 2001. Prevention of type 2 diabetes by changes in lifestyle among subjects with impaired glucose tolerance. N Engl J Med 344:1343–1350.
44. Knowler WC, Barrett-Connor E, Fowler SE, et al for The Diabetes Prevention Program Group. Reduction in the incidence of type 2 diabetes with lifestyle intervention or metformin. N Engl J Med 2002;346: 393–403.
45. Yip J, Facchini FS, Reaven GM. Resistance to insulin-mediated glucose disposal as a predictor of cardiovascular disease. J Clin Endocrinol Metab 1998;83:2773–2776.
46. Facchini, FS, Hua, N, Abbasi, F, et al. Insulin resistance as a predictor of age-related diseases. J Clin Endocrinol Metab 2001;86:3574–3578.
47. McLaughlin T, Allison G, Abbasi F, et al. Prevalence of insulin resistance and associated cardiovascular disease risk factors among normal weight, overweight, and obese individuals. Metabolism 2004;53:495–499.
48. McLaughlin T, Abbasi F, Cheal K, et al. Use of metabolic markers to identify overweight individuals who are insulin resistant. Ann Intern Med 2003;139:802–809.
49. Kim SH, Abbasi F, Reaven G. Impact of degree of obesity on surrogate estimates of insulin resistance. Diabetes Care 2004;27:1998–2002.
50. Valdez R, Mitchell BD, Haffner SM, et al. Predictors of weight change in a bi- ethnic population. The San Antonio Heart Study. Int J Obes 1984;18:85–91.

51. Swinburn BA, Nyomba BL, Saad MF, et al. Insulin resistance associated with lower rates of weight gain in Pima Indians. J Clin Invest 1991;88: 168–173.
52. Hoag S, Marshall JA, Jones RH, et al. High fasting insulin levels associated with lower rates of weight gain in persons with normal glucose tolerance: The San Luis Valley Diabetes Study. Int J Obes 1995;19: 175–180.
53. Schwartz MW, Boyko EJ, Kahn SE, et al. Reduced insulin secretion: An independent predictor of body weight gain. J Clin Endocrinol Metab 1995;80: 1571–1576.
54. Zavaroni I, Zuccarelli A, Gasparini P, et al. Can weight gain in healthy, nonobese volunteers be predicted by differences in baseline plasma insulin concentrations? J Clin Endocrinol Metab. 1998;83: 3498–3500.
55. McLaughlin T, Abbasi F, Carantoni M, et al. Differences in insulin resistance do not predict weight loss in response to hypocaloric diets in healthy obese women. J Clin Endocrinol Metab 1999;84:578–581.
56. McLaughlin T, Abbasi F, Lamendola C, et al. Metabolic changes following sibutramine-assisted weight loss in obese individuals: role of plasma free fatty acids in the insulin resistance of obesity. Metabolism 2001;50:819–882.
57. McLaughlin T, Abbasi F, Lamendola C, et al. Differentiation between obesity and insulin resistance in the association with C-reactive protein. Circulation 2002;106:2908–2912.
58. McLaughlin T, Stuhlinger M, Lamendola C, et al. Plasma asymmetric dimethylarginine concentrations are elevated in obese insulin resistant women and fall with weight loss. J Clin Endocrinol Metab 2006;91: 1896–2000.
59. Wu M-S, Johnston P, Sheu W H-H, et al. Effect of metformin on carbohydrate and lipoprotein metabolism in NIDDM patients. Diabetes Care 1990;13:1–8.
60. Hollenbeck CB, Johnston P, Varasteh, BB, et al. Effects of metformin on glucose insulin and lipid metabolism in patients with mild hypertryglyceridaemia and non-insulin dependent diabetes by glucose tolerance test criteria. Diabete Metab 1991;17:483–489.
61. Reaven GM. Effect of metformin on various aspects of glucose, insulin and lipid metabolism in patients with non-insulin-dependent diabetes mellitus with varying degrees of hyperglycemia. Diab/Metab Rev 1995;11:S97–S108.
62. Chu JW Abbasi F Lamendola C, et al. Effect of rosiglitazone treatment on circulating vascular and inflammatory markers in insulin-resistant subjects. Diabetes Vasc Dis Res 2005;2:37–41.
63. Kim SH, Abbasi F, Chu, et al. Rosiglitazone reduces glucose-stimulated insulin secretion and increases insulin clearance in nondiabetic, insulin resistant individuals. Diabetes 2005;54:2447–2452.
64. Abbasi F, Chang S-A, Chu JW, GM, Improvements in insulin resistance with weight loss, in contrast to rosiglitazone, is not correlated with changes in plasma adiponectin or adiponectin multimeric complexes. Am J Physiol Integr Comp Physiol 2006;290: R 139–144, 47.
65. Promrat K, Lutchman G, Uwaifo GI, et al. A pilot study of pioglitazone treatment for nonalcoholic steatohepatitis. Hepatology 2004;39:188–196.
66. Cataldo NA, Abbasi F, Mclaughlin TL, et al. Metabolic and ovarian effects of rosiglitazone treatment for 12 weeks in insulin-resistant women with polycystic ovary syndrome. Hum Repro 2006;1: 109–120.
67. The Diabetes Prevention Program Research Group. Effects of withdrawal from metformin on the development of diabetes in the Diabetes Prevention Program. Diabetes Care 2003;26:977–980.
68. The DREAM (Diabetes REduction Assessment with ramipril and rosiglitazone Medication) trial investigators. Effect of rosiglitazone on the frequency of diabetes in patients with impaired glucose tolerance or impaired fasting glucose: a randomized controlled trial. Lancet 2006;368: 1096–1105.
69. Reaven GM. Compensatory hyperinsulinemia and the development of an atherogenic lipoprotein profile: the price paid to maintain glucose homeostasis in insulin-resistant individuals. Endocrinol Metab Clin N Am. 2005;34:49–62.
70. Austin MA, Breslow JL, Hennekens CH, et al. Low-density lipoprotein subclass patterns and risk of myocardial infarction. JAMA 1988;260:1917–1921.
71. Patsch JR, Miesenbock G, Hopferwieser T, et al. Relation of triglyceride metabolism and coronary artery disease: studies in the postprandial state. Arterioscler Thromb 1992;12:1336–1345.
72. Manninen V, Tenkanen L, Koskinen P, et al. Joint effects of serum triglyceride and LDL and HDL cholesterol concentrations on coronary heart disease risk in the Helsinki Heart Study: implications for treatment. Circulation 1992;85:37–45.
73. Robins SJ, Collins D, Wittes, JT. et al. Relation of gemfibrozil and lipid levels with major coronary events: VA-HIT: a randomized control trial. JAMA 2001;285:1585–1591.
74. Robins SJ, Rubins HB, Fass FH, et al. Insulin resistance and cardiovascular events with low HDL cholesterol: the Veterans Affairs HDL Intervention Trial (VA-HIT). Diabetes Care 2003;26:1513–1517.

75. Zavaroni I, Mazza S, Dall'Aglio E, et al. Prevalence of hyperinsulinaemia in patients with high blood pressure. J Intern Med 1992; 231:235–240.
76. Reaven GM. Insulin resistance/compensatory hyperinsulinemia, essential hypertension, and cardiovascular disease. J Clin Endocrinol Metab 2003;88: 2399–2403.
77. Sheuh WH-H, Jeng C-Y, Shieh S-M, et al. Insulin resistance and abnormal electrocardiograms in patients with high blood pressure Am J Hypertens 1992;5:444–448.
78. Jeppesen J, Hein HO, Suadicani P, et al. High triglycerides and low HDL cholesterol and blood pressure and risk of ischemic heart disease. Hypertension 2000;36:226–239.
79. Jeppesen J, Hein HO, Suadicani P, et al. Low triglycerides-high high-density lipoprotein cholesterol and risk of ischemic heart disease. Arch Int Med 2001;161:361–366.

4
Medical Emergencies – Diabetic Ketoacidosis and Hyperosmolar Hyperglycaemia

Niels Møller and K. George M.M. Alberti

Keywords: Diabetic ketoacidosis, hyperosmolar hyperglycemia, ketone bodies, glucose, insulin, fluid and electrolyte therapy.

Diabetic ketoacidosis (DKA) and hyperosmolar non-ketotic hyperglycaemia (HH) are acute, life threatening conditions, which represent the ultimate metabolic consequences of deranged type 1 and type 2 diabetes [1–4]. The hallmark of DKA is metabolic acidosis caused by rapid excess of ketoacids (3-hydroxybutyrate and acetoacetate) while hyperosmolarity caused by hyperglycaemia is the most notable feature of HH. The distinction is not clear-cut as DKA patients may be very hyperosmolar and ketone body levels are generally modestly elevated in HH. Although the clinical picture may vary considerably depending on co-morbidities, differential diagnosis seldom poses major problems and in the rare cases in which distinction is difficult, treatment generally follows the same principles, regardless of aetiology.

Mortality rates have been steadily declining over the recent years [5], but remain close to 5% for DKA and between 10% and 15% for HH [1]. The decline in mortality may be a consequence of lower incidence of DKA and HH, earlier diagnosis, improved treatment or – more plausibly – all combined. It is likely that improved education schedules and self-monitoring (e.g. blood ketone testing), organisation of specialised diabetes clinics and the use of standardised low-dose insulin regimens [1,6] have contributed to this favourable trend.

Diabetic Ketoacidosis

DKA is the most important and demanding medical emergency within the fields of diabetology and endocrinology. There is no generally accepted definition of DKA and in particular very mild cases may be problematic. As a minimum it seems reasonable to require that pH is below normal range and that levels of ketoacids (ketone bodies) in blood or urine are markedly elevated. As outlined in Table 1 there is a continuous deterioration from clinically insignificant *stress ketosis* to full blown *severe ketoacidosis*. In the US population it has been estimated that between 2% and 8% of hospital admissions in children with diabetes are due to DKA [7] and that the annual incidence rate of DKA in children is around 5 per 1,000 patients [8].

Pathogenesis and Pathophysiology

In DKA the major culprit is insulin deficiency. Insulin deficiency may be relative, for example, in the setting of severe infection, where normal amounts of insulin are insufficient or absolute when insulin therapy is neglected. At some stage insulin deficiency becomes coupled with an excess of counter-regulatory hormones and cytokines [9,10]. The traditional catabolic (stress) hormones include glucagon, epinephrine,

TABLE 1. Classification of clinical pictures and diagnostic criteria (adapted from Standards of Medical Care in Diabetes – 2004/2006 POSITION STATEMENT Diabetes Care 27:S94–S101, 2004, 2006 by the American Diabetes Association, Inc.).

	Stress ketosis	Compensated DKA	Diabetic ketoacidosis			Hyperosmolar hyperglycaemia
			Mild	Moderate	Severe	
Plasma glucose	Variable	Generally increased	Generally increased	Generally increased	Generally increased	>35–40 mmol/L
Arterial pH	Normal	Normal	Decreased >7.25	7.0–7.25	<7.0	Generally normal
Serum bicarbonate	Normal	Marginally decreased	15–18 mmol/L	10–15 mmol/L	<10 mmol/L	>15 mmol/L
Urine ketones	Increased	Increased	Increased	Increased	Increased	Normal/ marginally increased
Blood ketones	Increased	Increased	Increased	Increased	Increased	Normal/ marginally increased
Anion gap[a]	Normal/ marginally increased	Marginally increased	>10	>12	>12	Variable
Mental status	Normal	Normal	Normal	Normal/ drowsy	Drowsy–coma	Drowsy–coma

[a]Can be calculated as: $[Na^+]–([Cl^-] + [HCO_3^-])$.

growth hormone and cortisol, all of which have well-described metabolic actions. The metabolic actions of cytokines are in general not so well understood and it is possible that many of these actions are mediated by hypothalamo-pituitary activation and subsequent elevation of catabolic hormones.

Lipid Metabolism

Contrary to popular belief deranged *lipid* – not carbohydrate – metabolism is the main cause of DKA. In essence DKA is caused by uncontrolled lipolysis in adipose tissue and uncontrolled ketogenesis in liver.

Adipose tissue is present in regional depots such as subcutaneous upper and lower body and visceral fat [11]. Apart from these classic depots fat is present in most other tissues, for example, connective tissue, bone marrow, liver and muscle. The picture is further complicated by the fact that within each tissue fat is distributed in compartments. In muscle for instance fat is present intramyocellularly, intermyocellularly and intermuscularly. Under physiological conditions lipolysis is tightly controlled by lipases. Hormone-sensitive lipase and probably also adipose triglyceride lipase stimulate release of free fatty acids and glycerol into the circulation. This process is inhibited by insulin and low insulin levels increase lipolysis swiftly. The stress hormones, such as epinephrine, growth hormone and cortisol, stimulate lipolysis. It is plausible that dehydration per se also participates in the stimulation of lipolysis [12]. These events take place in the course of hours and may rapidly triple or quadruple blood concentrations of free fatty acids.

Ketogenesis occurs in the liver by oxidation of free fatty acids to ketoacids/ketone bodies. Ketone bodies, in particular 3-hydroxybutyrate, are phylogenetically ancient fuel compounds, which are present and prominent in very primitive species [13], suggesting that they have played an important role throughout evolution over the past 2–3 billion years. Physiologically ketone bodies provide important fuel energy for the brain and other tissues under fasting, prolonged exercise and other conditions of fuel shortage. In DKA ketogenesis becomes uncontrolled and circulating levels of ketone bodies rise manifold. This occurs because of both increased supply of fatty acids to the liver and because low levels of insulin and high levels of glucagon in the liver promote ketogenesis [14]. In normal individuals this unrestrained process is prevented by compensatory rises in insulin secretion, but this does not occur in type 1 diabetes.

Glucose Metabolism

Hyperglycaemia is usually present in DKA, but it is important to realise that DKA not infrequently presents with normal or modestly elevated glucose concentrations [15]. This may particularly be the case during caloric deprivation due to, for example, gastrointestinal disease. Hyperglycaemia is caused by a combination of lack of insulin and excess of stress hormones, leading to insulin resistance. In the liver this increases gluconeogenesis and hepatic glucose production. It is unlikely that the kidney plays any significant role in the initial stages of DKA [16]. The ensuing high glucose levels generate a high flux state with increased peripheral glucose disposal, but the increased mass action of glucose is generally insufficient to compensate fully. Muscle glucose metabolism is characterised by low insulin levels and insulin resistance because of high levels of stress hormones, high levels of free fatty acids and varying degrees of dehydration.

Precipitating Factors

Unless related to omission of insulin therapy, DKA is usually precipitated by coexisting illness. The most common factor is infection ranging from trivial viral infections to full-blown septicaemia. Other precipitating factors are cardiovascular events (myocardial infarction, stroke), gastrointestinal disease, inflammatory diseases, pancreatitis, trauma and major surgery, alcohol abuse and drugs (e.g. glucocorticoids). All of these factors induce insulin resistance due to stress hormone responses. Furthermore, poor appetite and food deprivation will often lead the patient to take less insulin, erroneously of course. In this context gastrointestinal disease with nausea and vomiting poses a specific problem and it may be necessary to admit such patients to hospital for intravenous glucose and insulin therapy.

Psychological factors also play an important role. Poor compliance is commonly seen in younger patients, patients with psychiatric illnesses and in minority groups with poor understanding of diabetes care principles for linguistic or cultural reasons.

Diagnosis and Clinical Presentation

DKA usually develops over a short period of time, generally in less than 24 h. There may have been some antecedent days with general malaise and poor metabolic control. Depending on the degree of hyperglycaemia, the history will include symptoms of polydipsia and polyuria. Specific symptoms depend on precipitating factors and co-morbidity. Physical examination may reveal poor skin turgor, hyperventilation (Kussmaul), hypotension, tachycardia and impairment of mental status. Many patients have infection, but patients may present with normothermia or even hypothermia due to peripheral vasodilation caused by the acidemia.

Prompt diagnosis and initial treatment rests on: (i) careful clinical examination, (ii) determination of plasma glucose, (iii) measurement of ketones in blood or urine, (iv) measurement of plasma potassium and other electrolytes and (v) assessment of acidemia. If glucose is high and blood/urine ketones are markedly elevated, DKA is likely and fluid and insulin therapy can usually be initiated, unless the patient is severely hypokalaemic (<3.5 mmol/L). If potassium is very low supplementation must be given before insulin therapy. However, rehydration should not be delayed whilst waiting for a potassium measurement.

The next diagnostic steps usually include arterial gas analysis, blood electrolytes (including anion gap), serum lactate (if there is doubt about the cause of the acidemia), complete blood cell count, biochemical assessment of liver and renal function, blood and urine cultures, myocardial biomarkers (if there is suspicion of a myocardial infarction), ECG and chest X-ray. In this context it is advantageous that most modern gas analysers also readily provide potassium concentrations. Another recent advantage is the advent of bedside ketone body monitors. It is thus nowadays possible to have quick and reliable measures of 3-hydroxybutyrate concentrations in blood [17], as opposed to unreliable measurements of acetoacetate in urine or time-consuming conventional laboratory methodology of the past. Diagnostic criteria are shown in Table 1.

Despite potassium depletion, serum potassium is typically either normal or elevated due to water deficiency and an intra- to extracellular shift caused by insulin deficiency and acidemia. Patients with potassium in the low range have severe total body potassium deficiency and should receive vigorous replacement therapy guided by cardiac monitoring. Sodium concentrations can be normal or low, due to osmotic shifts. It can be calculated that for every 3 mmol/L rise in plasma glucose the plasma sodium falls by 1 mmol/L. Thus there is often a real hypernatremia and the sodium levels will always rise as the glucose is brought under control. A majority of patients will have leukocytosis, which correlates with ketone body levels rather than with the presence of infection. There is also a water deficit of around 10% of body weight. Non-specific elevations of amylase and liver enzymes are common.

Differential diagnoses include all other causes of acidosis. It should be emphasised that many acute medical conditions induce stress ketosis and may be associated with acidosis. DKA is a metabolic acidosis characterised by a high anion gap and varying degrees of respiratory compensation. It is therefore crucial to obtain measures of ketone body concentrations and arterial gas analysis. If there is a major discrepancy between the extent of the ketonaemia and the acidemia, then lactate measurements are warranted. Starvation ketosis and alcoholic ketoacidosis can usually be identified by clinical history. Other conditions causing metabolic acidosis include lactic acidosis and intoxication with salicylate, methanol, ethylene glycol (antifreeze) and paraldehyde. The clinical picture may be blurred whenever the acidosis is aggravated by renal failure or respiratory failure. In addition DKA may imitate other diseases. High levels of potassium may cause ECG changes suggestive of myocardial infarction, and elevation of myocardial enzymes and biomarkers may occur in the absence of clear myocardial infarction [18]. DKA may also mimic an acute abdomen, particularly in younger patients.

Management

Management and treatment of DKA rests on four pillars:

1. Fluid and electrolyte therapy.
2. Intravenous insulin therapy.
3. Treatment of co-morbidities.
4. Careful monitoring of the clinical course.

It is particularly important that treatment is initiated without delay and that the patient is monitored frequently and carefully, preferably in a highly specialised unit. Severe cases should be treated and monitored in intensive care unit, where possible. Useful algorithms for treatment are available from many sources including the American Diabetes Association. In general the overall goal is a controlled, gradual correction of metabolic abnormalities and fluid and electrolyte deficiencies in the course of around 24 h.

Treatment of DKA in children and young adolescents follows slightly different guidelines than those presented here [19]. It is recommended that insulin is given continuously intravenously (0.1 IU/kg BW/h) *after* initiation of fluid and electrolyte therapy in order to minimise the risk of cerebral oedema. Otherwise children are in general treated with weight-reduced doses as indicated later.

Fluid/Saline Therapy

The first priority is to start to replace fluids. Water and sodium deficits typically are around 10% of body weight and 10 mmol/kg and isotonic saline (0.154 mmol/L; 0.9% NaCl) is given at a rate of approximately 15–20 mL/kg/h or 1 L/h initially, followed by 250 mL/h after the first 2–3 h depending on the state of dehydration. Depending on prevailing sodium concentrations and hydration hypotonic saline may also be used, but this is rarely necessary. Urine production and cardiovascular, renal and mental performance should be monitored frequently.

Insulin

Lack of insulin is the culprit in DKA and insulin treatment is mandatory. Insulin therapy in adults is given by infusion of 0.1 IU/kg BW/h or more simply as 6 units/h. An i.v. bolus of 0.15 IU/kg BW (or 10 IU) of regular insulin can be given initially but is not really required, as most of the initial improvement in metabolic status is due to rehydration. Alternatively a bolus of 0.15 IU/kg BW (or 10 IU) may be given every hour or a 20 unit bolus IM followed by 6 units every hour. If the patient is very insulin resistant (e.g. assessed by daily insulin requirements) dosage can be increased and vice versa if the patient is insulin sensitive. Considering the short half-life of i.v.-administered insulin, it is imperative that insulin is given with at least hourly intervals, regardless of prevailing blood glucose.

Insulin therapy is adjusted based on hourly measurements of blood glucose and – if possible – blood ketones, the overall aim being a gradual decline in both. The initial decline is to a large extent due to rehydration and expansion of the extracellular volume. Repeated analysis of arterial blood gases may be indicated but only in those patients with very low pH values and/or poor clinical condition. Measurements of ketone levels in urine is in general unreliable in this phase; these methods measure acetoacetate, which is quantitatively of minor importance compared with 3-hydroxybutyrate, and acetoacetate in urine may exhibit a paradoxical initial increase due to increasing blood concentrations (and low urine production), despite successful treatment. In particular, acetone is also measured by standard urine dipstick methods and may continue to be excreted for up to 48 h after the onset of treatment as it is fat-soluble and leaches out slowly during treatment.

When glucose concentrations are between 10 and 15 mmol/L, glucose is given i.v. and/or orally to avoid hypoglycaemia. It is usually possible to taper i.v. insulin treatment when 3-hydroxybutyrate concentrations are well below 3 mmol/L. Ten percent of glucose should be used for i.v. replacement as this provides some extra anabolic substrate. If the patient is still dehydrated, then the saline infusion should be continued.

Potassium, Bicarbonate and Phosphate

Even though the body is *potassium* depleted, with a typical deficit of around 5 mmol/kg, initial potassium values are usually normal or elevated. Insulin therapy, rehydration and correction of acidosis all cause a decrease in serum potassium and 20–30 mmol potassium/h may be administered once potassium levels are below 5.0 mmol/L, provided renal function is intact. Subsequent potassium administration is guided by frequent concentration measurements; adjuvant oral administration may be used in very mild cases of DKA. It is a frequent practical problem that there may be some delay before values are available from the laboratory; gas analysers that provide instant bedside potassium concentrations greatly facilitate this process.

Bicarbonate use in DKA is a matter of controversy, but it is empirically recommended that 25–50 mmol sodium bicarbonate is given hourly for 1–2 h, if pH is below 7.0. *Phosphate* deficiency of around 1 mmol/kg is typically present in DKA, but there is no evidence that phosphate supplementation should be given routinely. In patients with severe hypophosphataemia and/or cardiac and skeletal muscle/respiratory weakness, 20–30 mmol of potassium phosphate can be given hourly for 1–2 h.

Co-morbidity

Coexisting diseases precipitate DKA and DKA precipitates coexisting disease. Most often patients with DKA suffer from infectious disease and signs of infection should be vigorously sought for and treatment should be instituted on wide indications. Other prominent co-morbidities include cardiovascular events (myocardial infarction, stroke, thrombophlebitis, pulmonary embolism), acute gastrointestinal disorders and a variety of intoxications.

Complications

Iatrogenic hypoglycaemia and hypokalaemia are common and preventable, provided there is access to rapid analysis of glucose and potassium and – not less important – a competent and experienced medical team. Another frequent complication is recurrence of DKA or unnecessary protraction of the course, typically due to insufficient insulin therapy. Thrombotic events are also not uncommon although more often in HH than DKA.

Cerebral oedema is a rare, but often fatal, complication preponderant in children and adolescents. The pathophysiology is poorly understood, but may relate to overly aggressive therapy, the use of hypotonic replacement fluids, local cerebral overhydration and abnormalities of vasogenic function [19]. Symptoms frequently develop 4–12 h after initiation of therapy and include headache, altered mental status, specific neurological deficits and signs of increased intracranial pressure. Treatment with mannitol or hypertonic saline may be beneficial.

Prevention

Implementation of self-care and shared-care principles is crucial. Patients should learn about symptoms of DKA and be able to measure ketones in blood or urine. A common lapse is omission/reduction of insulin during episodes with impaired well-being and poor appetite. Persistent ketosis should be treated with extra insulin, fluid and carbohydrate, when necessary. Furthermore, it is very important that the individual patient had ready, 24-h access to diabetological expertise, preferably in a specialised diabetes centre.

Hyperosmolar Hyperglycaemia

Hyperosmolar hyperglycaemia (HH) is generally the fulminant result of poorly treated type 2 diabetes or delayed diagnosis of previously unknown type 2 diabetes. HH is less frequent than DKA, but mortality is higher and remains close to 15% in many centres [1,20]. As implied hyperosmolality is the primary clinical problem and there will be hyperglycaemia of >35–40 mmol/L and an effective serum osmolality of >320 mOsm/kg (Table 1). HH most often occurs in frail patients in combination with other potentially fatal conditions. Strict differentiation between DKA and HH can be difficult, because some degree of ketosis may be present in HH and because, for example, lactic acidosis, respiratory and renal failure may also be present. In practise this dilemma is mainly ornamental, since diagnostic and therapeutic efforts follow the same principles.

In line with DKA, HH is most often precipitated by infectious diseases or cardiovascular events and symptoms of hyperglycaemia usually have been present for some days. Hyperglycaemia is caused by a vicious cycle, in which relative insulin deficiency and high levels of stress hormones lead to increased endogenous glucose production and decreased peripheral glucose utilisation; hyperglycaemia in turn induces hyperosmolality and dehydration, which amplifies the stress hormone response and further impairs insulin secretion and vice versa.

At presentation the clinical condition is poor and the patient is very dehydrated with poor skin turgor and often exhibits altered level of consciousness (ranging from drowsiness to coma) and signs of hypovolaemic shock. In general the diagnostic procedures are similar to DKA. Typically, there will be a water deficit of 10–20% of body weight together with sodium, chloride and potassium deficits between 5 and 10 mmol/kg body weight.

Treatment of HH also follows the same guidelines as for DKA, the main aim being a controlled correction of hyperglycaemia, hyperosmolality and water and electrolyte deficits over 24 h. Patients are generally more sensitive to insulin and an infusion of 0.1 IU/kg BW/h is more than adequate in most cases. Repeated hourly boluses of 0.15 IU/kg BW (or 10 IU) may also be used. As with DKA dosage should be adjusted according to normal daily insulin needs and depending on therapeutic response. Usually 1L of isotonic saline is infused in the first hour but after that slower rehydration is advisable. Haemodynamic performance should be monitored carefully and it should be borne in mind that many of the patients have pre- or coexisting cardiac disease. The use of a central venous pressure line is helpful. It should be noted that a significant proportion of HH patients are hypernatraemic. In this case hypotonic saline can be used but more slowly. Potassium is administered along the same lines as with DKA and it is often wise to monitor the patient in the intensive care unit.

References

1. Standards of Medical Care in Diabetes – 2004/2006 POSITION STATEMENT Diabetes Care. 27: S94–S101, 2004, 2006 by the American Diabetes Association, Inc.
2. Kitabchi AE, Umpierrez GE, Murphy MB, Kreisberg RA. Hyperglycemic crises in adult patients with diabetes: a consensus statement from the American

Diabetes Association. Diabetes Care. 2006;29(12): 2739–2748.

3. Kitabchi AE, Nyenwe EA. Hyperglycemic crises in diabetes mellitus: diabetic ketoacidosis and hyperglycemic hyperosmolar state. Endocrinol Metab Clin North Am. 2006;35(4):725–751, viii.
4. Eledrisi MS, Alshanti MS, Shah F, Brolosy B, Jaha N. Overview of the diagnosis and management of diabetic ketoacidosis. Am J Med Sci. 2006;331: 243–251.
5. Wang J, Narayan KMV, Williams DE, Geiss LS. Declining death rates from hyperglycaemic crisis among adults with diabetes, U.S. 1985–2002. Diabetes Care. 2006;29:2018–2022.
6. Alberti KG. Low-dose insulin in the treatment of diabetic ketoacidosis. Arch Intern Med. 1977;137(10): 1367–1376.
7. White NH. Diabetic ketoacidosis in children. Endocrinol Metab Clin North Am. 2000;29: 659–682.
8. Kaufman FR, Halvorson M. The treatment and prevention of diabetic ketoacidosis in children and adolescents with type 1 diabetes mellitus. Pediatr Ann. 1999;28:576–582.
9. Barnes AJ, Kohner EM, Bloom SR, Johnston DG, Alberti KG, Smythe F. Importance of pituitary hormones in aetiology of diabetic ketoacidosis. Lancet. 1978;1(8075):1171–1174.
10. Stentz FB, Umpierrez GE, Cuervo R, Kitabchi AE. Proinflammatory cytokines, markers of cardiovascular risks, oxidative stress, and lipid peroxidation in patients with hyperglycemic crisis. Diabetes. 2004;53:2079–2086.
11. Koutsari C, Jensen MD. Thematic review series: patient-oriented research. Free fatty acid metabolism in human obesity. J Lipid Res. 2006;47(8): 1643–1650. Epub 2006 May 9.
12. Keller U, Szinnai G, Bilz S, Berneis K. Effects of changes in hydration on protein, glucose and lipid metabolism in man: impact on health. Eur J Clin Nutr. 2003;57(Suppl 2):S69–S74.
13. Cahill GF. Fuel metabolism in starvation. Annu Rev Nutr. 2006;26:1–22.
14. Foster DW, McGarry JD. The metabolic derangements and treatment of diabetic ketoacidosis. N Engl J Med. 1983;309(3):159–169.
15. Burge MR, Hardy KJ, Schade DS. Short-term fasting is a mechanism for the development of euglycemic ketoacidosis during periods of insulin deficiency. J Clin Endocrinol Metab. 1993;76(5):1192–1198.
16. Moller N, Jensen MD, Rizza RA, Andrews JC, Nair KS. Renal amino acid, fat and glucose metabolism in type 1 diabetic and non-diabetic humans: effects of acute insulin withdrawal. Diabetologia. 2006;49(8): 1901–1908. Epub 2006 May 23.
17. Federici MO, Benedetti MM. Ketone bodies monitoring. Diabetes Res Clin Pract. 2006;74(Suppl 2): S77–S81.
18. Moller N, Foss AC, Gravholt CH, Mortensen UM, Poulsen SH, Mogensen CE. Myocardial injury with biomarker elevation in diabetic ketoacidosis. J Diabetes Complications. 2005;19(6):361–363.
19. Wolfsdorf J, Glaser N, Sperling MA; American Diabetes Association. Diabetic ketoacidosis in infants, children, and adolescents: a consensus statement from the American Diabetes Association. Diabetes Care. 2006;29(5):1150–1159.
20. Gaglia JL, Wyckoff J, Abrahamson MJ. Acute hyperglycemic crisis in the elderly. Med Clin North Am. 2004;88(4):1063–1084, xii.

5
Notes on the Use of Glucagon in Type 1 Diabetes

Carl Erik Mogensen

Keywords: Glucagon, hypoglycaemia.

Hypoglycaemia may be an important complication in the treatment of type 1 diabetes. When intravenous glucose is available, glucagon has no place in the treatment and certainly also many patients may be treated with glucose or sweet foods given orally. However, if the patients are not conscious or acting negatively, glucagon used intramuscularly or subcutaneously is important in a dose of 1–2 mg [1–3].

Glucagon acts by activating the enzymes in hepatic cells that increase glycogenolysis and thereby increase the hepatic glucose production. Quite often, immediate clinical improvement is necessary to avoid the risk of neurological damage associated with severely low blood glucose. One problem might be that glucagon can be useless if hepatic stores of glycogen are depleted.

Relatives of patients with type 1 diabetes are quite often keen to use this kind of treatment. Glucagon is a safe and reliable alternative to intravenous glucose, which is, as mentioned, the most important and rapid restoration of blood glucose.

A glucagon emergency kit should be available in homes and family members should be instructed in the use of the kit in case of hypoglycaemia. It should be followed by the use of glucose as soon as possible.

References

1. Kahn CR, Schechter Y. Insulin, oral hyperglycaemic agents, and the pharmacology of the endocrine pancreas. In *Goodman and Gilman's the Pharmacological Basis of Therapeutics,* Goodman AG, Rall TW, Nies AS, Taylor P, Eds., 8th ed., New York, McGraw-Hill, 1990, pp. 1463–1495.
2. Howell MA, Guly HR. A comparison of glucagons and glucose in prehospital hypoglycaemia. *J Accid Emerg* 1997;14:30–32.
3. Carstens S, Sprehn M. Prehospital treatment of severe hypoglycaemia: a comparison of intramuscular glucagon and intravenous glucose. *Prehospital Disaster Med* 1998;13:44–50.

6 Insulin and New Insulin Analogues, Insulin Pumps and Inhaled Insulin in Type 1 Diabetes

Kjeld Hermansen

Keywords: Insulin, insulin analogues, basal bolus insulin treatment, continuous subcutaneous insulin infusion, insulin pump, inhaled insulin, type 1 diabetes mellitus.

The microvascular complications of type 1 diabetes mellitus (T1DM) were rarely noted before the discovery of insulin. The introduction of insulin therapy allowed patients to live long enough to develop diabetic retinopathy and diabetic nephropathy [1]. It was discussed extensively whether these complications were caused by hyperglycaemia, and whether they could therefore be prevented or delayed by improved blood glucose control. The Diabetes Control and Complication Trial (DCCT) [2] followed up in the Epidemiology of Diabetes Intervention and Complications (DCCT/EDIT) [3] showed that there was a clear-cut relationship between the degree of glycaemic control measured by HbA1C and the onset or progression of microvascular complications in T1DM [2,3]. The DCCT ended in 1993, after a mean duration of follow-up of 6.5 years [2]. Interestingly, the DCCT/EDIT extension study [3] clearly demonstrated that the risk reduction has been maintained through 7 years of EDIT, even though the difference in mean HbA1C levels between the intensive and conventional T1DM groups was only 0.4% at 1 year (8.3% in the former conventional treatment group vs. 7.9% in the former intensive treatment group), continued to narrow, and became statistically non-significant by 5 years (8.1% vs. 8.2%). Thus, the benefits of 6.5 years of intensive treatment extend well beyond the period of its most intensive implementation. Intensive treatment should be started as soon as possible after the onset of T1DM and maintained thereafter, aiming at as low HbA1C as practicable. However, there is an inverse relation between glycaemic control and the risk of severe hypoglycaemia in T1DM [2]. In the DCCT, severe hypoglycaemia occurred about 2.5–3 times more frequently in the intensive therapy group compared with the conventional therapy group. Thus, hypoglycaemia is a major limiting factor to achieving optimal control for many subjects with T1DM. There are several reasons why it is difficult in T1DM to mimic the physiological insulin secretion. This is in part due to the unfavourable pharmacokinetics and pharmacodynamics of subcutaneously injected insulin. As demonstrated by Binder et al. [4] more than 20 years ago, the coefficient of variation for conventional insulin preparations is as much as 25% intrasubject and 50% between subjects. The resulting unpredictability of glycaemic responses is most prominent with delayed-acting preparations. In addition, the administration of subcutaneous insulin in the periphery rather than into the portal circulation results in hyperinsulinaemia in the systemic circulation. Insulin absorption is influenced by the anatomical site of injection, being faster from the abdomen than from the thigh. The absorption is faster during exercise and after intramuscular injection rather than subcutaneous injection. Injecting into the abdomen rather than the thigh can attenuate the effect of exercise.

There are three main types of insulin preparations: (i) short acting, which have a relatively rapid onset of action and are injected just before meals ('preprandial' injections), (ii) intermediate acting, and (iii) long acting, which have a slower onset of action and act for long periods, meeting an individual's background (round-the-clock) needs. The duration of action of a particular type of insulin varies considerably from one patient to another and needs to be assessed individually. Insulin is given by subcutaneous injection into the layer of tissue immediately beneath the skin. Short-acting insulins can also be given by continuous subcutaneous infusion using a portable infusion pump. This device delivers a continuous basal insulin infusion and patient-activated bolus doses at meal times.

Treatments using insulin analogues or insulin pump treatment with continuous subcutaneous insulin infusion (CSII) have less variability and a lower incidence of hypoglycaemia than seen with traditional insulins and delivery systems.

This chapter deals first with the therapeutic use of insulin and its analogues in T1DM as well as different ways of insulin administration, that is, by conventional intensified insulin therapy with multiple injections (MDI), pump treatment (CSII) and inhalation (INHI).

Insulin and New Insulin Analogues

The Need for Physiological Insulin Delivery

Physiologically, insulin secretion is characterized by rapid increases at meal times together with a lower and constant basal output during interprandial intervals, including during the night. Secretion falls acutely during exercise and prolonged fasting. These dynamic responses maintain euglycaemia (4.0–5.0 mM) at all times, except for 1–1.5 h after eating, consequently avoiding the damaging effects of hyperglycaemia. Insulin therapy in T1DM should aim to mimic nature, that is, limiting postprandial hyperglycaemia and preventing hypoglycaemia during interprandial intervals in T1DM.

Conventional Intensified Insulin Therapy or Multiple Daily Insulin Injections (MDI)

In conventional intensified insulin therapy (MDI) using the basal-bolus approach with MDI, continuous basal insulin supply is obtained by once- or twice-daily subcutaneous injections of longer-acting preparations, supplemented by mealtime injections of more rapid-acting formulations.

Rapid-Acting (Mealtime) Insulins

These include structurally unchanged regular insulin preparations and short-acting insulin analogues (SIAs), which dissociate more rapidly than regular insulins and are absorbed faster. The glucose-lowering effect of rapid-acting insulins is enhanced by exercise within 1–3 h after the meal and by reducing the carbohydrate content of the meals.

Regular (Soluble) Insulins

Following subcutaneous injection of structurally unchanged regular insulin preparations, the native insulin tends to associate a hexameric form, which is slowly dissociated to single molecules and absorbed, thereby interfering with recreation of the physiological prandial insulin response (Table 1).

TABLE 1. Time course of action in T1DM of currently available subcutaneously injected insulin preparations.

	Appearence	Onset	Peak	Duration
Mealtime insulins				
Human regular insulin	Clear	0.5–1 h	2–3 h	5–8 h
Short-acting analogues				
Insulin Lispro	Clear	5–10 min	0.5–2 h	3–5 h
Insulin Aspart	Clear	5–10 min	0.5–2 h	3–5 h
Insulin Glusiline	Clear	5–10 min	0.5–2 h	3–5 h
Basal insulins				
Intermediate acting isophane insulin (NPH)	Cloudy	0.5–1.5 h	4–6 h	8–16 h
Long-acting insulin analogues				
Glargine	Clear	0.5–1 h	Peakless?	16–24 h
Detemir (0.3–0.8 U/kg)	Clear	1–2 h	8–12 h	17–23 h

Regular insulin needs to be injected 20–30 min before eating, or exaggerated postprandial hyperglycaemia will result. Subcutaneous absorption of regular insulin continues well beyond the postprandial glycaemic response with a peak 2–3 h after injection (Table 1), resulting in continued elevated circulating insulin levels, which tend to cause hypoglycaemia 3–5 h after the injection. Insulin dosages should be adjusted to optimize blood glucose levels 3–5 h after the injection, rather than 2 h postprandially. To avoid hypoglycaemia it will often be needed for the patients to snack between meals.

Short-Acting Insulin Analogues: Insulin Lispro, Insulin Aspart and Insulin Glusiline

Much attention has been devoted to develop SIA with pharmacokinetic profiles that mimic prandial insulin responses. In the SIA Lispro (Humalog), lysine at position 28 and proline at position 29 of the B-region of regular human insulin were interchanged. In the SIA Aspart (NovoRapid), proline at position 29 of the B-region was replaced by aspartic acid, and in the SIA Glusiline (Apidra), the amino acid, asparagine was replaced by lysine at position 3 and lysine with glutamic acid at position 29 of the B-chain.

SIAs have lesser tendency toward self-association and are therefore absorbed more quickly, achieving peak plasma concentrations about twice as high and within approximately half the time compared with regular insulin (Table 1). When injected at the start of the meal, the pharmacokinetic profile of SIA leads to lower glucose levels after meals than with regular insulins given up to 30 min beforehand. Another advantage is the possibility of injecting SIA up to 15 min after starting to eat without deterioration of prandial glycaemic control [5]. SIAs also have a shorter duration of action than regular insulin (Table 1), which reduces the need to snack between meals.

In a recent Cochrane review [6], the meta-analysis showed in adults with T1DM a small decrease in HbA1C of –0.1% with SIA compared with regular human insulin. Assuming that a reduction in HbA1C with SIA would result in a relative benefit similar to that found in DCCT [2], 650 patients would have to be treated with SIA for 1 year to prevent the development of retinopathy in one patient [6]. In terms of overall hypoglycaemia, comparable results were obtained with SIA and regular insulin; however, severe hypoglycaemia occurred less frequently in the SIA group than in the regular group [6]. Regarding quality of life (QOL), SIA showed improvement due to changes in the convenience, flexibility and continuation of treatment [6]. However, SIAs have higher cost than regular insulin. SIAs are judged safe during pregnancy. The short duration of action of SIA causes periods of hypoinsulinaemia between meals if the intervals between mealtime injections are long. Obtaining the potential benefits of SIA fully depends on the application of optimized basal insulin.

Basal Insulin Replacement

Basal Insulin Replacement with Intermediate Acting Neutral Protamine Hagedorn (NPH) Insulin

The most widely prescribed basal insulin globally is insulin combined with protamine [7], the so-called NPH insulin. The action profile of this preparation is, however, not optimal, with a peak effect at about 4–6 h and a duration of action of 8–16 h (Table 1). At a common dose of 0.3 U/kg, NPH insulin has been found to have a duration of around 13 h [8,9], which is insufficient to control hepatic glucose output to physiological levels. The peak of action of NPH insulin gives a potential risk of hypoglycaemia; however, it is the large variability in absorption of NPH insulin that poses the greatest problem. Thus, NPH insulin provides a considerable within-subject variability in T1DM assessed by the coefficient of variation (CV) for pharmacodynamic endpoints attaining 46–68% [10]. Variability of absorption arises from local changes at the injection sites in combination with the process of absorption after injection. In addition, there is often inadequate suspension and mixing of NPH insulin in pens before injection.

Basal Insulin Replacement with Long-Acting Analogues: Insulin Glargine and Insulin Detemir

The first of the long-acting insulin analogues to be used was insulin glargine (Fig. 1). This analogue is produced by the substitution of glycine for asparagine at position A21 of the insulin molecule and by the addition of two arginine molecules at position B30. These changes lead to a shift in the isoelectric point toward a neutral pH, which results

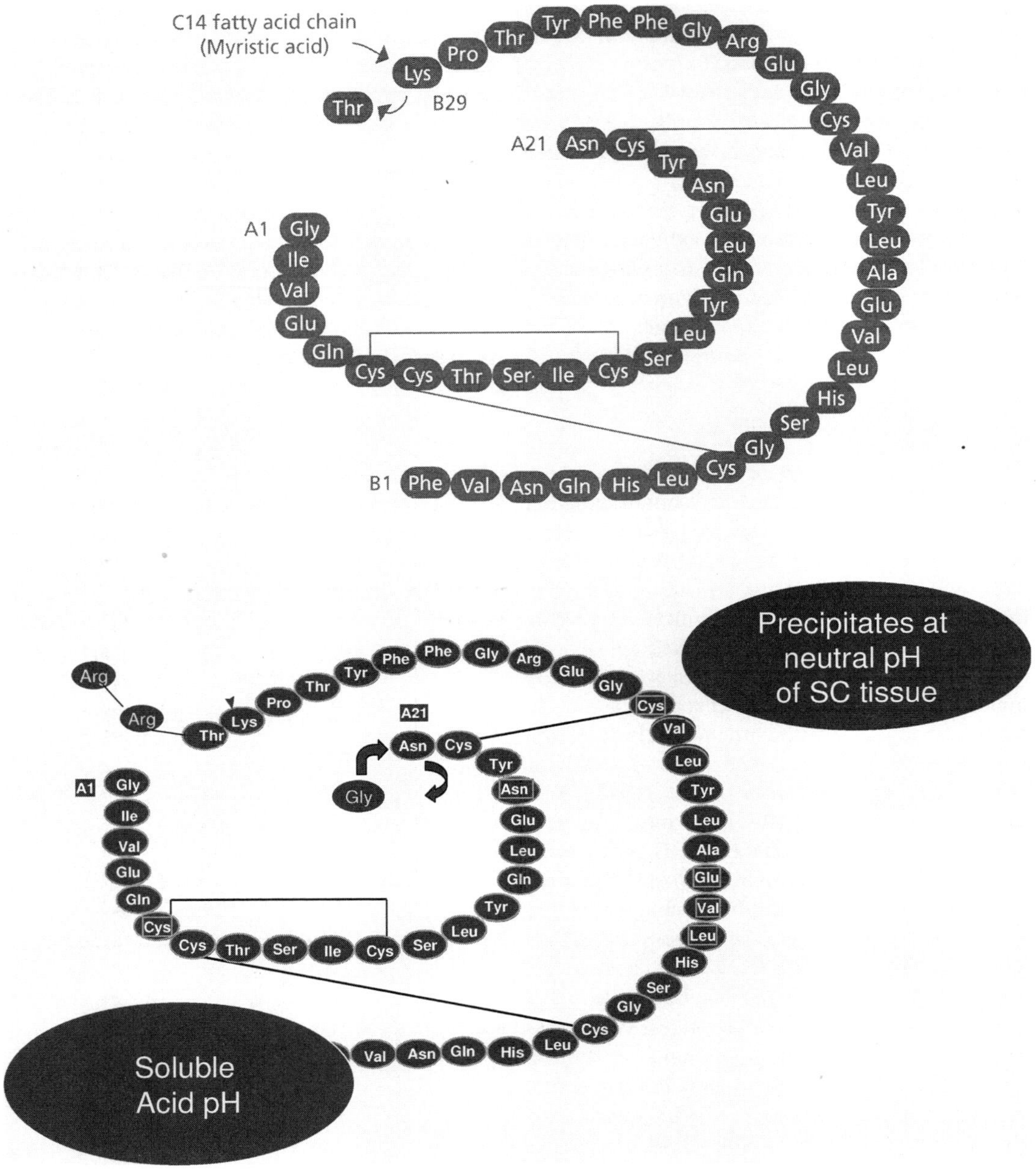

FIG. 1. Molecular structures of the long-acting insulin analogues, detemir (upper part) and glargine (lower part).

in an insulin molecule that is less soluble at the injection site and that precipitates in the subcutaneous tissue to form a depot from which insulin is slowly released [11]. As compared with NPH insulin, insulin glargine results in prolonged insulin absorption and shows little peak activity, as demonstrated by differences in disappearance curves (Table 1). Rates of absorption of insulin glargine at various sites do not differ. In the study of Lepore et al. [9] insulin glargine was found to have no peak and to have a mean (±SE) duration of action of 22 ± 4 h. It is important not to over-interpret the pharmacodynamic studies, because the data presented are simply averages of the results obtained in a relatively small number of subjects. The onset or duration of action may be substantially longer or shorter in individual patients and especially the profiles of action are dependent on the dose of insulin. In studies in T1DM the effect of only one glargine dose on pharmacokinetic and pharmacodynamic has been reported [9,10], which does not give a legitimate impression of the action profile. In this context it is of interest to note that the time-action profiles of glargine and the other long-acting insulin analogue, detemir, are comparable in T2DM and vary critically with the insulin dose [12]. Glargine did not show the 'ideal' peakless profile with an equal distribution of the metabolic effect over 24 h in some studies [10,12]. Thus, a low glargine dose does not have a duration of action that covers 24 h in T1DM. Recently, it was found that using insulin glargine twice daily at breakfast and before dinner compared with glargine once daily at dinner time – taken with a rapid-acting insulin analogue at meal times – gave a better glycaemic profile with reduced pre-dinner hyperglycaemia in T1DM [13]. However, besides this study [13], all clinical studies have been carried out with only one daily glargine injection. Most clinical studies in T1DM, except two [14,15], have failed to show any clinically significant improvement in HbA1C with insulin glargine compared with NPH insulin [16–18], whereas the pre-breakfast blood glucose level in general is lower. Compared with NPH insulin + unmodified human insulin, the combination of insulin glargine plus the SAI lispro, however, caused an overall improved glycaemic control in T1DM including HbA1C [14]. It is possible that experience in using the insulin analogues with adequate titration may allow improvement of HbA1C in T1DM to a relevant degree. Importantly, a reduction in the risk of hypoglycaemia, especially nocturnal hypoglycaemia, has been the rule with insulin glargine when compared with NPH insulin [14,16,17].

Insulin detemir is the second basal insulin that has been registered (Fig. 1). Its extended action is achieved by an entirely different principle from that attempted previously. Thus, a 14-C fatty acid, myristic acid, has been attached to the lysine residue at position B29, the threonine having been removed from position B30. The myristic acid side chain binds to albumin in the interstitium at the injection site and in the circulation providing the longer action profile. Insulin detemir has a lower in vivo potency compared with NPH insulin and glargine. Consequently, the commercial preparation of insulin detemir is formulated as 2,400 nM concentration (insulin NPH and insulin glargine both 600 nM) as has proven adequate in clinical studies. In T1DM insulin detemir (0.1–1.6 U/kg) has a linear dose–response relationship for both pharmacokinetic and pharmacodynamic measures [10]. Compared to NPH, detemir shows longer duration and lower maximum effect (Table 1). A recent study in T1DM using glucose clamp has demonstrated a lower within-subject variability of insulin detemir (CV 27%) than of insulin NPH (CV 68%) and insulin glargine (CV 48%) [10]. In most clinical studies twice-daily insulin detemir has been compared with twice-daily insulin NPH [19–24]. Regardless of whether detemir was administered at equal 12-h interval (morning + dinner) or with a longer interval (morning + bedtime), this improved overnight control with lower pre-breakfast glucose levels together with a lower risk of nocturnal hypoglycaemic events was seen [23,24]. The study of Home et al. [23] suggests that where nocturnal hypoglycaemia is a dominant problem, bedtime detemir may be a better choice than dinner detemir. Similar improvement in glycaemic control and hypoglycaemia as seen with twice-daily insulin detemir can be obtained when it is only given once daily in T1DM [25]. Thus, insulin detemir administered once daily at bedtime resulted in lower fasting blood glucose, less day-to-day variability in blood glucose and lower risk of nocturnal hypoglycaemia than NPH insulin [25]. Hermansen et al. [21], comparing the combination of insulin detemir + insulin aspart with the combination of NPH insulin + human regular insulin, found that the analogue regimen caused improvement in prandial glucose increments (Fig. 2, upper part), reduced plasma glucose variability at all pre-meal time points and lowered HbA1C more and caused less nocturnal hypoglycaemia than the human insulin regimen.

There is clinical evidence in favour of both insulin glargine and insulin detemir over NPH insulin in T1DM with reduced nocturnal hypoglycaemia and lower pre-breakfast blood glucose levels. Data indicate that the combination of SIA and one of the long-acting analogues compared with regular insulin + NPH insulin may even provide a small gain in overall glycaemic control

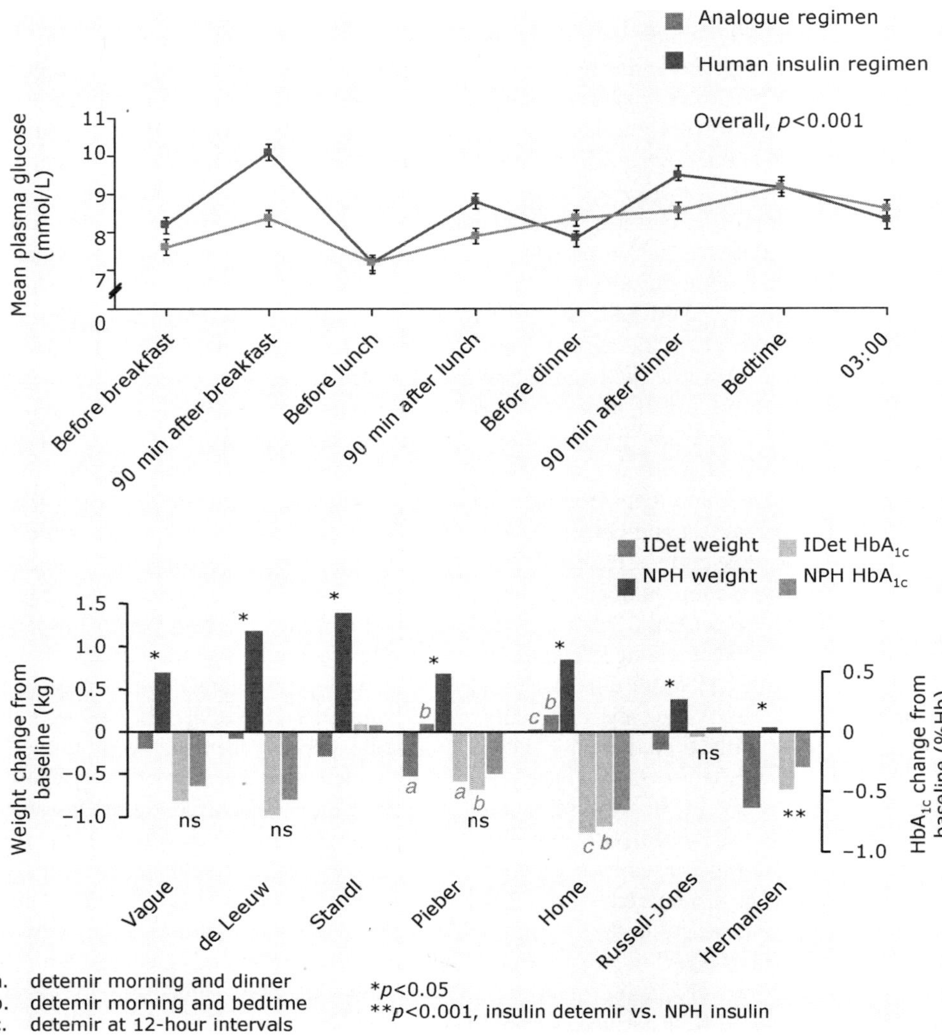

FIG. 2. Upper panel: Effects on 8-point plasma glucose profiles at the end of an 18 weeks study period of insulin analogues (insulin detemir + insulin aspart) versus traditional human insulin (NPH insulin + regular insulin) in T1DM (adapted with permission from Hermansen et al. Diabetologia 2004;47:622–629 [21]). Lower panel: Changes in weight and HbA1C with insulin detemir and NPH insulin in T1DM trials [19–25].

with lowering of HbA1C and self-monitored glucose profiles [14,21] (Fig. 2, upper part). It should be underlined, however, that the direct cost of long-acting analogues is higher than that of NPH insulin. Furthermore, the published clinical studies on insulin glargine and insulin detemir are all open-label, which may cause bias. Uniquely, there is a further advantage of insulin detemir over NPH insulin in body weight control [26]. In all studies published to date, insulin detemir shows a consistent weight sparing effect compared with NPH insulin in both T1DM [19–25] (Fig. 2, lower part) and in T2DM. This may have important implications for treatment, as weight gain can be a barrier to compliance and thus jeopardize glycaemic control [26]. A weight sparing effect has not been reported with any consistency for any other insulin, including insulin glargine. The long-acting insulin analogues, insulin glargine or insulin detemir, should be considered in subjects with

T1DM with problems with hypoglycaemia, unawareness of hypoglycaemia or large plasma glucose variations on standard treatment with NPH insulin as basal insulin.

There are potential problems with insulin therapy in T1DM. In addition to hypoglycaemia and weight gain, there are a few more rare conditions after starting insulin therapy, for example, insulin oedema, and local reactions to insulin injection. Insulin oedema is a rare phenomenon seen at the start of insulin treatment in poorly controlled or previously untreated patients. Oedema is due to acute sodium and water retention. It usually disappears after a few days. At the injection sites a localized overgrowth of subcutaneous adipose tissue can develop in response to high local insulin concentrations (lipohypertrophy). It is a more frequent problem in patients in MDI regimen who inject repeatedly at the same site, for example, in the abdomen. Injection into the lipohypertrophic area may worsen the glycaemic control due to impaired insulin absorption. Lipoatrophy is loss of subcutaneous fat at the injection site, causing pitting of the skin. In addition, local reactions at the injection sites can occur with erythema, burning or tender subcutaneous nodules.

Self-Monitoring of Plasma Glucose (HBGM)

Self-monitoring of plasma glucose (HBGM) is fundamental to diabetes care [27,28]. Frequent monitoring facilitates improved glycaemic control, avoidance of hypoglycaemia and lifestyle flexibility when results are used to assist the individual in their dietary choices, physical activity and insulin doses. HBGM should be carried out three or more times daily in T1DM on MDI and at least four times daily on insulin pump treatment. To achieve postprandial glucose targets, postprandial HBGM may be appropriate. Obviously, it is important to instruct subjects with T1DM in HBGM and routinely evaluate the patient's technique and ability to adjust therapy. Glucose monitors are now much smaller than previously, require very small amounts of blood (2–10 μL), are faster at providing a result (5–15 s) and can be used at sites other than fingertips. Most metres incorporate data management systems; however, keeping a blood glucose logbook is needed to detect patterns of glucose control and make appropriate dose adjustments [27]. Continuous glucose monitoring technologies using subcutaneous sensors are being used in clinical care as a means of accessing more complete glycaemic data than are available with traditional self-monitoring.

Treatment Targets

Glycaemic control is fundamental to the management of diabetes. Glycaemic control is best judged by the combination of the results of the patient's HBGM measurements and the current HbA1C value. The HbA1C should be used not only to assess the patient's control over the preceding 2–3 months but also as a check on the accuracy of the metre and the self-reported measurements as well as the adequacy of the HBGM testing schedule [28]. The goal is to achieve an HbA1C as close to normal as possible – representing normal fasting and postprandial glucose concentrations – in the absence of hypoglycaemia. However, the goal can be difficult to achieve. According to the American Diabetes Association (ADA), treatment regimens that reduce average HbA1C to <7.0%, preprandial plasma glucose between 5.0 and 7.3 mM and peak postprandial plasma glucose <10 mM in nonpregnant individuals are recommendable [28] (Table 2). As seen in Table 2 the recommended targets for the glycaemic control judged by HbA1C is slightly lower for the International Diabetes Federation (IDF) and American Association for Clinical Endocrinology than for ADA. Less-stringent treatment goals are appropriate in people with severe or frequent hypoglycaemia and in people with limited life expectancy or older adults.

TABLE 2. Targets for the glycaemic control according to the American Diabetes Association (ADA), the International Diabetes Federation (IDF) and the American Association of Clinical Endocrinologists (AAEC).

	ADA	IDF	AAEC
HbA1C %	<7.0	≤6.5	≤6.5
F-PG mM	5.0–7.3	≤6.0	<6.0
PP-PG mM	<10.0	<7.5	<7.8

F-PG mM, fasting plasma glucose in mM; PP-PG mM, postprandial plasma glucose in mM

Insulin Pump Treatment or Continuous Subcutaneous Insulin Infusion

Insulin pump therapy started in UK in 1976. Insulin pumps deliver a continuous basal insulin infusion (CSII) and patient-activated bolus doses at meal times. The pump is attached to the patients by an infusion set consisting of long flexible tubing with a needle or catheter on the end and is inserted subcutaneously in the patient. In two meta-analysis CSII was compared with conventional insulin treatment [29,30], which is not the actually used MDI. CSII caused a significant reduction in HbA1C of the size of 0.4–0.8% [29,30]. This degree of improvement in glycaemic control for 10 years would reduce the number of patients developing retinopathy by about 5% [29]. Using SIA for CSII provides a further small, but statistically significant improvement in glycaemic control (– 0.19% in HbA1C) as compared with regular insulin [31]. Therefore, the insulin of choice for CSII is now SIA. The frequency of hypoglycaemia is less after CSII treatment rather than after MDI treatment in more recent studies but is not affected if SIA is used instead of regular insulin [31]. With proper education and pump practice, the frequency of ketoacidosis is the same on CSII and MDI. A marked rise in blood glucose before breakfast, the so-called 'dawn phenomenon', occurs quite often in T1DM. It is due to a combination of waning of the circulating insulin concentration from the previous basal insulin injection and an increase in insulin resistance caused by nocturnal rise in growth hormone. If moving of the injection time of the previous basal insulin or a dose increase does not solve this problem, the modern CSII treatment with pre-programmed increase in the late night/early morning can minimize the dawn blood glucose increase. Clinical guidelines are the first step in making standards of care explicit. Table 3 gives the indications for CSII in T1DM suggested by a Danish expert committee [32]. CSII should be cancelled in case of recurrent ketoacidosis, if HbA1C increases, recurrent local infections/reactions, and when lacking compliance [32,33]. There ought to be demands on the CSII treatment teams about knowledge and education, experience and organization and monitoring [32,33]. The total insulin requirement per 24 h usually decreases 15–20% after starting with CSII. Approximately 40–50% of the daily insulin doses are given as the basal rate, but some patients require up to 60%. The remainder is given as premeal bolus doses. The insulin requirement in adults is about 20% lower between 01 and 03 A.M. compared with that between 05 and 07 A.M.. Standard advice is to decrease the basal rate during the night and after physical exercise and to increase in case of intercurrent illness with a rise in plasma glucose levels. Approaches with carbohydrate counting to the nutritional management of T1DM allow adjustment of premeal insulin boluses to both the premeal glucose levels as well as the carbohydrate content of the meal. Calculation of insulin to carbohydrate ratios allows increased flexibility in meal planning. Testing for ketones is mandatory if plasma glucose is >15 mM for more than a couple of hours or if the patient is ill or is nauseous/vomiting. The evidence suggests that the expanding use of CSII is justified. Despite the fact that a number of patients could greatly benefit

TABLE 3. Indications for insulin pump treatment (CSII) in T1DM.

CSII should be offered to subjects with T1DM who are not satisfactorily controlled on MDI, that is having HbA1C >7.5% (>7.0% for women who want to become pregnant) in case this is due to one or more of the following reasons:
If the patient despite optimized treatment inclusive of a dose increase of insulin experiences recurrent and/or unpredictable hypoglycaemic events
If the patient has hypoglycaemic unawareness
If the patient has erratic swings of blood glucose concentrations or an erratic lifestyle with delayed or missed meals and/or unpredictable activity
If the patient cannot control night time blood glucose levels on MDI even after having tried a long-acting insulin analogue, for example, patients with dawn phenomenon where the dose of basal insulin cannot be increased due to nocturnal hypoglycaemia
And under the prerequisite that the unacceptable treatment with MDI is not due to:
Not wanting to measure HBGM to a sufficient degree (≥4 times daily)
Insufficient compliance and/or understanding of the interplay between insulin, diet and exercise

for an affordable cost, there is still unwillingness in some countries to fund and reimburse insulin pump therapy [32]. CSII in T1DM is therefore very unevenly used and available in Western countries where, for example, only a few percent of T1DM in Denmark, around 10% of T1DM in Norway and Sweden and maybe up to 20–25% of T1DM in USA, are on this treatment [32].

Inhaled Insulin

Subcutaneous injection has been the only route of insulin administration for daily use by patients with T1DM for the past 80 years. A barrier to insulin therapy relates among other things to patient fears and anxiety about insulin injections. Although needles have become smaller and sharper, thereby causing less painful injections some people consider needles and injections a perceived stigma for diabetic subjects. It is only recently that alternative routes of insulin administration are becoming viable. Many avenues of insulin administration have been explored including oral, buccal and pulmonary routes [34,35]. Among non-invasive candidates, inhaled insulin (INH) appears to be the most promising. The lung offers a large surface area (75 m^2) and the alveolar epithelium is approximately 0.1–0.5 μm thick, allowing rapid absorption of inhaled drugs.

A number of pharmaceutical companies are developing INH delivery systems using both liquid and dry-powder insulin formulations [34,35]. Table 4 briefly indicates those arrived at in phase III studies. A few companies have developed systems based on liquid formulations, which utilize relatively complex pressurized metred-dose devices or nebulization systems to generate appropriately sized aerosolized doses. In the AERx system inhalation flow rate, inhaled volume and duration are patient-controlled variables that need to be regulated for successful deep-lung peptide delivery [34]. These systems are relatively less susceptible to environmental humidity compared with dry-powdered formulations. However, the majority of INH delivery systems being developed employ human insulin inhalation powder formulations that do not require sterile manufacturing conditions (Table 4) [35]. Because of its pharmacokinetic profile, inhaled insulin has been studied as a premeal non-invasive alternative to subcutaneous regular insulin or SIA [36,37]. The bioavailability of INH is low, that is, as compared with subcutaneous insulin only about 10–15%. It should be stressed that using injected insulin is not usually a major concern for the majority of people with T1DM, given the availability of patient support and education, modern small needles and insulin pens. Furthermore, the availability of inhaled insulin will not completely replace the need for injections of insulin in T1DM because the inhaled formulation is intended only to replace the need for preprandial injected insulin and not the basal insulin. Combining studies that compared INH and subcutaneous insulin in T1DM showed no difference [37] or a small difference in the decrease in HbA1C levels from baseline favouring subcutaneous insulin [36]. There was no difference between INH and subcutaneous insulin in the proportion of patients with T1DM reporting hypoglycemia and there was no difference in weight gain [36,37]. The overall patient satisfaction for INH versus subcutaneous insulin was higher [36,37]. This included ease of administration, comfort, convenience, mealtime flexibility and ease of taking insulin many times a day [36,37]. The question naturally arises concerning immunogenicity with delivering peptides to the deep lung with inhaled insulin devices. In T1DM higher levels of insulin antibodies were seen after INH versus subcutaneous insulin, however, the level of insulin antibodies was not associated with altered dosing requirements for

TABLE 4. Insulin inhalation systems in phase III studies.

Trade name	Delivery system
Exubera (Pfizer)	Dry-powder, single-dose blister packs (1–3 mg); breath-activated inhaler
AERx iDMS (Novo Nordisk)	Liquid aerosol; patient guided by microprocessor feedback inhaler system
Technosphere (MannKind)	Dry-powder, encapsulated in microspheres with diketopiperzine derivative; breath-actuated inhaler
AIR [Alkermes (Eli Lilly)]	Dry-powder phospholipid matrix; small mechanical and breath-actuated inhaler

INH, glycaemic control or adverse outcomes (allergic events, pulmonary side effects or hypoglycaemia) [36,37]. However, there are several potential problems to be overcome with patients who smoke and patients with impaired pulmonary function conditions that could affect the kinetics of INH. Previously, it has been demonstrated that smoking as well as chronic obstructive lung disease can increase pulmonary absorption of INH whereas asthma decreases it. Mild to moderate cough is seen with INH [34,36,37]. A major concern with INH is the potential for pulmonary toxicity because of the growth-promoting properties of insulin. Small decreases in lung function as judged by FEV_1 and DL_{CO} have been found to develop early in the treatment with INH but, however, it does not progress over 2 years. At present it can be concluded that INH offers an alternative non-invasive route for premeal insulin administration with glycaemic efficacy in T1DM [36,37]. INH should be a treatment option for people who have poor glycaemic control despite other appropriate therapeutic interventions and adequate educational support and who are unable to initiate or intensify preprandial subcutaneous insulin therapy because of (i) a marked and persistent fear of injections or (ii) severe and persistent problems with injection sites, for example as a consequence of lipohypertrophy despite support with injection site rotation [37]. In patients receiving inhaled insulin, treatments should only be continued beyond 6 months if there is evidence of a sustained improvement in HbA1C [37]. Initiation of inhaled insulin treatment and monitoring of response should be carried out at a specialist diabetes centre [37]. INH is contraindicated in people with poorly controlled, unstable or severe asthma or severe chronic obstructive pulmonary disease and in patients who smoke because of the unpredictable absorption with changes in smoking behaviour.

References

1. Nathan DM. Long-term complications of diabetes mellitus. N Engl J Med 1993;328:1676–1685.
2. The DCCT Research Group. The effect of intensive treatment of diabetes on the development and progression of long-term complications in insulin-dependent diabetes mellitus. N Engl J Med 1993;329:977–986.
3. The writing group for the Diabetes Control and Complication Trial/Epidemiology of Diabetes Interventions and Complications Research Group. JAMA 2002;287:2563–2569.
4. Binder C, Lauritzen T, Faber O, Pramming S. Insulin pharmacokinetics. Diabetes Care 1984;7:188–199.
5. Brunner GA, Hirschberger S, Sendlhofer G, Wutte A, Ellmerer M, Balent B, Schaupp L, Krejs GJ, Pieber TR. Post-prandial administration of the insulin analogue insulin aspart in patients with Type 1 diabetes mellitus. Diabet Med 2000;17(5):371–375.
6. Siebenhofer A, Plank J, Berghold A, Jeitler K, Horvath K, Narath M, Gfrerer R, Pieber TR. Short acting insulin analogues versus regular human insulin in patients with diabetes mellitus. Cochrane Database Syst Rev 2006;(2):CD003287. DOI:10.1002/14651858.CD003287.pub4.
7. Hagedorn HC, Jensen BN, Krarup NB, Wodstrup I. Protamine insulinate. JAMA 1936;106:177–180.
8. Plank J, Bodenlenz M, Sinner F, Magnes C, Gorzer E, Regittnig W, Endahl LA, Draeger E, Zdravkovic M, Pieber TR. A double-blind, randomized, dose–response study investigating the pharmacodynamic and pharmacokinetic properties of the long-acting insulin analog detemir. Diabetes Care 2005;28(5):1107–1112.
9. Lepore M, Pampanelli S, Fanelli C, Porcellati F, Bartocci L, Di Vincenzo A, Cordoni C, Costa E, Brunetti P, Bolli GB. Pharmacokinetics and pharmacodynamics of subcutaneous injection of long-acting human insulin analog glargine, NPH insulin, and ultralente human insulin and continuous subcutaneous infusion of insulin lispro. Diabetes 2000;49(12):2142–2148.
10. Heise T, Nosek L, Ronn BB, Endahl L, Heinemann L, Kapitza C, Draeger E. Lower within-subject variability of insulin detemir in comparison to NPH insulin and insulin glargine in people with type 1 diabetes. Diabetes 2004;53(6):1614–1620.
11. Bolli GB, Di Marchi RD, Park GD, Pramming S, Koivisto VA. Insulin analogues and their potential in the management of diabetes mellitus. Diabetologia 1999;42:1151–1167.
12. Klein O, Lynge J, Endahl L, Damholt B, Nosek L, Heise T. Albumin bound basal insulin analogues (insulin detemir and NN344): comparable time-action profiles but less variability than insulin glargine in type 2 diabetes. Diabetes Obes Metab 2007;9(3):290–299.
13. Ashwell SG, Gebbie J, Home PD. Twice-daily compared with once-daily insulin glargine in people with Type 1 diabetes using meal-time insulin aspart. Diabet Med 2006;23(8):879–886.
14. Ashwell SG, Amiel SA, Bilous RW, Dashora U, Heller SR, Hepburn DA, Shutler SD, Stephens JW, Home PD. Improved glycaemic control with insulin glargine plus insulin lispro: a multicentre, randomized, cross-over trial in people with Type 1 diabetes. Diabet Med 2006;23(3):285–292.

15. Rossetti P, Pampanelli S, Fanelli C, Porcellati F, Costa E, Torlone E, Scionti L, Bolli GB. Intensive replacement of basal insulin in patients with Type 1 diabetes given rapid-acting insulin analog at mealtime. Diabetes Care 2003;26:1490–1496.
16. Ratner RE, Hirsch IB, Neifing JL, Garg SK, Mecca TE, Wilson CA. Less hypoglycaemia with insulin glargine in intensive insulin therapy for Type 1 diabetes. Diabetes Care 2000;23:639–643.
17. Pieber TR, Eugene-Jolchine I, Derobert E. Efficacy and safety of HOE 901 versus NPH insulin in patients with Type 1 diabetes. Diabetes Care 2000;23:157–162.
18. Rosenstock J, Park G, Zimmerman J. Basal insulin glargine (HOE 901) versus NPH insulin in patients with Type 1 diabetes on multiple daily insulin regimens. Diabetes Care 2000;23:1137–1142.
19. Hermansen K, Madsbad S, Perrild H, Kristensen A, Axelsen M. Comparison of the soluble basal insulin analog insulin detemir with NPH insulin. Diabetes Care 2001;24:296–301.
20. Vague P, Selam, J-L, Skeie S, De Leeuw I, Elte JW, Haahr H, Kristensen A, Draeger E. Insulin detemir is associated with more predictable glycemic control and reduced risk of hypoglycemia than NPH insulin in patients with type 1 diabetes on a basal-bolus regimen with premeal insulin aspart. Diabetes Care 2003;26:590–596.
21. Hermansen K, Fontaine P, Kukolja KK, Peterkova V, Leth G, Gall MA. Insulin analogues (insulin detemir and insulin aspart) versus traditional human insulins (NPH insulin and regular insulin) in a basal bolus therapy for patients with type 1 diabetes. Diabetologia 2004;47:622–629.
22. De Leeuw I, Vague P, Selam JL, Skeie S, Lang H, Draeger E, Elte JW. Insulin detemir used in basal-bolus therapy in people with type 1 diabetes is associated with a lower risk of nocturnal hypoglycaemia and less weight gain over 12 months in comparison to NPH insulin. Diabetes Obes Metab 2005;7(1):73–82.
23. Home P, Bartley P, Russell-Jones D, Hanaire-Broutin H, Heeg JE, Abrams P, Landin-Olsson M, Hylleberg B, Lang H, Draeger E. Study to Evaluate the Administration of Detemir Insulin Efficacy, Safety and Suitability (STEADINESS) Study Group. Insulin detemir offers improved glycemic control compared with NPH insulin in people with type 1 diabetes: a randomized clinical trial. Diabetes Care 2004;27(5):1081–1087.
24. Pieber TR, Draeger E, Kristensen A, Grill V. Comparison of three multiple injection regimens for Type 1 diabetes: morning plus dinner or bedtime administration of insulin detemir vs. morning plus bedtime NPH insulin. Diabet Med 2005;22(7):850–857.
25. Russell-Jones D, Draeger E, Esimpson R, Bolinder J, Hylleberg B. Effects of once daily Insulin Detemir or NPH insulin on blood glucose control in people using a basal bolus regimen. Clin Ther 2004;26:724–736.
26. Hermansen K, Davies M. Does insulin detemir have a role in reducing risk of insulin-associated weight gain? Diabetes Obes Metab 2007;9(3):209–217.
27. Daneman D. Type 1 diabetes. Lancet 2006;367: 847–858.
28. ADA. Standards of medical care in diabetes – 2006. Diabetes Care 2006;29(Suppl 1):S4–S42.
29. Pickup J, Mattock M, Kerry S. Glycaemic control with continuous subcutaneous insulin infusion compared with intensive insulin injections in patients with type 1 diabetes: meta-analysis of randomised controlled trials. BMJ 2002;324:705–708.
30. Benchell-Weissberg J, Antisdel-Lomaglio J, Sehadri R. Insulin pump therapy. Diabetes Care 2003;26:1079–1087.
31. Siebenhofer A, Plank J, Berghold A, Horvath K, Sawicki PT, Beck P, Pieber TR. Meta-analysis of short-acting insulin analogues in adult patients with type 1 diabetes: continuous subcutaneous insulin infusion versus injection therapy. Diabetologia 2004;47(11):1895–1905.
32. Hermansen K, Bendtson I, Borch-Johnsen K, Christiansen JS, Henriksen JE, Lervang HH, Nørgaard K. Insulin pump treatment in Denmark (in Danish). Ugeskr Laeger 2004;166(42):3685–3689.
33. National Institute for Clinical Excellence. Technology Appraisal Guidance No 57. Guidance on the use of continuous subcutaneous insulin infusion for diabetes. February 2003 (www.NICE.org.UK).
34. Hermansen K. Waiting to inhale: non-injectable insulin, are we there yet? Curr Diab Rep 2004;4(5):335–341.
35. Muchmore DB, Gates JR. Inhaled insulin delivery – where are we now? Diabetes Obes Metab 2006;8:634–642.
36. Ceglia L, Lau J, Pittas AG. Meta-analysis: efficacy and safety of inhaled insulin therapy in adults with diabetes mellitus. Ann Int Med 2006;145:665–675.
37. National Institute for Clinical Excellence. Inhaled insulin for the treatment of diabetes (types 1 and 2). NICE technology appraisal guidance 113 (2006). Available from www.nice.org.uk/TA113

7
Insulin and New Insulin Analogues with Focus on Type 2 Diabetes

Sten Madsbad

Introduction

The underlying insulin resistance and impaired insulin secretion in patients with type 2 diabetes worsen over time, necessitating the use of antidiabetic drugs, often in combination, to control glycaemic levels [1]. From the UKPD study the main explanation for the progressive history of type 2 diabetes seems to be a failure of beta-cell function over time [2], while insulin resistance may be more constant from diagnosis [2]. Therefore, it is not surprising that insulin treatment is necessary in most patients 10–15 years after diagnosis to maintain of HbA1c level as close to normal as is safely possible [2]. A consensus recommendation for the treatment of type 2 diabetes has recently been published [1]. The algorithm for treatment strategy includes early and aggressive use of insulin, the most powerful antidiabetic drug, to achieve treatment goals. Many patients and health care professionals delay insulin treatment due to concerns about injection-site pain, hypoglycaemia and weight gain, despite the fact that several studies have suggested that improvement of glycaemic control by insulin treatment improves the well-being and quality of life [3,4]. Furthermore, insulin treatment is often delayed because a traditional stepwise approach is applied, with a period of lifestyle modification followed by a slow process of uptitration of oral monotherapy and eventually combination therapy, despite failure to achieve glycaemic targets [5]. Moreover, there is no consensus about the most optimal insulin regimen for treatment of subjects with type 2 diabetes [1]. Of note, most of the studies on insulin treatment of subjects with type 2 diabetes have been initiated by the pharmaceutical companies and have not been investigator driven. The studies have often been performed for registration and promotion of the new insulin analogues.

The aim of insulin replacement therapy is to normalise or near-normalise blood glucose in order to reduce the complications of diabetes mellitus. Until a few years ago we only had fast-acting human insulin and the long-acting neutral protamin Hagedorn (NPH) insulin. The pharmacokinetics of the traditional insulin preparations does not match the profile of the normal physiological insulin secretion. Another problem is that some patients are characterised by a large day-to-day variation in glycaemic level, which in part is explained by a large day-to-day variation in insulin absorption [6]. The absorption rate of the fast-acting human insulin is with a peak action 2–4 h after injection and does not provide the early and quick rise in plasma insulin required to prevent exaggerated postprandial hyperglycaemia after a meal. The pharmacokinetic profile also increases the risk of hypoglycaemia 3–5 h after a meal, especially if snacks are omitted [6]. The intermediate acting NPH insulin cannot deliver insulin in a constant and reproducible low-level rate that characterises normal insulin secretion, but produces a peak in insulin concentration 4–6 h after injection, which increases the risk of nocturnal hypoglycaemia [6]. On this background the new insulin analogues were developed, making a more physiological insulin regimen realistic for many patients, since onset and duration of the action of these analogues more closely mimic human insulin secretion. At the moment we have three rapid-acting insulin analogues with similar pharmacokinetic profiles for targeting postprandial hyperglycaemia, two long-acting insulin analogues, and several biphasic premix analogues.

The present narrative review will discuss whether the new insulin analogues have improved the treatment of type 2 diabetic patients. First the two long-acting analogues glargine and detemir will be discussed, followed by a review of the biphasic premix insulins. Comments will be given on the rapid-acting insulin analogues used in combination with NPH insulin or the long-acting insulin analogues. The use of inhaled insulin in the treatment of type 2 diabetes will also be mentioned. Combination therapy with insulin plus oral antidiabetic drugs versus treatment with insulin alone and the comparison of human insulin versus insulin analogues are also a part of the present review. Lastly, it is helpful to distinguish between basal and postprandial hyperglycaemia caused by ingestion of food, since the strategies for treatment of diabetes primarily control one or the other of these aspects of hyperglycaemia. Recommended HbA1c targets for treatment of subjects with type 2 diabetes are between 6.5% and 7.0% [1]. The majority of individuals with type 2 diabetes in both the USA and Europe do not achieve a HbA1c <7.0 [7,8].

Treatment with NPH Insulin and the Long-Acting Insulin Analogues

One treatment concept has gained popularity in recent years following its success in clinical trials: the addition of a long-acting basal insulin formulation to an existing oral antidiabetic drug (OAD) treatment, followed by aggressive titration of the insulin dose to achieve target levels of glycemia. Adding basal insulin has been shown to lower the entire 24-h blood glucose profile, and in combination with metformin the increase in weight after initiation of insulin treatment has been significantly reduced [9,10].

Both long-acting insulin analogues – insulin glargine and insulin detemir – have been implemented in the “treat to target” approach used in type 2 diabetic patients. The analogues are injectable, clear solutions, but the mechanisms by which they achieve prolonged activity differ entirely as described in detail in Chapter 8 and in [11,12].

Insulin Glargine (Lantus)

Insulin glargine (Lantus) was the first available long-acting human insulin analogue [12]. Glargine is a clear solution and there is no need to thoroughly mix it before injection. Insulin glargine (21A-Gly-30Ba-L-Arg-30Bb-L-Arg-human insulin) differs from native insulin in that the 21 amino acid residue aspargine on the A chain has been substituted with a glycerine residue and 2 arginine residues have been added to the C terminus of the B chain, making glargine soluble in the acidic environment at pH of 4 [12]. Glargine precipitates in the neutral pH of subcutaneous tissue, which prolongs its absorption to the blood. The addition of zinc as a hexamer-stabilising agent further prolongs the duration of action. Insulin glargine must not be mixed with other insulins [12].

Clamp studies in normal subjects and type 1 diabetic patients have confirmed that the duration of glargine is longer than NPH insulin and the action profile is flatter. Median duration of action is 23 h for glargine versus 14 h for NPH insulin, and during the first 12 h intra-individual variability of the absorption rate is lower with glargine [13]. The pharmacokinetic suggests that glargine is more suitable than NPH human insulin to mimic the normal pattern of physiological basal insulin secretion.

Insulin glargine has been compared with NPH in type 2 patients. In theory, basal insulin supplementation with glargine offers the advantage of a simple once-daily injection regimen, which is easy to add to current oral glucose-lowering drugs.

In the “treat-to-target” studies glargine was administered once daily at bedtime and NPH was given once daily at bedtime or twice daily at bedtime and in the morning in combination with sulfonylurea (glimepiride)[14–19]. The overall conclusions from the studies are that the reduction in HbA1c was similar in the glargine and NPH groups and that the number of patients reaching the target of HbA1c <7.0% was not different. The fasting blood glucose was lower in the glargine groups than in the NPH groups. Except for one of the studies, comparing either bedtime or morning glargine versus bedtime NPH insulin, significantly more patients reached an HbA1c <7.5% with morning glargine than with bedtime glargine and bedtime NPH insulin [16]. In another study there was no difference in the reduction in HbA1c between morning and bedtime administration of glargine and similar proportion of patients achieved HbA1c <7.0 at the end of the study period [20].

In a recent 36-weeks study glargine or NPH insulin were combined with metformin [21]. HbA1c decreased similar values in the two groups, but the incidence of hypoglycaemia was lower in the glargine group the first 12 weeks of treatment. Thereafter, no difference was observed between the two treatments.

Treatment with glargine has also been compared with biphasic premix insulin. Once-daily morning glargine added to OADs induced a greater reduction in HbA1c and fasting blood glucose than twice-daily biphasic human premix (30% regular and 70% NPH) alone [22]. In three other studies, which are discussed later in detail, glargine once daily compared with twice-daily biphasic premix lispro (Mix 25) or biphasic premix aspart (BIAsp 30). The reduction in HbA1c was greater in the premix groups [23–25].

In 518 type 2 patients on basal-bolus regimen with glargine at bedtime plus a rapid acting analogue before meals or NPH once or twice daily in combination with fast-acting human insulin before meals [15], a similar HbA1c level was achieved in the two groups, and the decrease in fasting blood glucose and the number of hypoglycaemic episodes were the same.

The glargine studies (treat-to-target) are very important landmark studies. The studies illustrate for the first time the importance of using a forced titration algorithm to optimise glycaemic control. The treat-to-target studies have shown that it is possible to obtain HbA1c below 7.0% in approximately 50% of subjects with type 2 diabetes using one injection and one blood glucose measurement per day.

Hypoglycaemia

One of the greatest barriers to intensive insulin therapy is the risk of hypoglycaemia. A recent meta-analysis indicates that the incidence of symptomatic hypoglycaemia, nocturnal hypoglycaemia and severe hypoglycaemia is less (approximately 50%) during treatment with insulin glargine compared with NPH insulin [26]. In patients reaching an HbA1c below 7.0% the risk of moderate and severe nocturnal hypoglycaemia is reduced with 46% and 59%, respectively, with glargine compared with NPH insulin [26]. The reduction in nocturnal hypoglycaemia with glargine is most likely explained by its smooth time-action and less day-to-day variation in insulin absorption compared with NPH insulin.

Weight Gain

Weight changes have not been measured in most studies, but in two studies the weight changes were similar in the glargine and the NPH group when insulin was added to oral agents [14,17]. When subjects were randomised to prandial fast-acting human insulin with once-daily glargine or twice-daily NPH insulin, less weight gain was seen with glargine [15].

Comments on the Glargine Studies

Insulin glargine was the first candidate to challenge the position of NPH insulin as basal insulin. Glargine appears safe with a clinical benefit regarding risk reduction of hypoglycaemia. In most studies no differences have been observed between glargine and NPH insulin in the level of HbA1c at the end of the studies. Insulin glargine has a role in the treatment in type 2 diabetes in combination with metformin or sulphonylurea. Glargine can also be combined with prandial insulin including inhaled pulmonal insulin. Insulin glargine used in a simple once-daily injection regimen is easy to add to current oral glucose-lowering drugs. The low injection and monitoring frequency may increase the acceptance and compliance of insulin treatment. The disadvantage of basal insulin is that it does not address the key secretory defect (loss of first-phase insulin secretion) in type 2 diabetes and therefore provides inadequate insulin profile to the postprandial glucose excursions. As titration is focusing on fasting plasma glucose, this removes the focus from postprandial glucose control. As glycaemic control deteriorates, as a consequence of failing beta-cell function, more insulin injections are needed with fast-acting insulin or biphasic premix insulin before some of the meals. There are no clinical controlled studies of glargine in pregnant women, and glargine should not be used during pregnancy. Glargine is more expensive than the conventional insulins such as NPH insulin.

Insulin Detemir (Levemir)

In insulin detemir (B29lys(epsilon-tetradconoyl), des B30 human insulin) a 14-C fatty chain has been attached to position B29 and the amino residue at position B30 has been omitted [11,27]. When injected subcutaneous it dissociates exposing the fatty free acid chain, which subsequently binds to the free fatty acid binding sites on the albumin molecule [11,27]. Insulin detemir is 98–99% albumin bound in human plasma [11,27]. It is only the free fraction of detemir that is biologically active. The albumin binding and the ensuing slow release of detemir from albumin cause the prolonged blood glucose lowering effect of this insulin [27]. The soluble formulation ensures a homogenous concentration, with no need for resuspension before administration. The peak effect appears after 6–7 hours and the profile is more flat for detemir insulin compared with NPH insulin. The day-to-day variation in time action profile with detemir is much lower (CV 27%) than with insulin glargine (CV 48%) and NPH insulin (CV 68%). Insulin detemir may provide more consistent insulin levels and more predictable blood glucose concentrations than NPH insulin, which is one of the explanations for the reduced risk of hypoglycaemia during treatment with detemir.

Two studies have compared insulin detemir with NPH insulin in patients with type 2 diabetes [29,30]. Hermansen and coworkers in a treat-to-target protocol compared insulin detemir and NPH insulin added to oral therapy in patients with type 2 diabetes [29]. Approximately 65% received more than one oral glucose lowering drug. Totally 476 type 2 patients were randomised to addition of twice-daily insulin detemir or NPH insulin. Insulin doses were titrated towards a pre-breakfast and pre-dinner plasma glucose target of <6.0 mmol/L. At 24 weeks, HbA1c had decreased by 1.8% and 1.9% (from 8.6% to 6.8% and from 8.5% to 6.6%) for detemir and NPH insulin, respectively. A 10-point diurnal glucose profile was not different between the groups at the end of the study period, but the day-to-day variation in plasma glucose was lower in the insulin detemir group. In both groups 70% of the patients received HbA1c <7.0%, but the proportion achieving this goal without hypoglycaemia was higher with insulin detemir than with NPH insulin (26% vs. 16%). The risk for hypoglycaemia with insulin detemir was reduced by 47% and nocturnal hypoglycaemia by 55% compared with NPH insulin. Mean weight gain was 1.2 kg with detemir and 2.8 kg with NPH insulin. With increasing BMI patients gained less weight with detemir.

In the second study insulin detemir and NPH were administered to type 2 patients in poor control and they were treated with oral antidiabetic drugs [30]. It was a 20-week randomised, 3-arm, parallel-group trial including 504 patients treated with either insulin detemir before breakfast, or evening insulin detemir or NPH insulin during the evening. Evening was defined from 1 h before dinner to bedtime. The basal HbA1c was around 9.0% and the reductions in HbA1c were −1.58%, −1.48% and −1.74% in the three groups. As expected fasting plasma glucose was higher in the group treated with morning insulin detemir, whereas no difference was observed in the two groups treated with evening insulin. A nine-point glucose profile shows similar results with the lowest glycaemic values at day time in the morning detemir group and higher values overnight. Compared with NPH insulin overall risk of hypoglycaemia and nocturnal hypoglycaemia was reduced by 53% and 65%, respectively, with evening detemir. Nocturnal hypoglycaemia was reduced with 87% in the group treated with morning detemir compared with evening NPH insulin. Weight gain was 1.2, 0.7 and 1.6 kg, respectively, with morning and evening detemir and NPH insulin. The weight gain was significantly lower with evening detemir compared with NPH insulin.

The two studies comparing insulin detemir with NPH insulin support the results from the studies in type 1 diabetic patients, that detemir reduces the risk of hypoglycaemia, especially during night time compared with NPH insulin. A meta-analyses of insulin detemir versus NPH insulin in type 2 diabetic patients demonstrated a 39% reduction for hypoglycaemia with insulin detemir [31]. Furthermore, the weight gain during treatment with detemir was less than that in the groups treated with NPH insulin.

The explanation for the less weight gain with insulin detemir is unknown. It is not explained only by fewer hypoglycaemic events and thereby theoretically a reduced caloric intake. Potential explanations for the weight-sparing effect of insulin detemir could include improved hypothalamic insulin signalling and change in appetite regulation [32] or a relative reduction in peripheral lipogenesis [11,33].

The titration algorithms used in the studies with glargine and detemir were rather similar. The initial insulin dose has been low, approximately 10 units. Insulin dose was often titrated every third day by the mean of three self-measured plasma glucose levels. In patients receiving insulin in the morning, the dose was titrated to obtain a pre-dinner plasma glucose below 5–5 to 6.0 mmol/L, and in patients taking insulin in the evening, titration aimed at a fasting plasma glucose concentration of <6.0 mmol/L.

Comments on Insulin Detemir

The smooth time-action profile of detemir in combination with a low day-to-day variation of effect on glycaemic control seems to be translated into improved glycaemic control. If the average glucose levels are unchanged, then extreme high and low glucose excursions will be of lower frequency, and thus occurrence of hypo- and hyperglycaemia will be reduced. At the simple level improved glycaemic control should be possible without increasing the risk of hypoglycaemia by the use of insulin detemir. In type 2 diabetes weight gain is problematic when starting insulin treatment and can act as a barrier to acceptance of insulin therapy. An interesting observation from the studies is the weight advantage of levemir compared with NPH insulin. Thus, during a 6-month period the weight gain was only 50% of that observed with NPH insulin.

Treatment of Patients with Type 2 Diabetes with Biphasic Premix Insulin

A popular alternative to treatment with a long-acting basal insulin plus OAD – the "one pill, one shot" regimen discussed above in patients with type 2 diabetes is a twice-daily biphasic premixed insulin combined with OAD. Along with a beneficial effect on prandial glucose control, biphasic premix insulin may reduce the risk of diabetic complication and cardiovascular disease [34]. Twice-daily biphasic premix insulin is often used as an initial insulin regimen and also as a substitute if basal insulin fails to achieve the HbA1c goal. Biphasic premix insulin is convenient to patients, but titration of the fix ratio of prandial and basal insulin may be difficult.

Comparison of Biphasic Premix Insulin Analogues with Biphasic Premix Human Insulins

Several new biphasic premix insulin analogues have been introduced during the last years. Novomix 30, contains 30% rapid-acting aspart and 70% protamin – crystallised aspart. HumaLog (Mix 25), contains 25% rapid-acting lipro and 75% protamine-crystallised lispro. Biphasic premix analogues are available in other differently proportioned premix preparations, but these are used less frequently. The new premix insulin analogues can be injected immediately before a meal and the peak insulin concentration of the fast-acting component coincides with prandial glucose excursions [35]. The fast-acting component inhibits hepatic glucose production and promotes glucose uptake in the peripheral tissues and thereby reduces postprandial glucose excursions.

The new biphasic premix insulin analogues have been compared with biphasic premix human insulin [36–40]. The degree of glycaemic control obtained has been similar to the human premix insulins and the premix analogues. In McNally's study the incidence of nocturnal hypoglycaemia was reduced with the analogue, but in the other studies no significant difference was observed in hypoglycaemia with the premix human insulin and the new analogues [39]. Postprandial hyperglycaemia was, as expected, reduced more with the biphasic premix analogues.

Comparison of Premix Insulin Analogues with Long-Acting Insulin Analogues

In a 28-week study 209 subjects treated with OADs (except secretagogues) were randomised to BIasp 30/70 twice-daily or insulin glargine at bedtime and titrated to target blood glucose (4.0–5.5 mmol/L) before breakfast and dinner for biphasic premix aspart (BIasp) and before breakfast for insulin glargine by algorithm-directed titration [23]. At the end of the study HbA1c was lower in BIasp 30/70 than in the glargine group (6.9 ± 1.2 vs. 7.4 ± −1.2%), especially for subjects with baseline HbA1c >8.5%. More patients in the BIasp group reached target HbA1c below 7.0% than the glargine-treated patients (66 vs. 40%) [23]. Reduction in HbA1c was 3.1% versus 2.4%, respectively ($p < 0.05$). The reduction in fasting plasma glucose was comparable between the groups. The number of minor hypoglycaemic episodes, weight gain (5.4 kg vs. 3.5 kg) and insulin dose (79 vs. 51 units per day) were greater in the BIasp group than in the glargine group [23].

In another 26-week study insulin naïve type 2 patients were randomised to insulin BIasp 30/70 plus metformin or insulin glargine plus glimepiride [41]. Baseline mean HbA1c was about 9%. HbA1c reduction was 0.5% greater (1.6% vs. 1.1%) in the BIasp-treated subjects compared with the subjects treated with glargine. The mean plasma glucose values and the prandial glucose increments evaluated from seven-point diurnal plasma glucose profiles were significantly lower for BIasp 30 plus metformin compared with the glargine plus glimiperide-treated group. One major hypoglycaemic episode occurred in each group, and 20% and 9% displayed a minor hypoglycaemic episode in the two groups. The mean insulin doses in the two groups were not different at the end of the study (0.40 IU/kg BIasp and 0.39 IU/kg glargine). The weight gain was 0.7 kg in the BIasp group and 1.5 kg in the glargine group.

Similar results have been presented by Malone and coworkers [24,25] using biphasic lispro 25/75 versus once-daily insulin glargine. In 597 patients twice-daily biphasic insulin lispro 25/75 was compared with once daily insulin glargine. Both insulins were taken in combination with metformin. After 16 weeks of treatment more subjects reached target HbA1c <7.0% in the group receiving biphasic premix lispro than in those taking glargine (41% vs. 22%, $p < 0.001$).

The studies indicate that the degree of glycemic control obtained by biphasic premix insulin analogues is better than that with glargine in patients with type 2 diabetes mellitus.

A study of practical clinical interest is "The 1-2-3 study" using BIasp 30/70 [42]. The patients were treated with two OAD or one OAD plus once-daily basal insulin. Patients discontinued prior basal insulin and started insulin treatment with once daily BIasp 12 units before dinner, and at week 16 a pre-breakfast dose of BIasp was added, if HbA1c exceeded 6.5%. After additional 16 weeks a third dose of BIasp was added before lunch if HbA1c still exceeded 6.5%. Once-daily

BIasp enabled 21% of the patients to achieve HbA1c <6.5%. With two injections of BIasp 52% and with three daily injections 60% achieved HBA1c <6.5%, indicating that approximately 50% of patients with type 2 diabetes can obtain a HbA1c below 6.5% by the addition and vigorous titration of two daily injections of BIasp 30 to oral antidiabetic agents [42].

In a smaller study insulin treatment was given as once-daily BIasp 30 before dinner, human insulin premix 30 before dinner or NPH insulin at 10 P.M. [43]. After 12 weeks of treatment the reduction in HbA1c was 1.3%, 1.2% and 1.1% in the three groups.

Comments on the Treatment with Biphasic Premix Insulin

The explanation for the results with biphasic premix insulin versus basal insulins is that both postprandial and basal glycaemia are controlled by the biphasic premix insulin. In patients with high HbA1c, basal hyperglycemia plays a greater role for the HbA1c level than in a situation with low HbA1c, where postprandial hyperglycemia contributes more to overall glycaemic control [44]. The biphasic premix insulin analogues have an advantage over basal insulin alone because they provide the rapid-acting insulin component that covers mealtime hyperglycaemia. Therefore, it is not surprising that the premix insulin can reduce HbA1c more than intermediate-acting or the long-acting insulin analogues. Conversely, premixed regimens are relatively inflexible with their fixed ratio between the fast- and long-acting components. They can be difficult to intensify, because of risk of hypoglycaemia and weight gain.

Treating Subjects with Type 2 Diabetes with Multiple Injections (Basal-Bolus Therapy)

Multiple injections with fast-acting insulin before the meals and intermediate or long-acting insulin at bedtime (basal-bolus regimen) is the first choice insulin regimen in most type 1 patients, but is not used very much in patients with type 2 diabetes. Nevertheless, prandial glucose regulation is an emerging concept, since epidemiological and mechanistic studies indicate that postprandial glucose contributes significantly to overall glycaemic exposure and also contributes to the vascular complications in type 2 diabetes [34,45]. Adding prandial insulin to basal insulin is a logical approach when the target of HbA1c cannot be achieved by the combination of basal insulin and oral therapy. Basal-bolus therapy represents the most physiological insulin regimen, but is more complex and the patient needs to be more educated and motivated for glucose monitoring. A few studies have evaluated the efficacy of multiple injections in type 2 diabetic patients.

In the first study the efficacy and safety of a basal-bolus regimen compared insulin detemir or NPH insulin in combination with mealtime insulin aspart in 505 patients with type 2 diabetes (BMI 30.4 ± 5.3 kg/m^2, HbA1c 7.9 ± 1.3%) [46]. The patients were randomised 2:1 to insulin detemir or NPH insulin. After 26 weeks significant reduction in HbA1c was observed for both insulin detemir (0.2%) and NPH insulin (0.4%). HbA1c was comparable at study end (insulin detemir 7.6% and insulin NPH 7.5%). Nine points self-measured blood glucose profiles were similar for the two treatments as were reduction in fasting plasma glucose. The within-subject day-to-day variation in fasting plasma glucose was significantly lower with insulin detemir. Moreover, patients receiving insulin detemir gained significantly less body weight than those treated with NPH insulin (1.0 and 1.8 kg, respectively). The frequency of hypoglycaemia was similar in the two groups. Dose of basal insulin and insulin aspart was not different between the groups.

In a second study detemir plus aspart was compared with NPH and human fast-acting insulin [47]. Nocturnal hypoglycaemia weight gain and within-person variation in self-monitored plasma glucose were less in the analogue regimen, indicating, as found in patients with type 1 diabetes, that the use of analogue insulin reduces weight gain, hypoglycaemia and day-to-day variation in plasma glucose within subjects.

Three studies, including 722, 295 and 148 patients, compared lispro with human fast-acting insulin in combination with basal insulin found no difference in HbA1c. In one of the studies (n = 722) fewer episodes of hypoglycaemia were registered. In all studies postprandial plasma glucose was lower with the rapid-acting analogue than with human insulin [48–50].

In a fourth study the rapid-acting insulin analogue glulisine from Sanofi aventis was compared with fast-acting human insulin. NPH insulin was used as basal insulin in both arms (n = 876). After 26 weeks of treatment, 0.16% greater reduction in HbA1c and lower postprandial glucose excursions in favour of insulin glulisine were observed, but without any differences in episodes of hypoglycaemia [51].

Comments on Treatment with Basal-Bolus Regimen

It is still unknown whether it is essential to address postprandial hyperglycemia by using rapid-acting insulin before the meals to reduce the risk of a cardiovascular event and late diabetic complications. Nevertheless, in many patients, especially with a poor endogenous insulin secretion, treatment of both basal and postprandial hyperglycaemia with a basal-bolus regimen is necessary to reach a target of HbA1c less than 6.5–7.0%. The practical burden imposed by the frequency of injections and glucose testing may be taken into consideration before choosing multiple injections in a subject with type 2 diabetes mellitus.

Treatment of Subjects with Type 2 Diabetes Using Pulmonary Inhalation of Insulin

Several pharmaceutical companies have developed inhaled insulin, and exubera from Sanofi aventis and Pfizer has been approved in several countries.

The lungs with their large surface area and the thin alveolar epithelium allow rapid absorption of inhaled insulin [52]. The bioavailability has a range of 15–25% [52]. The exubera insulin is a fine powder insulin in doses of 1 or 3 mg, corresponding to approximately 3 and 9 units of human insulin. The clinical trials have shown that the insulin antibody levels increase with the use of inhaled insulin, but this has not been linked to any changes in glycemic control and episodes of hypoglycaemia or allergic reactions [53]. The pharmacokinetic profile of exubera is quite similar to that of rapid-acting insulin analogues, but with a duration of action between that of rapid-acting analogues and fast-acting human insulin [54].

The development of inhaled insulin must be seen in the light of a substantial resistance to insulin therapy in patients with type 2 diabetes and physicians who care for the patients. The reasons for this resistance include anticipated pain, inconvenience, fear of hypoglycaemia and weight gain [55,56].

Several clinical controlled trials have evaluated treatment with inhaled insulin. In 779 type 2 patients with an HbA1c >8% the availability of inhaled insulin as a treatment option significantly increased the proportion of patients who would theoretically choose insulin treatment [57]. Thus, patients were three times more likely to choose insulin when inhaled insulin was available compared with conventional insulin treatment [57].

In the first smaller randomised trial 68 type 2 patients with HbA1c between 8.1 and 11.9% despite treatment with sulfonylurea and/or metformin were randomised to receive inhaled insulin in addition to pre-study OHA (oral hypoglycaemic agents) or to continue to take OHA alone for 12 weeks [58]. After 12 weeks a mean reduction in HbA1c of 2.3% was found in the first group, compared with 0.1% in the group treated with OHA alone [58]. No long-acting insulin was used in the study.

In another study exubera was used in monotherapy or added to dual oral agent therapy in type 2 patients with an HbA1c between 8% and 11% [59]. The study design was a 12-week open label randomised trial. Exubera was used as a premeal insulin in the two insulin arms with either dual oral agents or as monotherapy. In the third treatment arm patients continued receiving dual oral agents [59]. At week 12 both inhaled insulin groups had a significantly greater reduction in HbA1c of 1.9% and 1.4%, respectively [59]. In the control group the decrease in HbA1c was 0.2%. Hypoglycaemia and cough were more often reported in the two groups treated with inhaled insulin. Pulmonary function tests showed no statistically significant differences between the groups, but increased insulin antibody titers were observed in the inhaled insulin groups [59].

In a 6-month study type 2 diabetic patients were randomised to treatment with premeal inhaled insulin plus bedtime ultralente or at least two injections of subcutaneous insulin (premix human/NPH insulin) [60]. HbA1c decreased similarly in both groups (0.7% vs. 0.6%), and no difference was found in the number of hypoglycaemic events. Insulin-binding antibodies increased more in the inhaled insulin group [60].

In the study by DeFronzo and coworkers, inhaled insulin was compared with rosiglitazone in 150 patients with suboptimal control on diet and exercise (HbA1c 9.4%) [61]. The HbA1c reduction was greater in the inhaled insulin group (2.3%) compared with 1.4% in the rosiglitazone group.

Lastly, Barnett et al. in a 24-week study randomised type 2 patients uncontrolled on sulfonylurea monotherapy to inhaled insulin before meals or metformin and demonstrated in subjects with HbA1c >9.5% at randomisation a greater reduction in HbA1c in the inhaled insulin-treated group (2.2% vs. 1.8%) [62]. In the patients with HbA1c <9.5% at randomisation, the decrease in HbA1c was not different between the two groups. More events of hypoglycaemia were observed in the inhaled insulin group [62].

Comments on Inhaled Insulin

In type 2 patients the effect of inhaled insulin before meals on HbA1c did not seem to differ from that of fast-acting human insulin. Adding three times inhaled insulin to existing oral therapy is generally more effective than adding another oral hypoglycaemic agent. In the trials, subjects have been more satisfied with inhaled insulin than with subcutaneous insulin treatment. Whether this outcome will be borne out in clinical practice remains to be determined. Inhaled insulin seems to be most suitable in patients with controlled fasting blood glucose using a basal insulin.

Smoking is a contraindication for inhaled insulin and inhaled insulin is not recommended in patients with asthma or chronic obstructive pulmonary disease. All candidates for inhaled insulin should have their lung function checked before and after 6 months and then every year. If lung function has declined more than 20% or by more than 500 ml from baseline, inhaled insulin should be discontinued. The long-term effect of inhaled insulin in the human lung and on neoplastic lung tissue is unknown. Pulmonary insulin is much more expensive than human insulin and still needs to be compared with the rapid-acting insulin analogues. In the UK, the NICE institute recommends that inhaled insulin should be only prescribed by diabetes specialists for patients with needle phobia or severe problems at injection sites.

Insulin Monotherapy versus Combinations of Insulin with Oral Hypoglycaemic Agents in Patients with Type 2 Diabetes

A Cochrane meta-analysis from 2004 of 20 studies including 1,811 patients with type 2 diabetes concluded that the quality of the studies was low, with no assessment of morbidity or mortality [63]. Insulin plus OHA combination therapy statistically had benefits on glycaemic control compared with insulin alone, but only when the latter was applied as once-daily injections of NPH insulin [63]. Conversely twice-daily biphasic premix or NPH insulin were superior to insulin plus OHA therapy regimens where insulin was administered as once-daily injection. Insulin plus OHA combination therapy was associated with a 43% relative reduction in total daily insulin requirement [63]. No significant differences in hypoglycaemia between insulin plus OHA and insulin alone were reported. Combination therapy with metformin and bedtime NPH insulin reported significantly less weight gain compared with insulin monotherapy. Insulin plus OHA combination therapy should be considered a suitable simple starting regimen for most insulin requiring type 2 diabetic patients [63]. Another comprehensive meta-analysis has reached similar conclusions [64].

Concluding Remarks

Type 2 diabetes mellitus is a progressive disease, where both fasting and postprandial blood glucose concentrations are elevated. Owing to the progressive nature of the disease, an evolving treatment strategy is necessary to maintain glycaemic control. A main problem in the treatment of subjects with type 2 diabetes is that physicians do not initiate and increase pharmacologic treatment in a timely fashion, but often wait until HbA1c has increased to above 8% [65]. Therefore, better definitions of the goals and method for initiating insulin therapy are needed.

The insulin regimen recommended for the individual patient will often depend on the state of the disease. If insulin treatment is started early, when the patient is treated with one or two OADs and HbA1c is about 7%, most patients can be treated with NPH insulin or one of the long-acting insulin analogues at bedtime. Later, when the endogenous insulin secretion has diminished treatment with a twice-daily biphasic premix insulin may be reliable to control glucose. Later treatment with multiple injections can be necessary in a subgroup of type 2 patients to control hyperglycaemia.

The regimen based on premixed insulin achieves good glycaemic control but with unwanted effects of more hypoglycaemia than the long-acting analogues. The place of inhaled insulin in the treatment of type 2 diabetes is at present unknown. Inhaled insulin can be an option in a few patients with needle phobia, but the degree of control obtained is comparable to that observed using fast-acting human insulin before main meals. The practical burdens imposed by the frequency of injections and glucose testing may be taken into consideration when choosing the insulin regimen.

It can be recommended that insulin treatment is combined with metformin. The combination improves glycaemic control and reduces the weight increase after starting up insulin when compared with treatment with insulin alone. The combination with metformin reduces the insulin dose.

An increasing number of type 2 diabetic subjects are treated with insulin, including insulin analogues. At present, there is no hard end point on mortality, morbidity or late diabetic complication, indicating the superiority of analogue insulins compared with conventional insulin treatment. HbA1c, fasting plasma glucose, postprandial glucose regulation, day-to-day variation in blood glucose control, risk of hypoglycaemia and change in weight have been the main outcome in the clinical randomised studies comparing the new and old insulin preparations. No major difference in HbA1c has been demonstrated between the analogue and human insulin-based regimens. The benefit of the long-acting analogues has been seen in relation to the reduction of risk of hypoglycaemia and in less weight gain with insulin detemir. It is still unknown whether it is essential to address the postprandial hyperglycemia by use of rapid-acting insulin or a biphasic premix insulin analogue before the meals to reduce the risk of cardiovascular events and late diabetic complications.

Lastly, the profile of adverse events and benefits, the relative costs of the different insulin preparations, and the complexity of insulin regimens together with the wishes of the individual patients should be considered when the treatment strategy is decided.

References

1. Nathan DM, Buse JB, Davidson MB, Heine RJ, Holman RR, Sherwin R et al. Management of hyperglycaemia in type 2 diabetes: a consensus algorithm for the initiation and adjustment of therapy. A consensus statement from the American Diabetes Association and the European Association for the Study of Diabetes. Diabetologia 2006;49(8):1711–1721.
2. Turner RC, Cull CA, Frighi V, Holman RR. Glycemic control with diet, sulfonylurea, metformin, or insulin in patients with type 2 diabetes mellitus: progressive requirement for multiple therapies (UKPDS 49). UK Prospective Diabetes Study (UKPDS) Group. JAMA 1999;281(21):2005–2012.
3. Taylor R, Davies R, Fox C, Sampson M, Weaver JU, Wood L. Appropriate insulin regimes for type 2 diabetes: a multicenter randomized crossover study. Diabetes Care 2000;23(11):1612–1618.
4. Chow CC, Tsang LW, Sorensen JP, Cockram CS. Comparison of insulin with or without continuation of oral hypoglycemic agents in the treatment of secondary failure in NIDDM patients. Diabetes Care 1995;18(3):307–314.
5. Harris SB, Ekoe JM, Zdanowicz Y, Webster-Bogaert S. Glycemic control and morbidity in the Canadian primary care setting (results of the diabetes in Canada evaluation study). Diabetes Res Clin Pract 2005;70(1):90–97.
6. Binder C, Lauritzen T, Faber O, Pramming S. Insulin pharmacokinetics. Diabetes Care 1984;7(2): 188–199.
7. Saydah SH, Fradkin J, Cowie CC. Poor control of risk factors for vascular disease among adults with previously diagnosed diabetes. JAMA 2004; 291(3): 335–342.
8. Liebl A, Mata M, Eschwege E. Evaluation of risk factors for development of complications in Type II diabetes in Europe. Diabetologia 2002; 45(7): S23–S28.
9. Yki-Jarvinen H, Kauppila M, Kujansuu E, Lahti J, Marjanen T, Niskanen L et al. Comparison of insulin regimens in patients with non-insulin-dependent diabetes mellitus. N Engl J Med 1992;327(20):1426–1433.
10. Yki-Jarvinen H, Nikkila K, Makimattila S. Metformin prevents weight gain by reducing dietary intake during insulin therapy in patients with type 2 diabetes mellitus. Drugs 1999;58(Suppl. 1):53–54.
11. Home P, Kurtzhals P. Insulin detemir: from concept to clinical experience. Expert Opin Pharmacother 2006;7(3):325–343.
12. Chatterjee S, Tringham JR, Davies MJ. Insulin glargine and its place in the treatment of Types 1 and 2 diabetes mellitus. Expert Opin Pharmacother 2006; 7(10):1357–1371.
13. Heinemann L, Linkeschova R, Rave K, Hompesch B, Sedlak M, Heise T. Time-action profile of the long-acting insulin analog insulin glargine (HOE901) in comparison with those of NPH insulin and placebo. Diabetes Care 2000;23(5):644–649.
14. Yki-Jarvinen H, Dressler A, Ziemen M. Less nocturnal hypoglycemia and better post-dinner glucose control with bedtime insulin glargine compared with bedtime NPH insulin during insulin combination therapy in type 2 diabetes. HOE 901/3002 Study Group. Diabetes Care 2000;23(8):1130–1136.
15. Rosenstock J, Schwartz SL, Clark CM, Jr., Park GD, Donley DW, Edwards MB. Basal insulin therapy in type 2 diabetes: 28-week comparison of insulin glargine (HOE 901) and NPH insulin. Diabetes Care 2001;24(4):631–636.
16. Fritsche A, Schweitzer MA, Haring HU. Glimepiride combined with morning insulin glargine, bedtime neutral protamine hagedorn insulin, or bedtime insulin glargine in patients with type 2 diabetes. A randomized, controlled trial. Ann Intern Med 2003; 138(12):952–959.
17. Riddle MC, Rosenstock J, Gerich J. The treat-to-target trial: randomized addition of glargine or human NPH insulin to oral therapy of type 2 diabetic patients. Diabetes Care 2003;26(11):3080–3086.
18. Eliaschewitz FG, Calvo C, Valbuena H, Ruiz M, Aschner P, Villena J et al. Latin American clinical

trial project on insulin glargine versus NPH insulin plus glimepiride in Type 2 diabetes. Diabetologia 2003;46:A272.
19. Massi BM, Humburg E, Dressler A, Ziemen M. A one-year, randomised, multicentre trial comparing insulin glargine with NPH insulin in combination with oral agents in patients with type 2 diabetes. Horm Metab Res 2003;35(3):189–196.
20. Standl E, Maxeiner S, Raptis S, Karimi-Anderesi Z, Schweitzer MA. Good glycemic control with flexibility in timing of basal insulin supply: a 24-week comparison of insulin glargine given once daily in the morning or at bedtime in combination with morning glimepiride. Diabetes Care 2005;28(2):419–420.
21. Yki-Jarvinen H, Kauppinen-Makelin R, Tiikkainen M, Vahatalo M, Virtamo H, Nikkila K et al. Insulin glargine or NPH combined with metformin in type 2 diabetes: the LANMET study. Diabetologia 2006; 49(3):442–451.
22. Janka HU, Plewe G, Riddle MC, Kliebe-Frisch C, Schweitzer MA, Yki-Jarvinen H. Comparison of basal insulin added to oral agents versus twice-daily premixed insulin as initial insulin therapy for type 2 diabetes. Diabetes Care 2005;28(2):254–259.
23. Raskin P, Allen E, Hollander P, Lewin A, Gabbay RA, Hu P et al. Initiating insulin therapy in type 2 Diabetes: a comparison of biphasic and basal insulin analogs. Diabetes Care 2005;28(2):260–265.
24. Malone JK, Kerr LF, Campaigne BN, Sachson RA, Holcombe JH. Combined therapy with insulin lispro Mix 75/25 plus metformin or insulin glargine plus metformin: a 16-week, randomized, open-label, crossover study in patients with type 2 diabetes beginning insulin therapy. Clin Ther 2004;26(12): 2034–2044.
25. Malone JK, Bai S, Campaigne BN, Reviriego J, Augendre-Ferrante B. Twice-daily pre-mixed insulin rather than basal insulin therapy alone results in better overall glycaemic control in patients with Type 2 diabetes. Diabet Med 2005;22(4):374–381.
26. Rosenstock J, Dailey G, Massi-Benedetti M, Fritsche A, Lin Z, Salzman A. Reduced hypoglycemia risk with insulin glargine: a meta-analysis comparing insulin glargine with human NPH insulin in type 2 diabetes. Diabetes Care 2005;28(4):950–955.
27. Kurtzhals P, Havelund S, Jonassen I, Kiehr B, Larsen UD, Ribel U et al. Albumin binding of insulins acylated with fatty acids: characterization of the ligand-protein interaction and correlation between binding affinity and timing of the insulin effect in vivo. Biochem J 1995;312(Pt 3):725–731.
28. Heise T, Nosek L, Ronn BB, Endahl L, Heinemann L, Kapitza C et al. Lower within-subject variability of insulin detemir in comparison to NPH insulin and insulin glargine in people with type 1 diabetes. Diabetes 2004;53(6):1614–1620.
29. Hermansen K, Davies M, Derezinski T, Martinez RG, Clauson P, Home P. A 26-week, randomized, parallel, treat-to-target trial comparing insulin detemir with NPH insulin as add-on therapy to oral glucose-lowering drugs in insulin-naive people with type 2 diabetes. Diabetes Care 2006; 29(6): 1269–1274.
30. Philis-Tsimikas A, Charpentier G, Clauson P, Ravn GM, Roberts VL, Thorsteinsson B. Comparison of once-daily insulin detemir with NPH insulin added to a regimen of oral antidiabetic drugs in poorly controlled type 2 diabetes. Clin Ther 2006; 28(10): 1569–1581.
31. Kolendorf K, Kim H. Lower risk of hypoglycemia at each level of glycemic control when insulin detemir is added to oral agents compared to NPH insulin in patients with type 2 diabetes. Diabetes 2005; 54:A121.
32. Fritsche A, Haring H. At last, a weight neutral insulin? Int J Obes Relat Metab Disord 2004; 28(Suppl. 2):S41–S46.
33. Hordern SV, Wright JE, Umpleby AM, Shojaee-Moradie F, Amiss J, Russell-Jones DL. Comparison of the effects on glucose and lipid metabolism of equipotent doses of insulin detemir and NPH insulin with a 16-h euglycaemic clamp. Diabetologia 2005; 48(3):420–426.
34. Ceriello A, Davidson J, Hanefeld M, Leiter L, Monnier L, Owens D et al. Postprandial hyperglycaemia and cardiovascular complications of diabetes: an update. Nutr Metab Cardiovasc Dis 2006; 16(7):453–456.
35. Hermansen K, Colombo M, Storgaard H, OStergaard A, Kolendorf K, Madsbad S. Improved postprandial glycemic control with biphasic insulin aspart relative to biphasic insulin lispro and biphasic human insulin in patients with type 2 diabetes. Diabetes Care 2002; 25(5):883–888.
36. Boehm BO, Home PD, Behrend C, Kamp NM, Lindholm A. Premixed insulin aspart 30 vs. premixed human insulin 30/70 twice daily: a randomized trial in Type 1 and Type 2 diabetic patients. Diabet Med 2002;19(5):393–399.
37. Boehm BO, Vaz JA, Brondsted L, Home PD. Long-term efficacy and safety of biphasic insulin aspart in patients with type 2 diabetes. Eur J Intern Med 2004; 15(8):496–502.
38. Roach P, Yue L, Arora V. Improved postprandial glycemic control during treatment with Humalog Mix25, a novel protamine-based insulin lispro formulation. Humalog Mix25 Study Group. Diabetes Care 1999;22(8):1258–1261.

39. McNally PG, Nelson G, Fitch M. Patients with Type 2 diabetes mellitus have lower rates of nocturnal hypoglycaemia on biphasic insulin aspart (BIAsp30) than on biphasic human insulin-30 (BHI30): data from the REACH study. Diabetologia 2004;47:A327.
40. Iwamoto Y. A randomised, multicentre trial of biphasic insulin aspart versus biphasic human insulin in Type 2 diabetes. Diabetologia 2003;46:A270.
41. Kann PH, Wascher T, Zackova V, Moeller J, Medding J, Szocs A et al. Starting insulin therapy in type 2 diabetes: twice-daily biphasic insulin Aspart 30 plus metformin versus once-daily insulin glargine plus glimepiride. Exp Clin Endocrinol Diabetes 2006;114(9):527–532.
42. Garber AJ, Wahlen J, Wahl T, Bressler P, Braceras R, Allen E et al. Attainment of glycaemic goals in type 2 diabetes with once-, twice-, or thrice-daily dosing with biphasic insulin aspart 70/30 (The 1-2-3 study). Diabetes Obes Metab 2006;8(1):58–66.
43. Kilo C, Mezitis N, Jain R, Mersey J, McGill J, Raskin P. Starting patients with type 2 diabetes on insulin therapy using once-daily injections of biphasic insulin aspart 70/30, biphasic human insulin 70/30, or NPH insulin in combination with metformin. J Diabetes Complicat 2003;17(6):307–313.
44. Monnier L, Lapinski H, Colette C. Contributions of fasting and postprandial plasma glucose increments to the overall diurnal hyperglycemia of type 2 diabetic patients: variations with increasing levels of HbA(1c). Diabetes Care 2003;26(3):881–885.
45. Ceriello A. Postprandial hyperglycemia and diabetes complications: is it time to treat? Diabetes 2005; 54(1):1–7.
46. Haak T, Tiengo A, Draeger E, Suntum M, Waldhausl W. Lower within-subject variability of fasting blood glucose and reduced weight gain with insulin detemir compared to NPH insulin in patients with type 2 diabetes. Diabetes Obes Metab 2005;7(1):56–64.
47. Raslova K, Bogoev M, Raz I, Leth G, Gall MA, Hancu N. Insulin detemir and insulin aspart: a promising basal-bolus regimen for type 2 diabetes. Diabetes Res Clin Pract 2004;66(2):193–201.
48. Anderson JH, Jr., Brunelle RL, Koivisto VA, Trautmann ME, Vignati L, DiMarchi R. Improved mealtime treatment of diabetes mellitus using an insulin analogue. Multicenter Insulin Lispro Study Group. Clin Ther 1997;19(1):62–72.
49. Anderson JH, Jr., Brunelle RL, Keohane P, Koivisto VA, Trautmann ME, Vignati L et al. Mealtime treatment with insulin analog improves postprandial hyperglycemia and hypoglycemia in patients with non-insulin-dependent diabetes mellitus. Multicenter Insulin Lispro Study Group. Arch Intern Med 1997; 157(11):1249–1255.
50. Ross SA, Zinman B, Campos RV, Strack T. A comparative study of insulin lispro and human regular insulin in patients with type 2 diabetes mellitus and secondary failure of oral hypoglycemic agents. Clin Invest Med 2001;24(6):292–298.
51. Dailey G, Rosenstock J, Moses RG, Ways K. Insulin glulisine provides improved glycemic control in patients with type 2 diabetes. Diabetes Care 2004; 27(10):2363–2368.
52. Hermansen K. Waiting to inhale: noninjectable insulin, are we there yet? Curr Diab Rep 2004; 4(5):335–341.
53. Fineberg SE, Kawabata T, Finco-Kent D, Liu C, Krasner A. Antibody response to inhaled insulin in patients with type 1 or type 2 diabetes. An analysis of initial phase II and III inhaled insulin (Exubera) trials and a two-year extension trial. J Clin Endocrinol Metab 2005;90(6):3287–3294.
54. Rave K, Bott S, Heinemann L, Sha S, Becker RH, Willavize SA et al. Time-action profile of inhaled insulin in comparison with subcutaneously injected insulin lispro and regular human insulin. Diabetes Care 2005;28(5):1077–1082.
55. Peyrot M, Rubin RR, Lauritzen T, Skovlund SE, Snoek FJ, Matthews DR et al. Resistance to insulin therapy among patients and providers: results of the cross-national Diabetes Attitudes, Wishes, and Needs (DAWN) study. Diabetes Care 2005;28(11): 2673–2679.
56. Zambanini A, Newson RB, Maisey M, Feher MD. Injection related anxiety in insulin-treated diabetes. Diabetes Res Clin Pract 1999;46(3):239–246.
57. Freemantle N, Blonde L, Duhot D, Hompesch M, Eggertsen R, Hobbs FD et al. Availability of inhaled insulin promotes greater perceived acceptance of insulin therapy in patients with type 2 diabetes. Diabetes Care 2005;28(2):427–428.
58. Weiss SR, Cheng SL, Kourides IA, Gelfand RA, Landschulz WH. Inhaled insulin provides improved glycemic control in patients with type 2 diabetes mellitus inadequately controlled with oral agents: a randomized controlled trial. Arch Intern Med 2003; 163(19):2277–2282.
59. Rosenstock J, Zinman B, Murphy LJ, Clement SC, Moore P, Bowering CK et al. Inhaled insulin improves glycemic control when substituted for or added to oral combination therapy in type 2 diabetes: a randomized, controlled trial. Ann Intern Med 2005;143(8):549–558.
60. Hollander PA, Blonde L, Rowe R, Mehta AE, Milburn JL, Hershon KS et al. Efficacy and safety of inhaled insulin (exubera) compared with subcutaneous insulin therapy in patients with type 2 diabetes: results of a 6-month, randomized, comparative trial. Diabetes Care 2004;27(10):2356–2362.

61. DeFronzo RA, Bergenstal RM, Cefalu WT, Pullman J, Lerman S, Bode BW et al. Efficacy of inhaled insulin in patients with type 2 diabetes not controlled with diet and exercise: a 12-week, randomized, comparative trial. Diabetes Care 2005; 28(8):1922–1928.
62. Barnett AH, Dreyer M, Lange P, Serdarevic-Pehar M. An open, randomized, parallel-group study to compare the efficacy and safety profile of inhaled human insulin (Exubera) with glibenclamide as adjunctive therapy in patients with type 2 diabetes poorly controlled on metformin. Diabetes Care 2006; 29(8):1818–1825.
63. Goudswaard AN FNVGSRRG. Insulin montherapy versus combinations of insulin with oral hypoglycaemic agents in patients with type 2 diabetes (review). 1–52. 2004. Cochrane Database Systematic Reviews 2004, Issue 4.Art NO.:CD003418.DOI: 10.1002/14651858.CD003418.pub2.
64. Yki-Jarvinen H. Combination therapies with insulin in type 2 diabetes. Diabetes Care 2001; 24(4): 758–767.
65. Brown JB, Nichols GA, Perry A. The burden of treatment failure in type 2 diabetes. Diabetes Care 2004; 27(7):1535–1540.

8
The Place of Insulin Secretagogues in the Treatment of Type 2 Diabetes in the Twenty-First Century

Harald Stingl and Guntram Schernthaner

Keywords: Sulfonylurea, glinides, insulin secretagogue, hypoglycaemia, cardiovascular, insulin resistance.

Introduction

Development of diabetes mellitus is closely related to development of insulin resistance [1]. However, insulin resistance itself cannot completely explain the development of hyperglycaemia, because impairment of beta-cell function is strongly involved in the pathogenesis of disease [2,3]. As fasting plasma glucose increases, it is overt that insulin secretion decreases progressively [4,5]. In particular, loss of first-phase insulin secretion seems to be the first and most important defect of the beta cell. In the UKPDS, the decline in insulin secretion was strongly associated with disease progression [6]. In Pima Indians, development of diabetes mellitus was associated with only a modest deterioration in insulin sensitivity, but a major decrease in acute insulin response to glucose [7]. In addition, loss of first-phase insulin secretion has been shown to be a predictor of impaired glucose tolerance in the San Antonio Heart Study [8].

Thus, effective treatment of diabetes mellitus will have to include drugs that improve insulin secretion.

History

Sulfonylurea

In 1942, the first sulfonylurea (SU) VK 57 was investigated in the Section of Infectious Diseases, Montpellier Hospital, France [9]. A few years later, that compound was shown to induce neoformation of insulin granules in rat beta cells. Since 1954 SUs (Fig. 1) have been available in the USA [10] and for many years they have been remained the most popular pharmacological drug in the treatment of diabetes mellitus. First-generation SUs include chlorpropamide, tolbutamide, tolazamide and acetohexamide and are now rarely used. They have a lower binding affinity to the sulfonylurea receptor and must therefore be given in higher doses than second-generation SUs like glibenclamide (=glyburide), glipizide, gliquidone, glimepiride and gliclazide (Table 1). In addition, the major side effect – hypoglycaemia – occurs more frequently in the longer-acting first-generation SUs [10–14].

Most guidelines like the 1999 IDF [15], the 2004 American Diabetes Association [16] as well as European national guidelines recommend SUs as first-choice monotherapy as well as combination-therapy with other antidiabetic drugs. As second-generation SUs seem to be safer, but essentially of equal efficacy [17], they have been preferred in most countries during the last years.

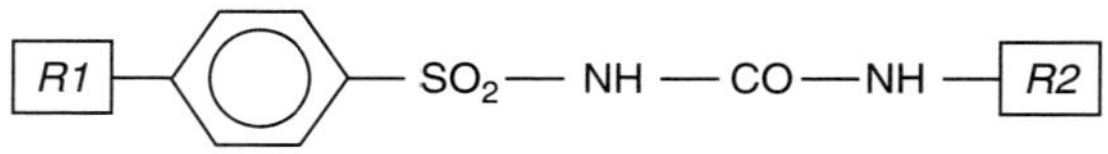

FIG. 1. Common chemical structure of sulfonylureas.

TABLE 1. Overview of first- and second-generation sulfonylureas as well as non-SU secretagogues.

Drug	Daily dosage (mg)	Ingestion per day	Duratio zn of action (h)
First-generation sulfonylureas			
Chlorpropamide	100–500	Once	60
Tolbutamide	500–2,000	Once	6–12
Tolazamide	100–1,000	Once	12–24
Acetohexamide	250–1,500	Once	12–18
Second-generation sulfonylureas			
Glibenclamide	2.5–20	Twice (or three times)	16–24
Glipizide	5–20 (40)	Once	12–24
Gliquidone	15–180	Twice	12–16
Glimepiride	1–8	Once (twice)	16–24
Gliclazide	40–240	Once (twice)	16–24
Gliclazide MR	30–120	Once	16–24
Non-SU secretagogues			
Repaglinide	1.5–12	Three times	1–2
Nateglinide	180–540	Three times	1–2

Non-SU Secretagogues

In order to improve postprandial glycaemic control, but to avoid hypoglycaemic episodes, the non-sulphonylurea moiety of glibenclamide, subsequently called meglitinide, was studied in the late 1970s and showed insulinotropic effects [18]. This finding led to the development of a relatively new class of medications: repaglinide, a benzoic acid derivative; and nateglinide, a phenyl-alanine derivative of meglitinide. Due to their short metabolic half-life and subsequent short stimulation of insulin secretion, postprandial hyperglycaemia is limited with a decreased risk of hypoglycaemia late postprandially [18–20]. However, when compared with one another, repaglinide was shown to be the more effective agent: In a 16-week randomized clinical trial in 150 type 2 diabetic patients previously treated with diet and exercise (HbA1c in both groups 8.9%), repaglinide monotherapy was more effective than nateglinide monotherapy in reduction of HbA1c (−1.57% vs. −1.04%, $p = 0.002$) and fasting blood glucose (−57 vs. −18 mg/dL; $p < 0.001$) [21].

Mechanism of Action

Insulin secretagogues bind to the so-called SU-receptors, which is a subunit of the voltage-dependent potassium adenosine triphosphate (K_{ATP}) channels on beta cells. Upon closure of those channels with subsequent inhibition of the efflux of potassium ions from the resting beta cell, the cell membrane is depolarized and voltage-dependent calcium channels are opened. The calcium entry into the cell leads to contraction of microtubules and thereby insulin exocytosis from vesicles, that is insulin secretion [10,22,23]. Thus, SUs induce insulin secretion at lower plasma glucose thresholds as normal. When given in maximally effective doses (Table 1), all available SUs seem to have equipotent capacity for stimulation of insulin secretion and lowering plasma glucose [24–27]. Similar results were obtained from the UKPDS comparing first- and second-generation SUs [11,12].

Glinides induce insulin secretion similarly (closure of the K_{ATP} channels), but they bind to the sulfonylurea receptor at a different site and with different kinetics [18]. Unlike conventional sulphonylureas, they are not internalized within the beta cell and have less stimulatory effect during postabsorptive conditions. Therefore, the risk of severe hypoglycaemic episodes has been shown to be markedly less than with classical SUs [28,29].

Treatment

There is huge variation in optimal dosing of each member of the SUs and the glinides (Table 1). If starting with monotherapy, it is best to start with the lowest recommended dose and to titrate upward every 7–14 days to achieve the desired glycaemic control without hypoglycaemia [23]. In some cases, the titration interval can be increased to 3–4 weeks, but there is no therapeutic advantage in waiting more than 4 weeks to increase the SU-dose [4]. About two thirds of the glucose lowering action of insulin secretagogues is already achieved at about half the maximal daily dose [24,30]. During SU monotherapy, most studies report a reduction in HbA1c of about 1–2% [10,11,24,25] compared with placebo.

After initiation of therapy, only ~25% of patients will achieve sufficient glycaemic control with HbA1c levels ≤7%. Those patients can be classified as complete responders [4]. Recently diagnosed diabetes mellitus, only moderate fasting hyperglycaemia at diagnosis (<~12 mmol/L or 220 mg/dL), absence of glutamic acid decarboxylase antibodies, no history of insulin therapy and good beta-cell function are predictors of good SU response [31]. Most of the diabetic patients (~50–60%) show good initial response, but do not achieve the desired treatment goals (fasting plasma glucose <7.8 mmol/L or <140 mg/dL) [4]. In such cases of partial response, a combination-therapy with other oral agents or even with basal insulin ("bed time insulin") will be necessary. In the rest of the patients (~15–25%) SUs or glinides will not be able to decrease fasting plasma glucose concentrations significantly (primary failure) [26]. Very high fasting plasma glucose concentrations (up to 17 mmol/L or >300 mg/dL) and low fasting C-peptide concentrations are predictors of primary failure. Some of those cases finally can be diagnosed as late onset autoimmune diabetes (LADA) [32] and need insulin treatment.

Although SUs are very effective in lowering blood glucose and HbA1c, this effect vanishes after some years. In the UKPDS, net HbA1c reduction after 10 years was only 0.9% [11]. After good initial response to SU therapy, the yearly secondary failure rate is about 5–7% [6,11,12]. After 10–12 years, most patients require additional oral medications or insulin therapy. The reasons for treatment failure are manifold: progression of disease-related factors (insulin resistance, weight gain), lack of exercise and concomitant medication (beta blockers and thiazide diuretics) [33,34]. In addition, beta cells lose their ability to maintain augmented insulin secretion continuously over the years [6]. That decline in beta-cell function parallels the progressive deterioration of glycaemic control, leading to the hypothesis that long-term SU exposure might cause desensitization and/or exhaustion of beta cells [9]. That concern was supported by studies that showed apoptosis in beta-cell lines and rodent islets [35]. In a recent study [36], repaglinide and nateglinide were compared with glibenclamide in isolated human islets with regard to cell apoptosis. In that study, only small advantages for the non-SU secretagogues could be shown at low concentrations. However, at 4-day exposure of the islets to secretagogues, beta-cell apoptosis was similar for all secretagogues [36]. In addition, hyperglycaemia per se as well as increased concentrations of plasma free fatty acids [37,38] could have toxic effects on beta cells [39].

Differences between first- and second-generation SUs have been studied recently and indicate preserved insulin responsiveness in islets incubated with glimepiride in contrast to glibenclamide or chlorpropamide [40]. Another second-generation SU, gliclazide, could even have protective effects on beta cells by reducing free radicals and thereby protecting the cells from oxidative stress [41].

On the other hand, in large clinical trials like the UKPDS or the recently published ADOPT-study [42], the loss of beta-cell function was not unique for therapy with insulin secretagogues, but occurred at the same rate of decline during therapy with metformin or diet, suggesting that progressive reduction of insulin secretion is peculiar for diabetes mellitus type 2. In the ADOPT-study, the yearly loss of beta-cell function 3–5 years after diagnosis of diabetes mellitus was similar when comparing glibenclamide, metformin or rosiglitazone treatment. In that study, progression of disease, that is, increase in HbA1c and fasting plasma glucose,

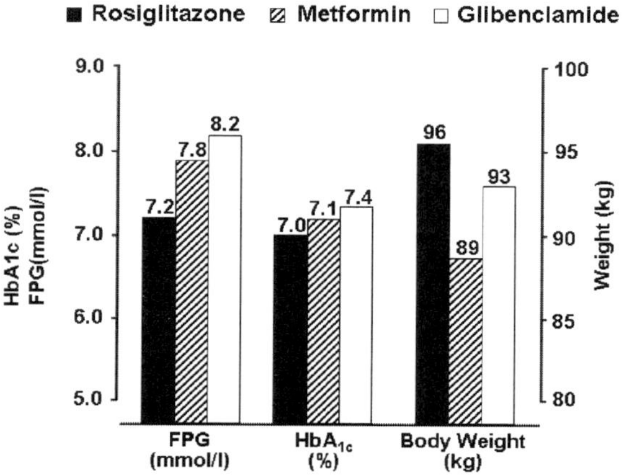

FIG. 2. Changes of fasting plasma glucose (FPG), HbA1c and body weight after 4 years treatment with either rosiglitazone, metformin or glibenclamide in the ADOPT-study population (for details see text and ref. 42).

was lower during treatment with rosiglitazone or metformin than during treatment with glibenclamide (Fig. 2). However, the increase in HbA1c levels was less pronounced than the increase in fasting plasma glucose, indicating that postprandial glucose concentrations were still effectively lowered by glibenclamide.

Side Effects

Hypoglycaemia

The main and most frequent side effect during therapy with insulin secretagogues is hypoglycaemia. Given the large number of patients treated with SUs, hypoglycaemia remains a major clinical concern even if the incidence is relatively low [4,9] and side effects are reversible when therapy is discontinued or reduced. Large variation of hypoglycaemic attacks has been reported depending on the pharmacological agent used and the metabolic control: from 2% [26] up to 38% in the glibenclamide-treated patients of the ADOPT-study [42]. The risk of major events was reported between 0.6% and 2% in the ADOPT-study and the UKPDS [11], being markedly lower than in intensively treated type 1 diabetic patients in the Diabetes Control and Complications Trial (DCCT) [43] despite similar metabolic control.

Hypoglycaemia induced by SUs is of particular concern in older diabetic patients, who very often are treated with polypharmacy and in many cases have reduced liver or kidney function [9]. In addition, higher incidence of hypoglycaemia has been observed for older long-acting first- and even second-generation SUs like glibenclamide, whereas new SUs like gliclazide and glimepiride seem to be less associated with hypoglycaemia, although given only once daily [10]. In a 100-min hyperglycaemic clamp study, glibenclamide suppressed hepatic glucose production more than glipizide [13], which could explain its higher incidence of hypoglycaemia. During treatment with glimepiride in a 1-year study markedly fewer hypoglycaemic episodes occurred with glimepiride than with glibenclamide [44]. Recently, a modified released derivative of gliclazide with different pharmacokinetic profiles has been introduced and studied under normal clinical practice in the GUIDE-study. In that double-blind, 27-week study, 845 type two diabetic patients were randomized to either gliclazide modified release (MR) 30–120 mg once daily or glimepiride 1–6 mg once daily as monotherapy or in combination with their current treatment (metformin or alpha-glucosidase inhibitor). HbA1c decreased similarly in both groups from 8.4% to 7.2% on gliclazide MR and from 8.2% to 7.2% on glimepiride. Throughout the study, no hypoglycaemia requiring external assistance occurred. Hypoglycaemia with blood glucose level <3 mmol/L occurred significantly less frequently ($p = 0.003$) with gliclazide MR (3.7% of patients) compared with glimepiride (8.9% of patients). The distribution of the sulphonylurea doses was similar in both groups [14]. As the availability of once-daily effective sulphonylurea with a good safety profile is of relevant clinical interest, many diabetes experts prefer treatment with the new second-generation SUs.

If adherence of patients is high, therapy with repaglinide and nateglinide can help to avoid hypoglycaemic episodes, especially in patients with renal diseases or older patients. A number of studies have shown markedly reduced risk of hypoglycaemia using glinides at similar glycaemic control compared with SUs [18,45]. In a study comparing repaglinide and nateglinide, 7% of subjects treated with repaglinide had minor hypoglycaemic episodes versus 0 patients for nateglinide [21].

Changes in Body Weight

SU treatment is usually associated with weight gain, usually from 2 to 5 kg, which is problematic in a group of patients already overweight [10,11,46]. However, this effect is also commonly seen during treatment with insulin and thiazolidinediones. Compared with the latter, the increase in body weight observed at SU treatment seems to be less [9,42]. In the UKPDS, mean body weight changes ranged from 1.7 kg (glibenclamide) to 2.6 kg (chlorpropamide). Nevertheless, this undesirable effect was paralleled by maintenance of good glycaemic control as well as reduction in diabetes related (micro-)vascular complications during intensive treatment. The results of the UKPDS were confirmed by the ADOPT-study, where body weight increased by 1.6 kg in the first year, but then remained stable during glibenclamide treatment [42].

Recently developed SUs seem to have only moderate impact on weight gain or even to be neutral: In Mexican Americans treated with diet and exercise, no difference in body weight gain between glimepiride and placebo treatment was reported within 14 weeks (+2.3 vs. +2.1 kg) [47]. In another study, even body weight reduction could be observed within 12 months compared with glibenclamide [48]. Similarly, treatment with gliclazide MR seems to be at least neutral on body weight: In the GUIDE-study, body weight was stable during 27 weeks with mean changes from 83.1 to 83.6 kg and 83.7 to 84.3 kg on gliclazide MR and glimepiride, respectively [14].

Repaglinide and nateglinide seem to increase body weight only slightly or to be at least neutral. During a 1-year monotherapy study, which compared repaglinide and gliclazide, no weight gain or serious hypoglycaemic events were reported in either treatment during the study [49]. In another study, when repaglinide and nateglinide were directly compared during 16 weeks of therapy, mean weight gain at the end of the study was 1.8 kg in the repaglinide group as compared with 0.7 kg for the nateglinide group [21].

Taken together, those data suggest that the relevance of body weight gain in response to therapy with insulin secretagogues may have been overestimated even when using older SUs [9].

Cardiovascular Implications

SUs bind to a subunit of the K_{ATP} channel complex inducing closure of the channel. In the past years, different cross-reactivity with cardiovascular K_{ATP} channels have been investigated [50]. Particular attention has been set on the phenomenon of ischemic preconditioning, which (self)protects the myocardial cells from ischemia and reduces infarct size [51]. As preconditioning is a result of opening the K_{ATP} channels, it could be opposed by closing these channels, a fact that raised concerns about possibly increased cardiovascular complications and mortality during SU therapy [9]. In a recent study, left ventricular myocardial function was determined in type 2 diabetic patients with known coronary artery disease after therapy with either insulin or glibenclamide. Stress conditions were provoked by dipyridamole infusion. Patients treated with glibenclamide showed much worse myocardial function assessed with echocardiography. This effect could be restored when therapy was changed to insulin [52].

Clinical and epidemiological data on the impact of SU use on myocardial infarction are controversial. In 1970, concerns about cardiovascular safety were raised upon results of the University Group Diabetes Program, in which treatment with tolbutamide increased cardiovascular mortality compared with insulin and placebo [53]. In diabetic patients undergoing direct balloon angioplasty for acute myocardial infarction, sulfonylurea drug use was associated with an increased risk of in-hospital mortality [54]. However, no detailed information on the specific SUs is given in that study. As data were collected between 1985 and 1994, probably first or early second-generation SUs have been used. In another study, treatment with glibenclamide or glipizide was associated with an attenuated magnitude of ST-elevation during myocardial infarction, resulting in failure to meet the criteria for thrombolytic therapy and as a consequence leading to inappropriate withholding therapy in those patients [55]. Some other studies yielded similar results [56,57], whereas others even suggested decreased cardiac mortality on treatment with SUs [58,59]. In the UKPDS and other studies, SU treatment seemed to be neutral [11,60,61]. It is of note that most of those data are based on the use of "older" SUs.

In the ADOPT-study [42] glibenclamide was associated with a lower risk of cardiovascular events (including congestive heart failure) than was rosiglitazone ($p < 0.05$), and the risk associated with metformin was similar to that with rosiglitazone (Table 2). This observation differs from the UKPDS findings, which suggested that metformin reduces overall mortality and may reduce coronary events. This difference may be related to the facts that patients in the ADOPT-study were younger and had a shorter follow-up period than did the British study. The lower cardiovascular risk associated with glibenclamide compared with rosiglitazone or metformin in the early phase of type 2 diabetes needs further confirmation, but could be related to better postprandial glucose lowering induced by glibenclamide, since HbA1c values were only slightly different, whereas fasting glucose levels were significantly higher in the SU group (Fig. 2).

Few data about new SU agents are available. Recently, in an epidemiologic study, the association between the use of SUs and other antidiabetic drugs and the risk of cardiovascular complications has been investigated [62] in a population-based case-control study. From those data, the risk of myocardial infarction appeared higher among users of "old" SUs like glibenclamide, glipizide and tolbutamide [adjusted odds ratio (OR), 2.07; 95% confidence interval (CI), 1.81–2.37] than among users of glimepiride and gliclazide (adjusted OR, 1.36; CI, 1.01–1.84). If diabetes was not treated with pharmacotherapy, the OR was 3.51 (CI 2.92–4.22).

In a study with type 2 diabetic patients undergoing coronary angioplasty, inhibition of ischemic preconditioning assessed by metabolic and electrocardiographic parameters was less severe during treatment with glimepiride than with glibenclamide. Restitution of a preconditioning response in glimepiride-treated patients may be the potential beneficial mechanism [63]. Other studies confirm different selectivity of SUs for beta cell versus cardiovascular K_{ATP} channels and therapeutic benefits of glimepiride in comparison with glibenclamide [64–66].

This epidemiological and observational approach evaluating the effect of "old" versus "new SUs" was recently enlarged in a Danish nationwide population-based study [67]. Altogether, 72,913 patients with first-time admissions with myocardial infarction were followed up including 6,644 patients with type 2 diabetes, 3,992 of them were treated with SUs (1,438 were on "new SUs" and 2,554 on "old SUs"). Remarkably, 30-day mortality was significantly lower in patients on "new SUs" (19%; gliclazide: 17.4%; glimepiride: 19.4%) compared with patients treated with old SUs (25.9%). The relative risk ratio for mortality after myocardial infarction associated with the use of "new SUs" was 0.75 ($p = 0.009$). The data observed in Danish patients with myocardial infarction are in agreement with a recent report from Italy [68], which evaluated the 3-year mortality in 696 diabetic patients treated with different combinations of insulin secretagogues and metformin. The yearly mortality was 8.7%, when metformin was combined with glibenclamide, but only 3.1%, 2.1% or 0.4% when the biguanide was combined with repaglinide, gliclazide or glimpiride. The risk ratio for mortality associated with glibenclamide versus other SUs was significantly increased: 2.09 (CI: 1.07; 4.11).

TABLE 2. Vascular serious adverse events during treatment with rosiglitazone, metformin or glibenclamide in the ADOPT-study population (for details see text and ref. 42).

	Rosiglitazone ($n = 1{,}456$)	Metformin ($n = 1{,}454$)	Glibenclamide ($n = 1{,}441$)
Cardiovascular disease, *n* (%)	49 (3.4%)	46 (3.2%)	26 (1.8%)[a]
Myocardial infarction			
Fatal, *n* (%)	2 (0.1%)	2 (0.1%)	3 (0.2%)
Non-fatal, *n* (%)	22 (1.5%)	18 (1.2%)	11 (0.8%)
CHF, *n* (%)	12 (0.8%)	12 (0.8%)	3 (0.2%)[a]
Stroke, *n* (%)	13 (0.9%)	17 (1.2%)	12 (0.8%)
Peripheral vascular disease, *n* (%)	7 (0.5%)	6 (0.4%)	4 (0.3%)

[a] $p < 0.05$ versus rosiglitazone.

In addition to coronary heart disease, other effects of modern SUs have been investigated: In a recent study, the effects of treatment with glibenclamide and gliclazide on forearm post-ischemic reactive hyperaemia were investigated. Four-week treatment with glibenclamide but not gliclazide resulted in sustained reduction of post-ischaemic reactive hyperaemia. The authors concluded that this difference was most probably based on different SU-receptor binding [69].

However, other mechanisms could contribute to such effects: gliclazide could also possess haemorrheologic properties [70,71]. It reduces platelet reactivity, increases prostacyclin synthesis and increases fibrinolysis [9]. In one study, administration of either modified release or standard gliclazide to type 2 diabetic patients resulted in a fall in 8-isoprostanes, a marker of lipid oxidation, and an increase in total plasma antioxidant capacity, superoxide dismutase and thiols, all of them antioxidant parameters [72]. In a similar study, where these data were confirmed, gliclazide, but not glibenclamide reduced systolic and diastolic blood pressure [73]. Following that data, gliclazide possesses antioxidant properties that produce measurable clinical effects at therapeutic doses. In another study, gliclazide, but not glibenclamide treatment was able to lower serum ICAM-1 levels in poorly controlled type 2 diabetic patients, which typically have elevated serum ICAM-1 as a marker of endothelial dysfunction [74].

Similarly, glimepiride, but not glibenclamide, has been shown to improve insulin resistance and TNF-alpha, interleukin-6, high sensitive-CRP, lipoprotein(a), homocystein and plasminogen activator inhibitor-1 (PAI-1) levels, all markers of atherosclerotic disorder [75,76]. In vitro studies suggest that glimepiride, and to a lesser extent gliclazide are more potent inhibitors of platelet aggregation than gliquidone and glibenclamide [77].

Conclusion

Although new therapeutic options for mellitus have been introduced during the last few years, sulfonylureas are still widely used for the treatment of diabetes mellitus. Despite the fact that all available SUs lower blood glucose effectively, new agents like glimepiride and gliclazide have much less interaction with the vascular system and patients suffer from less hypoglycaemic events. In addition, non-SU insulin secretagogues like repaglinide or nateglinide can help to avoid hypoglycaemia in patients with irregular food intake.

References

1. Reaven GM. Banting lecture 1988. Role of insulin resistance in human disease. Diabetes 1988;37(12): 1595–1607.
2. Polonsky KS. Lilly lecture 1994. The beta-cell in diabetes: from molecular genetics to clinical research. Diabetes 1995;44(6):705–717.
3. Weyer C, Tataranni PA, Bogardus C, Pratley RE. Insulin resistance and insulin secretory dysfunction are independent predictors of worsening of glucose tolerance during each stage of type 2 diabetes development. Diabetes Care 2001;24(1):89–94.
4. DeFronzo RA. Pharmacologic therapy for type 2 diabetes mellitus. Ann Intern Med 1999;131(4):281–303.
5. DeFronzo RA. Lilly lecture 1987. The triumvirate: beta-cell, muscle, liver. A collusion responsible for NIDDM. Diabetes 1988;37(6):667–687.
6. UKPDS. UK prospective diabetes study 16. Overview of 6 years' therapy of type II diabetes: a progressive disease. UK Prospective Diabetes Study Group. Diabetes 1995;44(11):1249–1258.
7. Weyer C, Bogardus C, Mott DM, Pratley RE. The natural history of insulin secretory dysfunction and insulin resistance in the pathogenesis of type 2 diabetes mellitus. J Clin Invest 1999;104(6):787–794.
8. Gastaldelli A, Ferrannini E, Miyazaki Y, Matsuda M, DeFronzo RA. Beta-cell dysfunction and glucose intolerance: results from the San Antonio metabolism (SAM) study. Diabetologia 2004;47(1): 31–39.
9. Del Prato S, Pulizzi N. The place of sulfonylureas in the therapy for type 2 diabetes mellitus. Metabolism 2006;55(5 Suppl 1):S20–S27.
10. Inzucchi SE. Oral antihyperglycemic therapy for type 2 diabetes: scientific review. JAMA 2002;287(3): 360–372.
11. UKPDS. Intensive blood-glucose control with sulphonylureas or insulin compared with conventional treatment and risk of complications in patients with type 2 diabetes (UKPDS 33). UK Prospective Diabetes Study (UKPDS) Group. Lancet 1998;352(9131):837–853.
12. UKPDS. Effect of intensive blood-glucose control with metformin on complications in overweight patients with type 2 diabetes (UKPDS 34). UK Prospective Diabetes Study (UKPDS) Group. Lancet 1998;352(9131):854–865.

13. Groop L, Luzi L, Melander A, Groop PH, Ratheiser K, Simonson DC, DeFronzo RA. Different effects of glyburide and glipizide on insulin secretion and hepatic glucose production in normal and NIDDM subjects. Diabetes 1987;36(11):1320–1328.
14. Schernthaner G, Grimaldi A, Di Mario U, Drzewoski J, Kempler P, Kvapil M, Novials A, Rottiers R, Rutten GE, Shaw KM. GUIDE study: double-blind comparison of once-daily gliclazide MR and glimepiride in type 2 diabetic patients. Eur J Clin Invest 2004; 34(8):535–542.
15. A desktop guide to Type 2 diabetes mellitus. European Diabetes Policy Group 1999. Diabet Med 1999;16(9):716–730.
16. Standards of medical care in diabetes. Diabetes Care 2004;27(Suppl 1):S15–S35.
17. Cohen KL, Harris S. Efficacy of glyburide in diabetics poorly controlled on first-generation oral hypoglycemics. Diabetes Care 1987;10(5):555–557.
18. Dornhorst A. Insulinotropic meglitinide analogues. Lancet 2001;358(9294):1709–1716.
19. Hirschberg Y, Karara AH, Pietri AO, McLeod JF. Improved control of mealtime glucose excursions with coadministration of nateglinide and metformin. Diabetes Care 2000;23(3):349–353.
20. Goldberg RB, Einhorn D, Lucas CP, Rendell MS, Damsbo P, Huang WC, Strange P, Brodows RG. A randomized placebo-controlled trial of repaglinide in the treatment of type 2 diabetes. Diabetes Care 1998;21(11):1897–1903.
21. Rosenstock J, Hassman DR, Madder RD, Brazinsky SA, Farrell J, Khutoryansky N, Hale PM. Repaglinide versus nateglinide monotherapy: a randomized, multicenter study. Diabetes Care 2004;27(6):1265–1270.
22. Zimmerman BR. Sulfonylureas. Endocrinol Metab Clin North Am 1997;26(3):511–522.
23. Cheng AY, Fantus IG. Oral antihyperglycemic therapy for type 2 diabetes mellitus. CMAJ 2005; 172(2):213–226.
24. Simonson DC, Kourides IA, Feinglos M, Shamoon H, Fischette CT. Efficacy, safety, and dose–response characteristics of glipizide gastrointestinal therapeutic system on glycemic control and insulin secretion in NIDDM. Results of two multicenter, randomized, placebo-controlled clinical trials. The Glipizide Gastrointestinal Therapeutic System Study Group. Diabetes Care 1997;20(4):597–606.
25. Rosenstock J, Samols E, Muchmore DB, Schneider J. Glimepiride, a new once-daily sulfonylurea. A double-blind placebo-controlled study of NIDDM patients. Glimepiride Study Group. Diabetes Care 1996;19(11):1194–1199.
26. Groop LC. Sulfonylureas in NIDDM. Diabetes Care 1992;15(6):737–754.
27. Groop L, Groop PH, Stenman S, Saloranta C, Totterman KJ, Fyhrquist F, Melander A. Comparison of pharmacokinetics, metabolic effects and mechanisms of action of glyburide and glipizide during long-term treatment. Diabetes Care 1987;10(6):71–78.
28. Moses RG, Gomis R, Frandsen KB, Schlienger JL, Dedov I. Flexible meal-related dosing with repaglinide facilitates glycemic control in therapy-naive type 2 diabetes. Diabetes Care 2001;24(1):11–15.
29. Hollander PA, Schwartz SL, Gatlin MR, Haas SJ, Zheng H, Foley JE, Dunning BE. Importance of early insulin secretion: comparison of nateglinide and glyburide in previously diet-treated patients with type 2 diabetes. Diabetes Care 2001;24(6):983–988.
30. Stenman S, Melander A, Groop PH, Groop LC. What is the benefit of increasing the sulfonylurea dose? Ann Intern Med 1993;118(3):169–172.
31. Blaum CS, Velez L, Hiss RG, Halter JB. Characteristics related to poor glycemic control in NIDDM patients in community practice. Diabetes Care 1997;20(1):7–11.
32. Leslie RD, Williams R, Pozzilli P. Clinical review: Type 1 diabetes and latent autoimmune diabetes in adults: one end of the rainbow. J Clin Endocrinol Metab 2006;91(5):1654–1659.
33. Fardoun RZ. Carvedilol versus cardioselective beta-blockers for the treatment of hypertension in patients with type 2 diabetes mellitus. Pharmacotherapy 2006;26(10):1491–1500.
34. Taylor EN, Hu FB, Curhan GC. Antihypertensive medications and the risk of incident type 2 diabetes. Diabetes Care 2006;29(5):1065–1070.
35. Efanova IB, Zaitsev SV, Zhivotovsky B, Kohler M, Efendic S, Orrenius S, Berggren PO. Glucose and tolbutamide induce apoptosis in pancreatic beta-cells. A process dependent on intracellular Ca^{2+} concentration. J Biol Chem 1998;273(50): 33501–33507.
36. Maedler K, Carr RD, Bosco D, Zuellig RA, Berney T, Donath MY. Sulfonylurea induced beta-cell apoptosis in cultured human islets. J Clin Endocrinol Metab 2005;90(1):501–506.
37. Sako Y, Grill VE. A 48-hour lipid infusion in the rat time-dependently inhibits glucose-induced insulin secretion and B cell oxidation through a process likely coupled to fatty acid oxidation. Endocrinology 1990;127(4):1580–1589.
38. Zhou YP, Grill VE. Long-term exposure of rat pancreatic islets to fatty acids inhibits glucose-induced insulin secretion and biosynthesis through a glucose fatty acid cycle. J Clin Invest 1994;93(2): 870–876.
39. Poitout V, Robertson RP. Minireview: Secondary beta-cell failure in type 2 diabetes–a convergence of

glucotoxicity and lipotoxicity. Endocrinology 2002;143(2):339–342.
40. Del Guerra S, Marselli L, Lupi R, Boggi U, Mosca F, Benzi L, Del Prato S, Marchetti P. Effects of prolonged in vitro exposure to sulphonylureas on the function and survival of human islets. J Diabetes Complications 2005;19(1):60–64.
41. McGavin JK, Perry CM, Goa KL. Gliclazide modified release. Drugs 2002;62(9):1357–1364; discussion 65–66.
42. Kahn SE, Haffner SM, Heise MA, Herman WH, Holman RR, Jones NP, Kravitz BG, Lachin JM, O'Neill MC, Zinman B, Viberti G. Glycemic durability of rosiglitazone, metformin, or glyburide monotherapy. N Engl J Med 2006;355(23):2427–2443.
43. DCCT. The effect of intensive treatment of diabetes on the development and progression of long-term complications in insulin-dependent diabetes mellitus. The Diabetes Control and Complications Trial Research Group. N Engl J Med 1993;329(14):977–986.
44. Draeger KE, Wernicke-Panten K, Lomp HJ, Schuler E, Rosskamp R. Long-term treatment of type 2 diabetic patients with the new oral antidiabetic agent glimepiride (Amaryl): a double-blind comparison with glibenclamide. Horm Metab Res 1996;28(9):419–425.
45. Hollingdal M, Sturis J, Gall MA, Damsbo P, Pincus S, Veldhuis JD, Porksen N, Schmitz O, Juhl CB. Repaglinide treatment amplifies first-phase insulin secretion and high-frequency pulsatile insulin release in Type 2 diabetes. Diabet Med 2005;22(10):1408–1413.
46. UKPDS. UK Prospective Diabetes Study 24: a 6-year, randomized, controlled trial comparing sulfonylurea, insulin, and metformin therapy in patients with newly diagnosed type 2 diabetes that could not be controlled with diet therapy. UK Prospective Diabetes Study Group. Ann Intern Med 1998;128(3):165–175.
47. Luis Bautista J, Bugos C, Dirnberger G, Atherton T. Efficacy and safety profile of glimepiride in Mexican American Patients with type 2 diabetes mellitus: a randomized, placebo-controlled study. Clin Ther 2003;25(1):194–209.
48. Martin S, Kolb H, Beuth J, van Leendert R, Schneider B, Scherbaum WA. Change in patients' body weight after 12 months of treatment with glimepiride or glibenclamide in Type 2 diabetes: a multicentre retrospective cohort study. Diabetologia 2003;46(12):1611–1617.
49. Madsbad S, Kilhovd B, Lager I, Mustajoki P, Dejgaard A. Comparison between repaglinide and glipizide in Type 2 diabetes mellitus: a 1-year multicentre study. Diabet Med 2001;18(5):395–401.
50. Lazdunski M. Ion channel effects of antidiabetic sulfonylureas. Horm Metab Res 1996;28(9):488–495.
51. Thisted H, Johnsen SP, Rungby J. Sulfonylureas and the risk of myocardial infarction. Metabolism 2006;55(5 Suppl 1):S16–S19.
52. Scognamiglio R, Avogaro A, Vigili de Kreutzenberg S, Negut C, Palisi M, Bagolin E, Tiengo A. Effects of treatment with sulfonylurea drugs or insulin on ischemia-induced myocardial dysfunction in type 2 diabetes. Diabetes 2002;51(3):808–812.
53. Meinert CL, Knatterud GL, Prout TE, Klimt CR. A study of the effects of hypoglycemic agents on vascular complications in patients with adult-onset diabetes. II. Mortality results. Diabetes 1970;19(Suppl):789–830.
54. Garratt KN, Brady PA, Hassinger NL, Grill DE, Terzic A, Holmes DR Jr. Sulfonylurea drugs increase early mortality in patients with diabetes mellitus after direct angioplasty for acute myocardial infarction. J Am Coll Cardiol 1999;33(1):119–124.
55. Huizar JF, Gonzalez LA, Alderman J, Smith HS. Sulfonylureas attenuate electrocardiographic ST-segment elevation during an acute myocardial infarction in diabetics. J Am Coll Cardiol 2003;42(6):1017–1021.
56. Rytter L, Troelsen S, Beck-Nielsen H. Prevalence and mortality of acute myocardial infarction in patients with diabetes. Diabetes Care 1985;8(3):230–234.
57. Gustafsson I, Hildebrandt P, Seibaek M, Melchior T, Torp-Pedersen C, Kober L, Kaiser-Nielsen P. Long-term prognosis of diabetic patients with myocardial infarction: relation to antidiabetic treatment regimen. The TRACE Study Group. Eur Heart J 2000; 21(23):1937–1943.
58. Knowler WC, Sartor G, Melander A, Schersten B. Glucose tolerance and mortality, including a substudy of tolbutamide treatment. Diabetologia 1997;40(6):680–686.
59. Sartor G, Schersten B, Carlstrom S, Melander A, Norden A, Persson G. Ten-year follow-up of subjects with impaired glucose tolerance: prevention of diabetes by tolbutamide and diet regulation. Diabetes 1980;29(1):41–49.
60. Halkin A, Roth A, Jonas M, Behar S. Sulfonylureas are not associated with increased mortality in diabetics treated with thrombolysis for acute myocardial infarction. J Thromb Thrombolysis 2001;12(2): 177–184.
61. Stevens RJ, Coleman RL, Adler AI, Stratton IM, Matthews DR, Holman RR. Risk factors for myocardial infarction case fatality and stroke case fatality in type 2 diabetes: UKPDS 66. Diabetes Care 2004;27(1):201–207.
62. Johnsen SP, Monster TB, Olsen ML, Thisted H, McLaughlin JK, Sorensen HT, Lervang HH, Rungby J. Risk and short-term prognosis of myocardial infarction among users of antidiabetic drugs. Am J Ther 2006;13(2):134–140.

63. Lee TM, Chou TF. Impairment of myocardial protection in type 2 diabetic patients. J Clin Endocrinol Metab 2003;88(2):531–537.
64. Geisen K, Vegh A, Krause E, Papp JG. Cardiovascular effects of conventional sulfonylureas and glimepiride. Horm Metab Res 1996;28(9):496–507.
65. Mocanu MM, Maddock HL, Baxter GF, Lawrence CL, Standen NB, Yellon DM. Glimepiride, a novel sulfonylurea, does not abolish myocardial protection afforded by either ischemic preconditioning or diazoxide. Circulation 2001;103(25):3111–3116.
66. Klepzig H, Kober G, Matter C, Luus H, Schneider H, Boedeker KH, Kiowski W, Amann FW, Gruber D, Harris S, Burger W. Sulfonylureas and ischaemic preconditioning; a double-blind, placebo-controlled evaluation of glimepiride and glibenclamide. Eur Heart J 1999;20(6):439–446.
67. Thisted H, Jacobsen J, Thomsen RW, Johnsen SP, Rungby J. Use of sulphonylureas and mortality after myocardial infarction in diabetic patients: a Danish nationwide population-based study. Diabetologia 2006;57(Suppl 1): Abstract 091.
68. Monami M, Luzzi C, Lamanna C, Chiasserini V, Addante F, Desideri CM, Masotti G, Marchionni N, Mannucci E. Three-year mortality in diabetic patients treated with different combinations of insulin secretagogues and metformin. Diabetes Metab Res Rev 2006;22(6):477–482.
69. Wascher TC, Boes U. Forearm vascular reactivity is differentially influenced by gliclazide and glibenclamide in chronically treated type 2 diabetic patients. Clin Physiol Funct Imaging 2005; 25(1):40–46.
70. Renier G, Mamputu JC, Serri O. Benefits of gliclazide in the atherosclerotic process: decrease in monocyte adhesion to endothelial cells. Metabolism 2003;52(8 Suppl 1):13–18.
71. Jennings PE. Vascular benefits of gliclazide beyond glycemic control. Metabolism 2000;49(10 Suppl 2): 17–20.
72. O'Brien RC, Luo M, Balazs N, Mercuri J. In vitro and in vivo antioxidant properties of gliclazide. J Diabetes Complications 2000;14(4):201–206.
73. Fava D, Cassone-Faldetta M, Laurenti O, De Luca O, Ghiselli A, De Mattia G. Gliclazide improves antioxidant status and nitric oxide-mediated vasodilation in Type 2 diabetes. Diabet Med 2002;19(9):752–757.
74. Papanas N, Tziakas D, Chalikias G, Floros D, Trypsianis G, Papadopoulou E, Kortsaris A, Symeonidis G, Souliou E, Maltezos E, Hatseras D. Gliclazide treatment lowers serum ICAM-1 levels in poorly controlled type 2 diabetic patients. Diabetes Metab 2006;32(4):344–349.
75. Koshiba K, Nomura M, Nakaya Y, Ito S. Efficacy of glimepiride on insulin resistance, adipocytokines, and atherosclerosis. J Med Invest 2006;53(1–2): 87–94.
76. Derosa G, Franzetti I, Gadaleta G, Ciccarelli L, Fogari R. Metabolic variations with oral antidiabetic drugs in patients with Type 2 diabetes: comparison between glimepiride and metformin. Diabetes Nutr Metab 2004;17(3):143–150.
77. Siluk D, Kaliszan R, Haber P, Petrusewicz J, Brzozowski Z, Sut G. Antiaggregatory activity of hypoglycaemic sulphonylureas. Diabetologia 2002;45(7):1034–1037.

9
Metformin – from Devil to Angel

Guntram Schernthaner and Gerit Holger Schernthaner

Keywords: Metformin, Weight loss, Cardioprotection, First-line Therapy, Insulin Resistance.

Introduction

Type 2 diabetes mellitus is a complex chronic metabolic disorder, which results from defects in both insulin secretion and insulin action. An elevated rate of basal hepatic glucose production in the presence of hyperinsulinemia is the primary cause of fasting hyperglycaemia. After a meal, impaired suppression of hepatic glucose production by insulin and decreased insulin-mediated glucose uptake by muscle contribute almost equally to postprandial hyperglycaemia.

Over 40 years ago various biguanides (e.g. metformin, phenformin, buformin) were used in different countries for the treatment of type 2 diabetes. All but metformin was removed from the international market in the 1970s because of the associated high risk of lactate acidosis [1]. In the late 1970s and early 1980s of the last century papers about this drug were rejected from leading journals, since it was felt that metformin is already historical. Since metformin had not been marketed in the USA at that time, it was only in 1995 that it was approved for use there, after safety concerns were satisfied by decades of experience in Canada, Europe and Asia. It is astonishing that metformin could only be used in Germany for decades in the late phase of type 2 diabetes in combination with sulfonylureas, when most patients had already contraindications. Remarkably, in the last 10 years the role of metformin changed from devil to angel and it is now recommended as first-line drug by almost all guideline committees worldwide (Fig. 1).

Mechanisms of Action of Metformin

The mechanism by which metformin exerts its antihyperglycaemic effects is still not entirely clear, but may be mediated by activation of hepatic and muscle adenosine monophosphate-activated protein kinase [2], which is a major regulator of lipid and glucose metabolism. Metformin improves fasting and postprandial glucose levels during an oral glucose tolerance test, whereas the plasma insulin response to glucose is unchanged or may be decreased in patients with hyperinsulinemia [3]. Metformin ameliorates hyperglycaemia by reducing hepatic glucose production and gastrointestinal glucose absorption and improving peripheral sensitivity to insulin [4–7]. Unlike sulfonylureas, it does not stimulate insulin secretion, aggravate hyperinsulinemia or cause hypoglycaemia [3–7]. However, the insulin-sensitizing effect of metformin is much smaller compared with that of thiazolidinediones [7]. The insulin-sensitizing action of metformin on peripheral tissues may be mainly explained by glucose toxicity. It is well known that chronic hyperglycaemia causes deterioration of both beta-cell function and insulin action and that these effects are reversed by improved glycaemic control.

The major action of metformin in patients with diabetes is to decrease hepatic glucose output, primarily by decreasing gluconeogenesis, but it may also, as a lesser effect, increase glucose uptake by skeletal muscles [6,7].

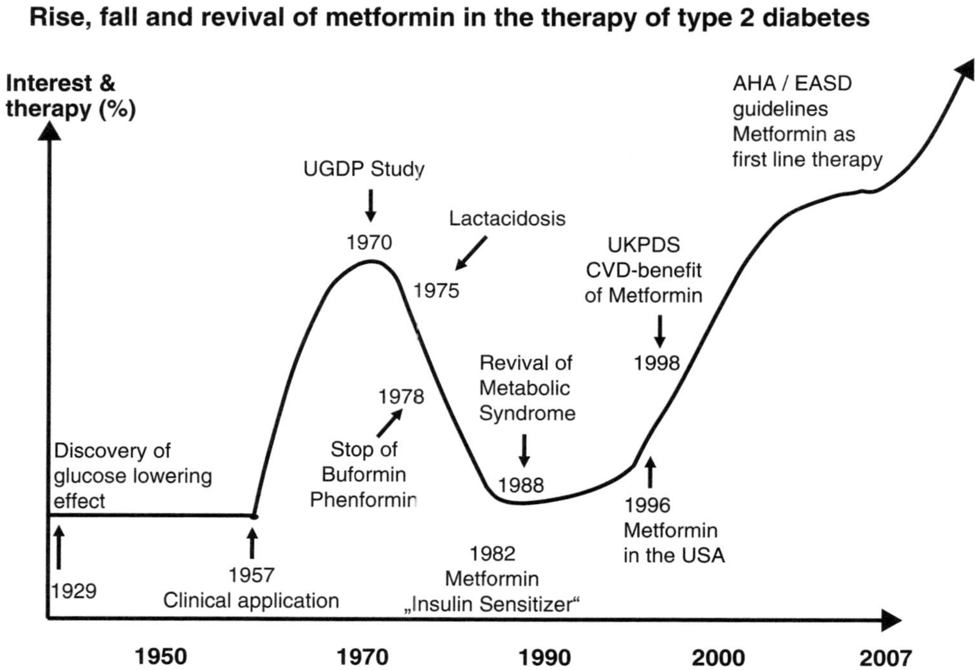

FIG. 1. Rise, fall and revival of metformin in the therapy of type 2 diabetes.

Clinical Efficacy of Metformin: HbA1c Lowering, But No Weight Gain

In placebo-controlled trials, metformin lowered HbA1c concentrations by about 1.0–2.0% [8,9]. The efficacy of metformin monotherapy was equivalent to the monotherapy of sulfonylurea or thiazolidendiones [10,11]. The greatest advantage of metformin compared with other anti-diabetic agents (insulin, sulfonylureas or thiazolidendiones) has been the fact that it is associated with weight loss but not with weight gain [1,9–14]. This has been shown for drug-naïve patients as well as for patients already receiving other oral anti-diabetic drugs. In the UKPDS, weight gain was modest with metformin and very similar to the diet group, whereas treatment with insulin and sulfonylureas was associated with a significant weight gain of 4–8 kg over 10 years [14]. The effect of metformin to pioglitazone or gliclazide in monotherapy or combination therapy was recently studied in large randomized head-to-head studies (QUARTET Studies) [11–13]. Table 1 shows that the HbA1c-lowering effect was very similar among the different oral anti-diabetic drugs, whereas weight change versus baseline and the frequency of symptomatic hypoglycaemic events was quite different. In the - head-to-head comparison of metformin with pioglitazone in 1,199 drug-naïve patients using a parallel-group, double-blind study design, HbA1c decreased similarly by 1.4% and 1.5% in both groups from baseline after 52 weeks [11]. However, the glycaemic improvement in the pioglitazone group was associated with an increase in body weight of 1.9 kg, whereas body weight decreased by 2.5 kg in the metformin group, resulting in a difference of 4.4 kg after 1 year.

Recently, the data of the ADOPT (A Diabetes Outcome Progression Trial) study confirmed the significant difference in weight loss or weight gain when either metformin, glibenclamide or rosiglitazone was used as first-line monotherapy in patients with recently diagnosed type 2 diabetes [15]. The mean HbA1c level at 4 years was only 0.13% less in the rosiglitazone group than in the metformin group and 0.42% less than in the glibenclamide

TABLE 1. Effects of oral anti-diabetic drugs on HbA1c, hypoglycaemic events and weight change in four randomized double-blind studies (QUARTET) results after 1 year.

	Number of Patients	HbA1c %	Hypoglycaemia %	Weight change (kg)	Weight difference (kg)
[a]Metformin	597	−1.5	1.3	−2.5	4.4
[a]Pioglitazone	597	−1.4	1.5	+1.9	
[b]Metformin + pioglitazone	317	−1.5	1.3	+1.5	0.1
[b]Metformin + SU	317	−1.4	11.2	+1.4	
[c]SU + pioglitazone	319	−1.35	10.7	+2.8	3.8
[c]SU + metformin	320	−1.43	14.1	−1.0	
SU = Sulfonylureas					

[a]Schernthaner et al. J Clin Endocrinol Metab 2004;89:6068 [11].
[b]Matthews et al. Diab Metab Res Rev 2005;21:167 [12].
[c]Hanefeld et al. Diabetes Care 2004;27:141 [13].

group. Over a period of 5 years, the mean weight increased from baseline by 4.8 kg in the rosiglitazone group, but decreased by 2.9 kg in the metformin group, resulting in a difference in body weight of 7.7 kg at the end of the study. Based on these data David Nathan concluded in his editorial [16] that metformin remains the logical choice when initiating pharmacotherapy for type 2 diabetes given the modest glycaemic benefit of rosiglitazone (with the risk of fluid retention and weight gain) and higher cost (including the need for more statins and diuretics). Surprisingly, the proportions of patients with cardiovascular events were similar in the rosiglitazone and metformin groups but were higher than in the glyburide group. This observation differs from the UKPDS findings, which suggested that metformin reduces overall mortality and may reduce coronary events [17]. This difference may be related to the shorter follow-up period of the ADOPT study compared with the UKPDS. In addition, the patients in ADOPT were younger and had better glycaemic control at study entry.

The mechanism for the weight loss associated with metformin therapy despite significant improvement of glycaemic control in contrast to other anti-diabetic drugs is not known, but an anorectic effect has been accused since many years. Several studies have shown that metformin reduces hunger and food intake [18,19]. Interestingly, metformin attenuates hypoglycaemia-induced hunger, but does not appear to influence post-hypoglycaemic food intake [18]. Recent studies may now explain why patients treated with metformin show weight loss or no weight gain despite significant lowering of glycosuria and HbA1c levels. Metformin enhances GLP-1 secretion in experimental animal studies [20] and inhibits DPP IV activity in type 2 diabetic patients [21], suggesting that the drug may have potential for future combination therapy with incretin hormones.

Metformin as First-Line Pharmacotherapy of Type 2 Diabetes

A recently published consensus statement from the American Diabetes Association (ADA) and the European Association for the Study of Diabetes (EASD) suggested using metformin as first-line pharmacotherapy not taking into account clinical characteristics such as obesity or body weight [22]. The authors recognized that for most individuals with type 2 diabetes, lifestyle interventions failed to achieve or maintain metabolic goals, either because of failure to lose weight, weight regain, progressive disease or a combination of factors. Therefore, they arrived at the consensus that (i) metformin therapy should be initiated concurrent with lifestyle intervention at diagnosis and (ii) metformin is recommended as the initial pharmacological therapy, in the absence of specific contraindications, for its effect on glycaemia, absence of weight gain and hypoglycaemia, generally low level of side effects, high level of acceptance and relatively low cost [22].

Metformin treatment should be titrated to its maximally effective dose over 1–2 months, as tolerated. Rapid addition of other glucose-lowering medications should be considered in the setting of persistent hyperglycaemia. In the ADA–EASD consensus statement the initial body weight is not given as a criterion for the use of metformin [22]. Recently, authors of an Australian study [23] concluded that metformin is at least as efficacious in the non-obese as it is in the obese type 2 diabetic patients and that their study provides evidence-based data to support metformin use in non-obese individuals who have type 2 diabetes.

Metformin in Combination Therapy

Many studies have shown that metformin can be used in combination with all available anti-diabetic drugs including sulfonylureas, glinides, α-glucosidase-inhibitors, thiazolidendiones, DPP-4 inhibitors as well as with injection of insulins and GLP-1 agonists [9,13,24–29]. The combination of metformin and sulfonylureas is the most common oral combination therapy and is used by about 50% of all type 2 diabetic patients. During the last years many other oral combination therapies were studied and are now in clinical use. In principal, most of the oral anti-diabetic drugs (metformin, sulfonylureas, thiazolidendiones and DPP-4 inhibitors) – with the exception of α-glucosidase-inhibitors – can lower HbA1c by about 1%. Since the action of the mechanism of the drugs are quite different, combination therapy is logical and helpful.

As already mentioned earlier metformin was recently recommended as first-line pharmacotherapy of type 2 diabetes by the ADA–EASD consensus group [22]. However, there was no strong consensus regarding the second medication added after metformin other than to choose among insulin, a sulfonylurea (SU) or a thiazolidendione.

A 1-year randomized double-blind study in 639 type 2 diabetic patients [13] showed clinically equivalent improvements in glycaemic control for the combination therapy of metformin and SU (HbA1c decrease 1.36%) or pioglitazone and SU (HbA1c decrease 1.20%). Pioglitazone addition to SU significantly reduced triglycerides (–16% vs. –9%; $p = 0.008$) and increased HDL-cholesterol (14% vs. 8%; $p < 0.001$) compared with metformin addition. LDL-cholesterol was increased by 2% with the addition of pioglitazone and decreased by 5% with the addition of metformin to SU ($p < 0.001$). Remarkably, urinary albumin-to-creatinine ratio was reduced by 15% in the SU plus pioglitazone group and increased by 2% in the SU plus metformin group ($p = 0.017$). In two 2-year, randomized, multicentre trials the long-term effects of three different oral anti-diabetic combination therapies were compared [25]. In the type 2 diabetic patients with inadequate glycaemic control (HbA1c 7.5–11%) studied, HbA1c was lowered similarly when either metformin or pioglitazone was added (HbA1c decrease 1.16% vs. 1.03%). Whereas weight decreased by 1.7 kg when metformin was added to SU, a significant weight gain of 3.7 kg was observed when pioglitazone was added to SU [25].

Several studies have evaluated the effect and safety of adding metformin to patients who had poor glycaemic control despite treatment with insulin [26,27]. In a study with 390 patients [26] metformin use compared to placebo, was associated with improved glycaemic control (mean HbA1c 6.9% vs. 7.6%, $p < 0.0001$), reduced insulin requirements (63.8 vs. 71.3 IU, $p < 0.0001$); reduced weight gain and decreased plasma LDL-cholesterol. Thus, in type 2 diabetic patients who are intensively treated with insulin, the combination of insulin and metformin results in superior glycaemic control compared with insulin therapy alone, whereas insulin requirements and weight gain are less. In another study [27] the addition of either metformin or troglitazone to insulin was compared with insulin monotherapy in 88 type 2 diabetic patients with a high baseline HbA1c value of 8.7%. Aggressive insulin therapy significantly improved glycaemic control in type 2 diabetic subjects to levels comparable with those achieved by adding metformin to insulin therapy. Although troglitazone was the most effective in lowering HbA1c, total daily insulin dose and triglyceride levels, treatment with insulin plus metformin was advantageous in avoiding weight gain and hypoglycaemia.

A recent study presented evidence that DPP-4 inhibition by vildagliptin when added to metformin in type 2 diabetes over 52 weeks improved beta-cell function along with improved postmeal insulin sensitivity [28]. When Exenatide (10 μg BID) was added to metformin instead of placebo [29],

HbA1c decreased by 0.78% from the baseline value of 8.2% associated with a further weight loss of 2.8 kg. Thus, the combination of metformin with injection of Exenatide seems to be superior to the combination therapy of metformin with insulin.

More recently, metformin has been used successfully in different forms of anti-diabetic triple therapy [30–34], which are becoming more and more popular to avoid insulin therapy. In these studies metformin was either combined with sulfonylureas and thiazolidendiones, or with sulfonylureas and Exenatide and in the end also with thiazolidendiones and insulin as proposed as the final step in the recently published ADA–EASD algorithm [22]. In a recent review [22] the triple therapy (metformin plus sulfonylurea plus thiazolidendione) was seen relatively critical. It should be considered only when patients are already close to target and when circumstances make it difficult to use insulin. Furthermore, the combination of three oral agents is more expensive than using insulin plus metformin, and no benefit has been shown.

Cardiovascular Endpoint Studies with Metformin

In a substudy of the UKPDS (with a median follow-up of 10.7 years), among overweight (54% with obesity) participants allocated to intensive blood glucose control, metformin ($n = 342$) showed a greater benefit [17] than chlorpropamide, glibenclamide or insulin ($n = 951$) for any diabetes-related outcomes [98 vs. 350, relative risk (RR) = 0.78; $p = 0.009$] and for all-cause mortality (50 vs. 190, RR = 0.73; $p = 0.03$). For the rest of the outcomes like diabetes-related death, myocardial infarction, stroke, peripheral vascular disease and microvascular disease, there were no significant differences between both comparison arms. Moreover, the overweight participants assigned to intensive blood glucose control with metformin ($n = 342$) showed a greater benefit than overweight patients on conventional treatment (non-intensive blood glucose control, mainly with diet) ($n = 411$), for any diabetes-related outcomes (98 vs. 160, RR = 0.74, $p = 0.004$), diabetes-related death (28 vs. 55, RR = 0.61, $p = 0.03$), all-cause mortality (50 vs. 89, RR = 0.68, $p = 0.01$) and myocardial infarction (39 vs. 73, RR = 0.64, $p = 0.02$). For the rest of the outcomes such as stroke, peripheral vascular disease and microvascular disease, there were no significant differences between both comparison arms. However, these results have been questioned because of findings in a substudy of 537 patients with poorly controlled type 2 diabetes who had been treated with sulfonylureas for 7.1 years and who were randomly assigned to receive either metformin with continued sulfonylurea treatment ($n = 268$) or continued sulfonylurea monotherapy ($n = 269$). After a mean follow-up of 4 years, a 96% increase in the risk for diabetes-related death ($p = 0.04$) in the group receiving sulfonylureas plus metformin was found compared with the group that continued receiving sulfonylurea monotherapy. Although the absolute numbers of heart attacks (33 and 31) and strokes (15 and 13) were very similar in the two groups, more patients in the sulfonylurea plus metformin group experienced a fatal heart attack or stroke. The authors pointed out that in the substudy, the number of patients and events was small and the duration of combination therapy was short. Furthermore, early addition of metformin in patients with suboptimal control while on maximum sulfonylurea therapy resulted in improved glycaemic control [3]. However, this early addition of metformin to sulfonylurea therapy was also associated with an increase in diabetes-related mortality compared with continued sulfonylurea alone [2]. Two recent observational studies also reported significantly increased mortality associated with metformin use, suggesting caution in the use of metformin for type 2 diabetes [4,5]. These discrepancies have left some questions regarding the overall benefit of metformin therapy, alone or in combination with sulfonylureas [6].

Observational Studies: Cardiovascular Death, Heart Failure and Outcome in Coronary Intervention

In a retrospective cohort study of patients newly treated with oral hypoglycaemic agents, Evans et al. [36] found that those treated with sulfonylureas only ($n = 3{,}331$), or combinations of sulfonylureas and metformin (n = 2,147), were at higher risk of adverse cardiovascular outcomes than those treated with metformin alone (n = 2,286).

In the metformin monotherapy cohort 4.7% of patients died (35.5% cardiovascular deaths), compared with 17.9% of patients in the SU monotherapy cohort (42.4% cardiovascular deaths). After adjusting for all available confounders, the risk for mortality and cardiovascular mortality in patients in the SU only cohort remained significantly increased with 1.43 and 1.70, respectively compared to the metformin monotherapy. Patients in the combination cohorts had significantly increased risk of mortality (2.47 and 2.16) and cardiovascular mortality (2.29 and 2.43) despite the adjustment for all available confounders and irrespective whether the patients started either with sulfonylureas or metformin and then added the other drug. A significantly reduced risk for overall mortality [odds ratio (OR) = 0.60] and cardiovascular mortality was already earlier observed in a Canadian observational study [37] of 1,150 users of metformin therapy in comparison with 3,033 users of sulfonylureas. By contrast, in that study sulfonylurea plus metformin combination therapy was also associated with reduced all-cause mortality (OR = 0.66).

Prospective controlled studies about the use of metformin in diabetic patients after acute myocardial infarction or heart failure are not available. Indirect information is coming from several large observational studies. In a retrospective cohort study of 24,953 diabetic patients [38] discharged after hospitalization with acute myocardial infarction, mortality rates after 1 year were not significantly different in patients treated with either metformin [Hazard ratio (HR) = 0.92] or a thiazolidendione (0.92) in comparison with patients who did not receive an insulin sensitizer but were lower in those prescribed both drugs (0.52).

In a retrospective cohort study [39] of 16,417 Medicare beneficiaries with diabetes discharged after hospitalization with the principal discharge diagnosis of heart failure. One-year mortality rates were lower in 2,226 patients treated with a thiazolidendione (30.1%) or in those 1,861 treated with metformin (24.7%) compared with 2,069 treated with neither insulin-sensitizing drug (36.0%, $p < 0.0001$ for both comparisons). In multivariable models, treatment with thiazolidendiones (HR = 0.87) or metformin (HR = 0.87) was associated with significantly lower risks of death, whereas no association was found between treatment with sulfonylureas (HR = 0.99) and mortality. However, there was a higher risk of readmission for heart failure thiazolidendiones treatment (HR = 1.06) and a lower risk with metformin treatment (HR = 0.92).

It is well known that diabetic patients undergoing coronary interventions have worse clinical and angiographic outcomes in comparison with non-diabetic patients. In the retrospective analysis of the PRESTO (Prevention of Restenosis with Tranilast and its Outcomes) trial the effect of different anti-diabetic treatment was analysed [40] in 1,110 diabetic patients who received non-sensitizer therapy (insulin and/or sulfonylureas) and in 887 patients who were treated with sensitizers (metformin with or without additional therapy). Compared with patients on non-sensitizer therapy, those on sensitizer therapy showed an adjusted OR of 0.72; $p = 0.005$ for any clinical event. The differences between the non-sensitizer therapy group and the sensitizer group were attributable mainly to decreased rates of death (OR = 0.39; $p = 0.007$) and myocardial infarction (OR = 0.31; $p = 0.002$). In this retrospective analysis, use of metformin in diabetics undergoing coronary interventions appeared to decrease adverse clinical events, especially death and myocardial infarction, compared with diabetic patients treated with non-sensitizer therapy.

Observational Studies: Cancer

In a population-based Canadian cohort study [41] of 10,309 new users of metformin or sulfonylureas with an average follow-up of 5.4 years it was found that patients with type 2 diabetes exposed to sulfonylureas and exogenous insulin had a significantly increased risk of cancer-related mortality compared with patients exposed to metformin. Cancer mortality 4.9% (162 of 3,340) for sulfonylurea monotherapy users, 3.5% (245 of 6,969) for metformin users and 5.8% (84 of 1,443) for subjects who used insulin. After multivariate adjustment, the sulfonylurea cohort had greater cancer-related mortality compared with the metformin cohort (adjusted HR = 1.3; $p = 0.012$). Insulin use was associated with an adjusted HR of cancer-related mortality of 1.9 ($p < 0.0001$). It is unclear whether this increased risk is related to a deleterious effect of sulfonylurea and insulin or a protective effect of metformin or due to some other unmeasured confounders.

Similar observations were made in a case-controlled study from Scotland [42] suggesting that the use of metformin may be associated with reduced risk of cancer (HR = 0.79). In line with these observational studies are new experimental data [43] demonstrating that metformin is an AMP kinase-dependent growth inhibitor for breast cancer cells.

Side Effects, Contraindications and Safety of Metformin

Gastrointestinal side effects, including abdominal discomfort and diarrhoea, are the most common adverse events, occurring 10–15% of patients, depending on the dose [1,8,11]. These side effects usually improve with continued use and are minimal if started at a low dose (e.g. 250–500 mg/d) and slowly titrated upward. Discontinuation of therapy because of side effects occurs in less than 4% of patients. Because metformin does not increase insulin secretion [3], biochemically documented hypoglycaemia is rare [11] in diabetic patients treated with metformin alone (Table 1). Metformin is contraindicated in patients with risk factors for lactate acidosis or drug accumulation, for example in those with moderate to severe kidney, liver or cardiac dysfunction. Metformin is contraindicated in renal failure because of the associated risk for lactate acidosis. It can be used at low dosages up to a creatinine clearance of 30–60 mL/min and should be avoided with clearances <30 mL/min [44]. There is increasing evidence that the risk of lactate acidosis associated with metformin treatment is a very low risk. A recent Cochrane Database Systematic Review [45] of the incidence of fatal and non-fatal lactate acidosis with metformin compared with placebo and other glucose-lowering therapies in patients with type 2 diabetes demonstrated no increased association, with an incidence of lactate acidosis of 8.4 cases per 100,000 patient-years in the metformin group and 9 cases per 100,000 patient-years in the non-metformin group [45]. Based on these and other findings, it has been proposed that advanced age per se, mild renal impairment and compensated heart failure can no longer be upheld as contraindications for metformin [46].

Improvement of Cardiovascular Risk Profile by Metformin

During the last two decades a number of studies showed beneficial effects of metformin on traditional and non-traditional cardiovascular risk factors [11,47–58]. Metformin reduces fasting and postprandial insulin levels [3], insulin resistance [4–6] and has beneficial effects on lipids, thrombosis and blood flow. Metformin has a weight-lowering effect [11,13,15] and reduces hypertriglyceridaemia [11], elevated levels of PAI-1 [47], factor VII [49], C-reactive protein [51,52,54] and intact proinsulin and des 31,32 proinsulin concentrations [48]. In randomized head-to-head comparisons (Fig. 2) of oral anti-diabetic drugs metformin treatment reduced triglycerides by 10% and increased HDL-cholesterol by 7%, whereas pioglitazone reduced triglycerides by 19% and increased HDL-cholesterol by 14% [11]. By contrast, LDL-cholesterol decreased by 4% under metformin therapy, but increased by 8% under pioglitazone. Remarkably, HbA1c improvement was very similar and the prognostically important total cholesterol/HDL-cholesterol ratio was reduced identical by 8% (Fig. 2) in both treatment arms [11]. Recent studies indicate that metformin has direct effects on fibrin structure/ function and stabilizes platelets, two important components of arterial thrombus [55]. In addition, metformin has been shown [56,57] to reduce soluble vascular cell adhesion molecule-1 (sVCAM-1) and migration inhibitory factor (MIF). Metformin also reduces methylglyoxal, a reactive alpha-dicarbonyl that is thought to contribute to diabetic complications in a dose-dependent fashion and minimizes the effect of worsening glycaemic control on methylglyoxal levels [50].

A recent Cochrane Systematic Review [59] about all available studies with metformin arrived at the following conclusion: Metformin may be the first therapeutic option in the diabetes mellitus type 2 with overweight or obesity, as it may prevent some vascular complications, and mortality. Metformin produces beneficial changes in glycaemia control, and moderated weight, lipids, insulinaemia and diastolic blood pressure. Sulfonylureas, alpha-glucosidase inhibitors, thiazolidendiones, meglitinides, insulin and diet fail to show more benefit for glycaemia control, body weight, or lipids, than metformin.

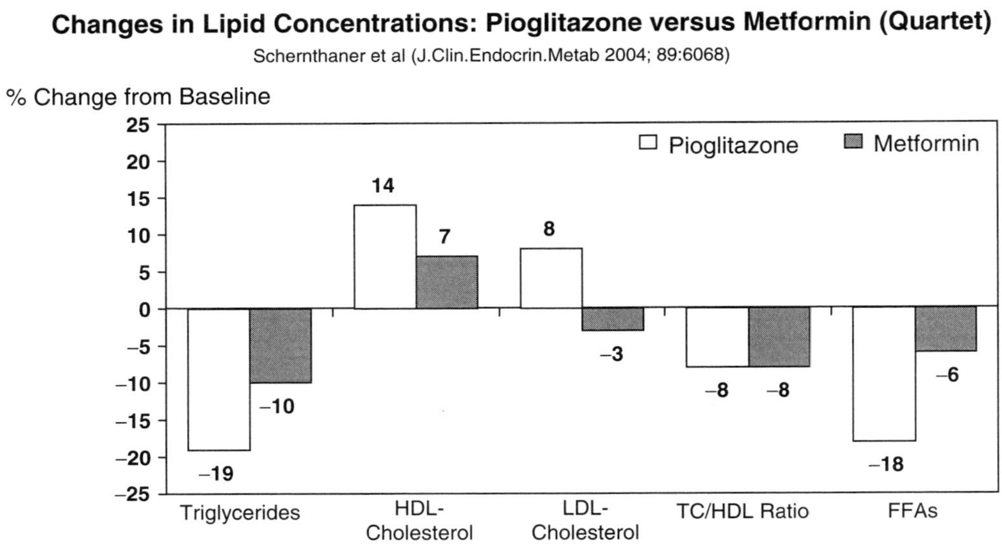

	mmol/L		mmol/L		mmol/L		Ratio		mmol/L	
	pio	met	pio	met	pio	met	pio	met	pio	met
Baseline	2.64	2.61	1.13	1.13	3.56	3.56	5.34	5.34	0.66	0.66
Week 52	2.03	2.31	1.29	1.21	3.83	3.44	4.92	4.92	0.54	0.62

FIG. 2. Changes in lipid concentrations: pioglitazone versus metformin (QUARTET) (Schernthaner et al. J Clin Endocrinol Metab 2004;89:6068 [11]).

References

1. Bailey CJ, Turner RC. Metformin. N Engl J Med 1996;334:574–579.
2. Zhou G, Myers R, Li Y et al. Role of AMP-activated protein kinase in mechanism of metformin action. J Clin Invest 2001;108:1167–1174.
3. Prager R, Schernthaner G. Insulin receptor binding to monocytes, insulin secretion, and glucose tolerance following metformin treatment. Results of a double-blind cross-over study in type II diabetics. Diabetes 1983;32:1083–1086.
4. Prager R, Schernthaner G, Graf H. Effect of metformin on peripheral insulin sensitivity in non insulin dependent diabetes mellitus. Diabete Metab 1986;12:346–350.
5. DeFronzo RA, Barzilai N, Simonson DC. Mechanism of metformin action in obese and lean noninsulin-dependent diabetic subjects. J Clin Endocrinol Metab 1991;73:1294–1301.
6. Stumvoll M, Nurjhan N, Perriello G et al. Metabolic effects of metformin in non-insulin-dependent diabetes mellitus. N Engl J Med 1995;333:550–554.
7. Natali A, Ferrannini E. Effects of metformin and thiazolidinediones on suppression of hepatic glucose production and stimulation of glucose uptake in type 2 diabetes: a systematic review. Diabetologia 2006; 49:434–441.
8. Garber AJ, Duncan TG, Goodman AM et al. Efficacy of metformin in type II diabetes: results of a double-blind, placebo-controlled, dose response trial. Am J Med 1997;103:491–497.
9. DeFronzo RA, Goodman AM. Efficacy of metformin in patients with noninsulin-dependent diabetes mellitus. The Multicenter Metformin Study Group. N Engl J Med 1995;333:541–549.
10. Clarke BF, Campbell IW. Comparison of metformin and chlorpropamide in non-obese, maturity-onset diabetics uncontrolled by diet. Br Med J 1977;2: 1576–1578.
11. Schernthaner G, Matthews DR, Charbonnel B et al. Efficacy and safety of pioglitazone versus metformin in patients with type 2 diabetes mellitus: a double blind randomized trial. J Clin Endocrinol Metab 2004;89:6068–6076.
12. Matthews DR, Charbonnel BH, Hanefeld M, Brunetti P, Schernthaner G. Long-term therapy with addition of pioglitazone to metformin compared with the addition of gliclazide to metformin in patients with type 2 diabetes: a randomized, comparative study. Diabetes Metab Res Rev. 2005;21:167–74.
13. Hanefeld M, Brunetti P, Schernthaner G et al. One-year glycemic control with a sulfonylurea plus pioglitazone versus a sulfonylurea plus metformin in patients with type 2 diabetes. Diabetes Care 2004;27:141–147.

14. United Kingdom Prospective Diabetes Study (UKPDS) Group. Relative efficacy of randomly allocated diet, sulphonylurea, insulin, or metformin in patients with newly diagnosed non-insulin dependent diabetes followed for three years (UKPDS 13). Br Med J 1995;310:83–88.
15. Kahn SE, Haffner SM, Heise MA et al. G. Glycemic durability of rosiglitazone, metformin, or glyburide monotherapy. N Engl J Med 2006;355:2427–2443.
16. Nathan DM. Thiazolidinediones for initial treatment of type 2 diabetes? N Engl J Med 2006;355:2477–2480.
17. United Kingdom Prospective Diabetes Study (UKPDS) Group. Effect of intensive blood-glucose control with metformin on complications in overweight patients with type 2 diabetes (UKPDS 34). Lancet 1998;352:854–865.
18. Lee A, Morley JE. Metformin decreases food consumption and induces weight loss in subjects with obesity with type II non-insulin-dependent diabetes. Obes Res 1998;6:47–53.
19. Schultes B, Oltmanns KM, Kern W et al. Modulation of hunger by plasma glucose and metformin. J Clin Endocrinol Metab 2003;88:1133–1141.
20. Yasuda N, Inoue T, Nagakura T et al. Enhanced secretion of glucagon-like peptide 1 by biguanide compounds. Biochem Biophys Res Commun 2002;298:779–784.
21. Lindsay JR, Duffy NA, McKillop AM et al. Inhibition of dipeptidyl peptidase IV activity by oral metformin in Type 2 diabetes. Diabet Med 2005;22:654–657.
22. Nathan DM, Buse JB, Davidson MB et al. B. Management of hyperglycaemia in type 2 diabetes: a consensus algorithm for the initiation and adjustment of therapy. A consensus statement from the American Diabetes Association and the European Association for the Study of Diabetes. Diabetologia 2006;49:1711–1721.
23. Ong CR, Molyneaux LM, Constantino MI et al. Long-term efficacy of metformin therapy in nonobese individuals with type 2 diabetes. Diabetes Care 2006;29:2361–2364.
24. Van Gaal L, Maislos M, Schernthaner G et al. Miglitol combined with metformin improves glycaemic control in type 2 diabetes. Diabetes Obes Metab 2001;3:326–331.
25. Charbonnel B, Schernthaner G, Brunetti P et al. Long-term efficacy and tolerability of add-on pioglitazone therapy to failing monotherapy compared with addition of gliclazide or metformin in patients with type 2 diabetes. Diabetologia 2005;48:1093–1104.
26. Wulffele MG, Kooy A, Lehert P et al. Combination of insulin and metformin in the treatment of type 2 diabetes. Diabetes Care 2002;25:2133–2140.
27. Strowig SM, Aviles-Santa ML, Raskin P. Comparison of insulin monotherapy and combination therapy with insulin and metformin or insulin and troglitazone in type 2 diabetes. Diabetes Care 2002;25:1691–1698.
28. Ahren B, Pacini G, Foley JE et al. Improved meal-related beta-cell function and insulin sensitivity by the dipeptidyl peptidase-IV inhibitor vildagliptin in metformin-treated patients with type 2 diabetes over 1 year. Diabetes Care 2005;28:1936–1940.
29. DeFronzo RA, Ratner RE, Han J et al. Effects of exenatide (exendin-4) on glycemic control and weight over 30 weeks in metformin-treated patients with type 2 diabetes. Diabetes Care 2005;28:1092–1100.
30. Strowig SM, Aviles-Santa ML, Raskin P. Improved glycemic control without weight gain using triple therapy in type 2 diabetes. Diabetes Care 2004;27:1577–1583.
31. Heine RJ, Van Gaal LF, Johns D et al. Exenatide versus insulin glargine in patients with suboptimally controlled type 2 diabetes: a randomized trial. Ann Intern Med 2005;143:559–569.
32. Rosenstock J, Sugimoto D, Strange P et al. Triple therapy in type 2 diabetes: insulin glargine or rosiglitazone added to combination therapy of sulfonylurea plus metformin in insulin-naive patients. Diabetes Care 2006;29:554–559.
33. Dailey GE III, Noor MA, Park JS et al. Glycemic control with glyburide/metformin tablets in combination with rosiglitazone in patients with type 2 diabetes: a randomized, double-blind trial. Am J Med 2004;116:223–229.
34. Dormandy JA, Charbonnel B, Eckland DJ et al. Secondary prevention of macrovascular events in patients with type 2 diabetes in the PROactive Study (PROspective pioglitAzone Clinical Trial In macroVascular Events): a randomised controlled trial. Lancet 2005;366:1279–1289.
35. Heine RJ, Diamant M, Mbanya JC et al. Management of hyperglycaemia in type 2 diabetes: the end of recurrent failure? Br Med J 2006;333:1200–1204.
36. Evans JM, Ogston SA, Emslie-Smith A et al. Risk of mortality and adverse cardiovascular outcomes in type 2 diabetes: a comparison of patients treated with sulfonylureas and metformin. Diabetologia 2006;49: 930–936.
37. Johnson JA, Simpson SH, Majumdar SR et al. Decreased mortality associated with the use of metformin compared with sulfonylurea monotherapy in type 2 diabetes. Diabetes Care 2002;25:2244–2248.
38. Inzucchi SE, Masoudi FA, Wang Y et al. Insulin-sensitizing antihyperglycemic drugs and mortality after acute myocardial infarction: insights from the National Heart Care Project. Diabetes Care 2005; 28:1680–1689.

39. Masoudi FA, Inzucchi SE, Wang Y et al. Thiazolidinediones, metformin, and outcomes in older patients with diabetes and heart failure: an observational study. Circulation 2005;111:583–590.
40. Kao J, Tobis J, McClelland RL et al. Relation of metformin treatment to clinical events in diabetic patients undergoing percutaneous intervention. Am J Cardiol 2004;93:1347–1350.
41. Bowker SL, Majumdar SR, Veugelers P et al. Increased cancer-related mortality for patients with type 2 diabetes who use sulfonylureas or insulin. Diabetes Care 2006;29:254–258.
42. Evans JM, Donnelly LA, Emslie-Smith AM et al. Metformin and reduced risk of cancer in diabetic patients. Br Med J 2005;330:1304–1305.
43. Zakikhani M, Dowling R, Fantus IG et al. Metformin is an AMP kinase-dependent growth inhibitor for breast cancer cells. Cancer Res 2006;66:10269–10273.
44. Yale JF. Oral antihyperglycemic agents and renal disease: new agents, new concepts. J Am Soc Nephrol 2005;16(Suppl 1):S7–S10.
45. Salpeter S, Greyber E, Pasternak G et al. Risk of fatal and nonfatal lactic acidosis with metformin use in type 2 diabetes mellitus. Cochrane Database Syst Rev 2006;25:CD002967. Review.
46. Holstein A, Stumvoll M. Contraindications can damage your health – is metformin a case in point? Diabetologia 2005;48:2454–2459.
47. Nagi DK, Yudkin JS. Effects of metformin on insulin resistance, risk factors for cardiovascular disease, and plasminogen activator inhibitor in NIDDM subjects. A study of two ethnic groups. Diabetes Care 1993:16:621–629.
48. Nagi DK, Ali VM, Yudkin JS. Effect of metformin on intact proinsulin and des 31,32 proinsulin concentrations in subjects with non-insulin-dependent (type 2) diabetes mellitus. Diabet Med 1996;13: 753–757.
49. Grant PJ. Metformin reduces circulating factor VII concentrations in patients with type 2 diabetes mellitus. Thromb Haemost 1998;80:209–210.
50. Beisswenger PJ, Howell SK, Touchette AD et al. Metformin reduces systemic methylglyoxal levels in type 2 diabetes. Diabetes 1999;48:198–202.
51. Morin-Papunen L, Rautio K, Ruokonen A et al. Metformin reduces serum C-reactive protein levels in women with polycystic ovary syndrome. J Clin Endocrinol Metab 2003;88:4649–4654.
52. Carter AM, Bennett CE, Bostock JA et al. Metformin reduces C-reactive protein but not complement factor C3 in overweight patients with Type 2 diabetes mellitus. Diabet Med 2005;22:1282–1284.
53. Li L, Mamputu JC, Wiernsperger N et al. Signaling pathways involved in human vascular smooth muscle cell proliferation and matrix metalloproteinase-2 expression induced by leptin: inhibitory effect of metformin. Diabetes 2005;54:2227–2234.
54. Stewart MW, Cirkel DT, Furuseth K et al. Effect of metformin plus rosiglitazone compared with metformin alone on glycaemic control in well-controlled Type 2 diabetes. Diabet Med 2006;23:1069–1078.
55. Standeven KF, Ariens RA, Whitaker P et al. The effect of dimethylbiguanide on thrombin activity, FXIII activation, fibrin polymerization, and fibrin clot formation. Diabetes 2002;51:189–197.
56. Abbasi F, Chu JW, McLaughlin T et al. Effect of metformin treatment on multiple cardiovascular disease risk factors in patients with type 2 diabetes mellitus. Metabolism 2004;53:159–164.
57. Dandona P, Aljada A, Ghanim H et al. Increased plasma concentration of macrophage migration inhibitory factor (MIF) and MIF mRNA in mononuclear cells in the obese and the suppressive action of metformin. J Clin Endocrinol Metab 2004;89:5043–5047.
58. De Jager J, Kooy A, Lehert P et al. Effects of short-term treatment with metformin on markers of endothelial function and inflammatory activity in type 2 diabetes. J Intern Med 2005;257:100–109.
59. Saenz A, Fernandez-Esteban I, Mataix A et al. Metformin monotherapy for type 2 diabetes mellitus. Cochrane Database Syst Rev 2005;20:CD002966. Review.

10
The Glitazones, Lessons So Far

Monika Shirodkar and Serge Jabbour

Keywords: Pioglitazone, Rosiglitazone, Giltazones, Diabetes, Thiazolidinediones, Insulin Resistance.

Thiazolidinediones (TZD) are known as insulin-sensitizing agents since they work by improving the action of insulin, independently of the pancreas. Rosiglitazone and pioglitazone are the two agents currently available and the pharmacology and use of these drugs will be discussed in this chapter.

Thiazolidinediones – Insulin Sensitizers

Thiazolidinediones are insulin-sensitizing agents used in the treatment of type 2 diabetes. Two of these agents are currently available for clinical use in the USA: pioglitazone (Actos), and rosiglitazone (Avandia), both of which were approved by the Food and Drug Administration (FDA) in 1999. Troglitazone (Rezulin), the first clinically available thiazolidinedione, was withdrawn in March 2000 due to concerns about severe liver toxicity and has now been replaced by these newer agents, which have demonstrated hepatic safety.

Mechanism of Action

Thiazolidinediones bind and activate the nuclear receptor peroxisome proliferator-activated receptor-γ (PPARγ). This receptor is expressed predominantly in adipocytes, where it regulates adipocyte differentiation and the expression of adipocyte-specific genes [1]. It is expressed in lower levels in muscle and liver tissue [2] and has also been identified in several other tissues (discussed below). Based on affinity for PPARγ, rosiglitazone is a more potent PPARγ ligand than pioglitazone.

The mechanism of action of thiazolidinediones has not been fully elucidated; however, the unique effects of this class of oral medications on glycemia as well as multiple vascular risk factors appear to be based on their amelioration of some of the pathogenetic links between visceral adiposity, insulin resistance, and type 2 diabetes (Fig. 1). The binding of PPARγ by a thiazolidinedione is known to affect the transcription of a number of genes [2]. Animal studies have offered some insight into the effects of thiazolidinediones on glucose and fat metabolism. Free fatty acids (FFA) are believed to be a major contributor to insulin resistance by inhibiting insulin action in skeletal muscle and the liver [3]. One of the main actions of the thiazolidinediones is to lower circulating levels of FFA by increasing their retention in certain adipose tissue depots [4]. Thiazolidinediones are potent inducers of the differentiation and proliferation of precursor cells into small, metabolically active adipocytes, which appear to take up and retain circulating FFA, primarily in a subcutaneous compartment.

Analogous to FFA, tumor necrosis factor-α (TNF-α) is a cytokine secreted by adipose tissue, which has also been implicated as a mediator of insulin resistance in skeletal muscle and the liver. Thiazolidinediones suppress the secretion of TNF-α as well as antagonize the effects of this cytokine at the cellular level in insulin target tissues [5]. Additional mechanisms of thiazolidinedione action have also been recently identified. For example, the levels of adiponectin, a recently described protein with insulin-sensitizing properties specifically secreted by adipose tissue that circulates in

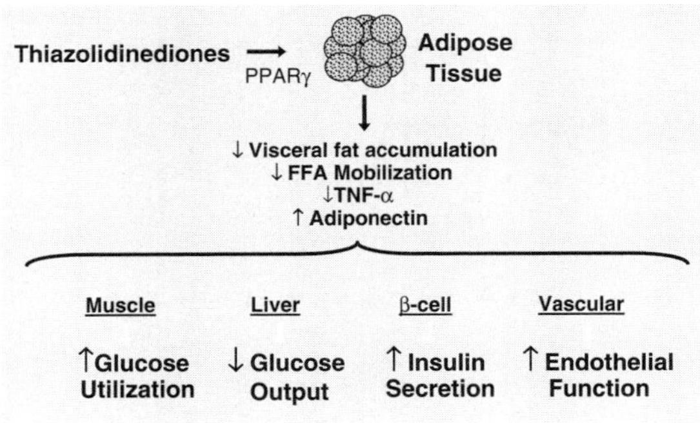

FIG. 1. Mechanism of the pleiotropic actions of the thiazolidinediones. Working *via* the PPAR-γ receptor system in adipose tissue, the thiazolidinediones interrupt the pathogenic signaling between the expanded visceral adipose mass in obesity, which leads to improved insulin sensitivity in skeletal muscle and liver, enhanced pancreatic β-cell insulin secretion, and improved vascular endothelial function. The processes affected by the thiazolidinediones include redistribution of adipose stores, reduced circulating levels of FFA, diminished levels and tissue effects of cytokines (TNF-α), and increased circulating levels of the insulin-sensitizing, anti-atherogenic plasma protein adiponectin, which also arises from adipose tissue. The thiazolidinediones have also been shown to have direct effects in muscle and endothelial cells, which is likely to also contribute to some of their pharmacologic activity.

relatively abundant quantities in the bloodstream, are dramatically increased by thiazolidinediones. Since adiponectin levels are reduced in patients with obesity and insulin resistance, the increased levels elicited by thiazolidinedione treatment may mediate some of the insulin-sensitizing properties of this class of drugs [6]. TZDs affect fat distribution by increasing subcutaneous peripheral fat depots and reducing intrahepatic and visceral fat, which, according to current views of the pathogenesis of insulin resistance, contributes to the improvement in insulin sensitivity and the decrease in circulating FFA and adipocytokines [7].

In human studies, thiazolidinediones improved insulin sensitivity by increasing glucose disposal in muscle and other tissues [8–10]. They also inhibited hepatic glucose production to a lesser extent [11]. Serum FFA and insulin levels are decreased with thiazolidinedione therapy.

Effects on Pancreatic Insulin Secretion

Clinical use of thiazolidinediones consistently results in reduced plasma insulin levels and reduced insulin requirements in patients with type 2 diabetes taking insulin, reflecting an increase in insulin sensitivity. Although these agents do not directly stimulate β-cell insulin secretion, studies indicate that they can restore aspects of defective glucose-coupled insulin responsiveness in humans and animals with type 2 diabetes.

There are several potential mechanisms whereby thiazolidinediones might enhance β-cell function, in addition to simply lowering ambient levels of glycemia and reducing "glucotoxic" signaling abnormalities in β-cells. Recently, abnormal β-cell secretory responsiveness and potential cell death (apoptosis) have been attributed to chronic effects of accumulated triglycerides and FFA derivatives in the pancreatic islet cells in obesity with insulin resistance, a phenomenon that has been dubbed "lipotoxicity" [12,13]. This hypothesis also postulates that the effect of thiazolidinediones to redistribute fat stores in the body, including from the pancreatic islets, and to reduce circulating levels of FFA, may improve β-cell function [14]. In diabetes-prone, obese rodents, pre-clinical data has shown a potent effect of thiazolidinediones to restore β-cell insulin content and preventing loss of β-cell mass in models of type 2 diabetes [12,15,16].

Effects on Glycemic Control

The US FDA has approved pioglitazone and rosiglitazone for use as monotherapy for type 2 diabetes or in combination with metformin, sulfonylureas, or insulin.

It is important to know that because of the drugs' effects on adipose tissue metabolism and the distribution of adipose stores in the body, several weeks to months are typically required to observe a clinical response. It is helpful to instruct patients that there is an expected delay in the glucose lowering effects on a thiazolidinedione, so they can anticipate the clinical outcome. In addition, patients should be followed on a starting dose for 3–4 months, before increasing the dose.

Pioglitazone

Pioglitazone monotherapy is effective in type 2 diabetes. In a study of 408 patients, pioglitazone reduced HbA1c in a dose-dependent fashion [17].

Mean HbA1c changes compared with baseline in all patients groups were as follows: +0.2%, –0.3%, –0.3%, and –0.9% with 7.5 mg, 15 mg, 30 mg, and 45 mg once-daily dosing, respectively, at 26 weeks of therapy. The groups were further analyzed with respect to previous antihyperglycemic therapy. In both drug-naïve and previously treated patients, HbA1c was decreased to the greatest extent by the 45-mg dose (−1.9% and –0.6% compared to baseline, respectively).

In combination studies with sulfonylureas or metformin, pioglitazone has resulted in an improvement in glycemic control. Five hundred and sixty patients who were receiving a stable dose of a sulfonylurea were randomized to receive pioglitazone 15 mg once daily, 30 mg once daily, or placebo [18]. After 16 weeks, HbA1c was 0.9% and 1.3% lower than placebo with the 15- and 30-mg doses, respectively. Another study assessed the effect of adding pioglitazone to stable therapy with metformin. Three hundred and twenty-eight subjects received pioglitazone 30 mg daily in combination with metformin or placebo. At 16 weeks, HbA1c was reduced by about 0.6% in the pioglitazone + metformin group compared with baseline. In contrast, HbA1c increased by almost 0.2% in the placebo + metformin group [19].

A 16-week trial compared the combination of insulin + pioglitazone with insulin alone. Five hundred and sixty-six patients with type 2 diabetes who were being treated with insulin received pioglitazone 15 mg or 30 mg once daily or placebo in addition to their pre-study insulin regimen. HbA1c was reduced by 0.73 and 1.0% in the 15-and 30-mg groups, respectively, compared with insulin + placebo [20].

Rosiglitazone

Rosiglitazone is effective as monotherapy in the treatment of type 2 diabetes. In a 26-week study of 959 patients with type 2 diabetes, rosiglitazone was given as 4 or 8 mg once daily, or 2 or 4 mg twice daily [21]. Drug-naïve patients had the greatest reductions in HbA1c. The effect was dose-dependent, and the 4-mg twice-daily dosing proved superior to the 8-mg once-daily dosing (ΔHbA1c –0.8% and −1.1% compared with baseline, respectively). In patients who were not drug-naïve, the 4-mg twice-daily dose was again the most effective, resulting in HbA1c decreases of –0.54% in patients who were previously treated with a single agent and –0.43% in patients who were previously treated with multiple agents. In this study, fasting plasma glucose declined starting at the fourth week of therapy and was maximally lowered at weeks 8–12. In another trial, rosiglitazone monotherapy in doses of 2 or 4 mg twice daily reduced HbA1c at 26 weeks by 1.1% or 1.5%, respectively, in patients with and without previous exposure to antihyperglycemic agents [22]. Both of these trials found that HbA1c decreased initially at 8 weeks and achieved maximal effects at weeks 18–26.

Rosiglitazone has been studied in combination with sulfonylureas and metformin. In a trial of 574 patients with type 2 diabetes who were receiving therapy with a sulphonylurea, low-dose rosiglitazone, or placebo was added to glibenclamide, gliclazide, or glipizide. The maximum dose of rosiglitazone in this study was 2 mg twice daily, which resulted in the greatest decrease in HbA1c (−1.0% compared with placebo + sulfonylurea) at 26 weeks [23]. The combination of metformin and rosiglitazone was also found to be effective therapy in a study of 348 patients with type 2 diabetes. These patients discontinued all antihyperglycemic agents except for metformin and were then randomized to receive placebo, rosiglitazone 4 mg once daily or 8 mg once daily. At week 26, HbA1c had decreased compared with baseline by 0.56% and 0.78% in the 4- and 8-mg groups, respectively and increased by 0.45% in the placebo group [24].

In a recent trial, the addition of rosiglitazone to insulin therapy was evaluated in patients with type 2 diabetes. Patients who were taking insulin were randomized to receive placebo or rosiglitazone 4 or 8 mg once daily. HbA1c was reduced by a greater degree in the rosiglitazone groups at 26 weeks of therapy (–0.6% and −1.2% in the 4- and 8-mg groups, respectively, compared with baseline). The placebo group exhibited an average increase of 0.1% in HbA1c [25].

Prevention of Diabetes

A recent study [26] examined the effects of rosiglitazone in the prevention of type 2 diabetes. The double-blind, randomized controlled trial consisted of 5,269 patients with either impaired fasting glucose or impaired glucose intolerance. They were assigned to receive rosiglitazone 8 mg daily versus placebo for approximately 3 years. The outcomes revealed a significant difference in the development of diabetes in the rosiglitazone-treated group (11%) versus placebo (26%). The rosiglitazone group also showed a significant regression to normoglycemia (50%) versus placebo (30%). There was, however, a small but statistically significant number of heart failure cases, which occurred in the rosiglitazone group (0.5%) versus placebo (0.1%). The trial concluded that an 8-mg dose of rosiglitazone daily, can prevent the development of diabetes in >60% of patients with impaired fasting glucose or impaired glucose tolerance.

Effects on Lipids

All of the thiazolidinediones sharply increase high-density lipoprotein (HDL) cholesterol and modestly increase low-density lipoprotein (LDL) cholesterol in patients with type 2 diabetes [27,28]. Pioglitazone also significantly decreases triglyceride levels [29].

In clinical trials, pioglitazone 45 mg raised HDL by 19.1% and LDL by 6.0% compared with baseline after 26 weeks of therapy [27]. Triglycerides fell by 9.3%. Pioglitazone was also reported to have dramatic effects on HDL in patients whose HDL levels fell into the lowest category. In a study of 408 patients with type 2 diabetes, Pioglitazone 45 mg increased HDL by 31.6% after 26 weeks in patients who had HDL levels less than 35 mg/dl. In contrast, HDL levels rose by 12.9% in patients who had baseline HDL levels greater than 45 mg/dl [30].

Compared with baseline, rosiglitazone 8 mg raised LDL and HDL by up to 18.6% and 14.2% at 26 weeks and by 12.1% and 18.5% at 52 weeks, respectively. These results show that LDL levels remained stable, whereas HDL levels continued to rise over time. Triglyceride levels in rosiglitazone-treated patients were variable and usually not statistically different from placebo controls [28]. Since reciprocal changes are almost invariably seen in HDL and triglyceride levels in most clinical trials, the mechanism of the relative lack of triglyceride lowering with rosiglitazone remains unexplained.

Cardiovascular Effects

The unique benefits demonstrated by the thiazolidinediones on vascular function appear to be mediated by direct (via PPARγ receptors in vascular cells) as well as indirect mechanisms (via changes in circulating factors, including adipokines, cytokines, and FFA). A summary of the effect of thiazolidinediones on vascular function and cardiovascular risk factors is presented in Table 1.

TABLE 1. Summary of effects of thiazolidinediones on cardiovascular risk factors and vascular function.

Lipids
↓ FFA
↓ Tiglyceride levels
↑ HDL-C and LDL-C
↓ LDL-C oxidation
↑ Buoyancy of LDL particles
Coagulation/fibrinolysis
↓ PAI-1 and fibrinogen
Vascular inflammation
↓ CRP, MCP-1, ROS
Δ Macrophage function in atherosclerotic lesions
↓ MMP-9
Vascular functional effects
↓ Intimal-media thickness
↓ BP
↓ Brachial arterial relaxation
↓ Microalbuminuria
↓ Migration and proliferation of vascular smooth-muscle cells
Platelet aggregation
↓ Platelet aggregation

Pioglitazone and Macrovascular Disease

A recent study [31] investigated the effects of intensive glycemic control on macrovascular disease. It was a prospective, randomized controlled trial involving over 5,000 type 2 diabetics with preexisting macrovascular complications. They were randomized to receive either 45-mg pioglitazone or placebo for approximately 2.5 years. Pioglitazone was shown to reduce the risk of all cause mortality, non-fatal myocardial infarction (excluding silent myocardial infarction), and stroke by approximately 16% as compared with placebo. There was, however, an increase in the rate of heart failure in the pioglitazone group (11%) versus placebo (8%). The study concluded that pioglitazone improved cardiovascular outcomes in type 2 diabetics with high cardiovascular risk profiles.

Effects on Atherogenesis

Rosiglitazone strongly inhibited the development of atherosclerosis in LDL receptor-deficient mice, a finding that correlated with increased insulin sensitivity [32]. In another study, rosiglitazone decreased atherosclerotic lesion area by 60% compared to controls in mice with angiotensin II-accelerated atherosclerosis [33]. Pioglitazone has also been shown to markedly decrease neointimal cross-sectional areas in air-injured rat carotid arteries relative to controls [34]. In human studies, troglitazone and pioglitazone treatment resulted in a significant decrease in common carotid arterial intimal and medial complex thickness (IMT) (–0.080 mm, N = 135 and –0.084 mm, N = 106, respectively) after 3–6 months of treatment as measured by carotid ultrasound. In contrast, control patients had a slight increase in IMT. There was not a significant correlation between this finding and HbA1c values [35,36]. A double-blind, placebo-controlled, prospective trial [37] enrolled 97 patients with diabetes in whom angiography had revealed coronary artery blockages. The patients were randomized to either a loading dose of 8 mg of rosiglitazone before angiography and stent placement, followed by 4 mg of rosiglitazone for 6 months or placebo on the same schedule. At the end of the 6-month period, coronary angiography was repeated: 11.4% of patients in the rosiglitazone arm had restenosis, compared with 44.7% of patients in the control group. Body weight and blood glucose levels were not significantly different between the 2 groups after 6 months but C-reactive protein levels were significantly lower in the rosiglitazone group.

Large randomized studies evaluating cardiovascular outcomes are necessary.

Cardiac Structure and Function

Thiazolidinediones were initially associated with increased cardiac weight in animal studies. However, human echocardiographic studies on rosiglitazone (4 mg twice daily) or pioglitazone (maximum 60 mg daily) for up to a year have shown no adverse effects on left ventricular mass or cardiac output [38,39].

TZD and Heart Failure

Diabetic patients often have significant cardiovascular risk factors, which may be exacerbated with TZD treatment. Congestive heart failure in diabetics treated concomitantly with insulin and TZDs has been reported. In placebo controlled trials the incidence of CHF was significantly higher in patients using pioglitazone and insulin (approximately 1%) versus patients on insulin alone [40].

Although the incidence of heart failure with pioglitazone or rosigliatoze monotherapy is low, <1%, the American Heart Association and American Diabetes Association have a joint consensus statement regarding the use of TZD in patients with cardiovascular disease. They recommend TZDs to be used cautiously and initiated at low doses in patients with class I or II NYHA category heart failure, and they are not recommended in class III or IV heart failure.

Effects on Blood Pressure

Thiazolidinediones have been shown to lower blood pressure in animal and human studies. Mechanisms for the blood-pressure lowering effect have not been fully elucidated. An improvement in insulin resistance is likely responsible, at least in part.

In insulin-resistant rats, rosiglitazone prevented the development of hypertension [41]. Pioglitazone was shown to lower blood pressure in rats to an extent that was not correlated with alterations in fasting insulin concentrations [42].

Renal Effects

PPARγ is expressed in the rat kidney, primarily in the collecting ducts [43]. Its presence in this location suggests that it may be involved in water and sodium retention [44]. It has also been detected in the mesangial cells of rats [45,46].

All of the thiazolidinediones used clinically have been shown to delay the onset of proteinuria or reduce established proteinuria [16,45–47]. In a small randomized study, pioglitazone significantly reduced urinary albumin excretion from 142.8 to 48.4 mcg/minute after 3 months of treatment in patients with type 2 diabetes and microalbuminuria [48]. Rosiglitazone also reduced albumin/creatinine ratio in patients with type 2 diabetes in a dose-dependent fashion [22]. Larger, longer-term studies are necessary to confirm the effects of thiazolidinediones on the delay and improvement of diabetic nephropathy.

Effects on Diabetic Retinopathy

PPARγ is expressed in bovine retinal endothelial cells [49]. In vitro studies found thiazolidinediones inhibited the effects of vascular endothelial growth factor on migration and proliferation of retinal endothelial cells. In vivo, intravitreous injection of both agents inhibited development of retinal neovascularization. These results indicate that thiazolidinediones may be effective in the treatment of diabetic retinopathy pending further research in humans [49].

Nonalcoholic Steatohepatosis

An uncontrolled trial included 30 adults with histologically confirmed steatohepatosis and treated with rosiglitazone (4 mg twice daily) for 48 weeks [50]. All patients were overweight. Paired biopsies before and after treatment were available in 26 patients, showing significant improvement. Mean serum ALT levels also showed corresponding improvement. Similar studies were done using pioglitazone [51,52]

Thiazolidinediones in Polycystic Ovary Syndrome

Polycystic ovary syndrome (PCOS) is characterized by menstrual irregularities, infertility, hyperandrogenism, obesity, and insulin resistance. In a study of rosiglitazone (4 mg twice daily for 2 months) with or without clomiphene in 25 women with PCOS who had not responded to clomiphene alone, ovulatory rates were higher in the combined versus monotherapy groups (77% and 33%, respectively) [53].

Pioglitazone has also been shown to improve ovulation rates and hyperadrogenism associated with PCOS. In a randomized controlled trial [54], 40 women were assigned to receive 30 mg pioglitazone versus placebo for 3 months. The results revealed that the pioglitazone group had a significant decrease in their free androgen index as well as higher ovulation rates (41% had normal ovulation in the pioglitazone group as compared with 5.6% in the placebo group).

These results point to an exciting new treatment option for PCOS; however, because of the effects of these agents on gene expression, there may be hazards in early pregnancy and are not recommended for that use.

Adverse Effects

The most commonly reported adverse events with both pioglitazone and rosiglitazone were upper respiratory tract infection and headache, although other side effects include abnormal liver function, edema, weight gain, and anemia.

Hepatic Effects

In combined North American clinical trials, troglitazone was associated with significant transaminase elevations (greater than three times the upper limit of normal) in about 2% of patients compared with 0.6% with placebo [55]. Troglitazone use led to liver failure and death in more than 20 cases [56], resulting in its withdrawal from the market by the FDA in March 2000.

Although premarketing trials revealed no cases of rosiglitazone- or pioglitazone-induced liver abnormalities, very few case reports have demonstrated possible associations between both drugs and moderate to severe hepatic toxicity [57–60]. Other patients have developed elevations in transaminases a few weeks after initiation of therapy with rosiglitazone; in each case, the abnormalities were reversible 4–7 weeks after discontinuation of therapy [58,60]. The FDA recommends periodic monitoring of ALT according to the clinical judgment of the health care professional.

Edema

Ankle edema occurred in about 5% of patients treated with both rosiglitazone and pioglitazone; in some cases, pulmonary edema can develop. Edema was more frequent in insulin combination therapy with either drug (about 15% compared with 5.4–7% with insulin alone). The reasons for fluid retention and peripheral edema with TZDs are multifactorial. The increase in plasma volume may result from a reduction in renal excretion of sodium and an increase in sodium and free water retention. TZDs may also interact synergistically with insulin to cause arterial vasodilatation, leading to sodium reabsorption and an increase in extracellular volume [61,62]. In case reports, the edema has not been responsive to diuretics [63,64].

Weight Gain

Pioglitazone and rosiglitazone are both associated with dose-dependent and time-dependent weight gain. The average weight gain ranged from 0.5 to 3.5 kg in patients treated with either drug as monotherapy. When either drug was combined with insulin or a sulfonylurea, the weight gain was more dramatic. Mechanisms for weight gain with thiazolidinediones may include increased adipogenesis resulting from PPAR-γ activation, fluid retention, and increased appetite [65]. In general, improvement in glycemic control with decreased glycosuria and caloric retention and storage may result in expanded adipose tissue and body weight. Several studies have shown that the weight gain with TZDs may be associated with an increase in subcutaneous fat. However, at the same time, there is a reduction in visceral fat and an overall decrease in the ratio of visceral to subcutaneous fat. This change in fat distribution seems to underlie the improvement in glycemic control despite an overall increase in body weight.

In a recent report, patients with a shorter duration of diabetes and higher body mass index were significantly more likely to gain weight on pioglitazone therapy [66].

Anemia

Anemia was reported in 1% of patients treated with pioglitazone and 1.9% with rosiglitazone. In pioglitazone-treated patients, hemoglobin decreased by 2–3% within the first 4–12 weeks and remained stable thereafter [27]. Rosiglitazone also caused a decrease in hemoglobin of up to 1 gm/dl [67]. This effect is most likely related to hemodilution secondary to a slight increase in plasma volume [68]. Studies have shown that thiazolidinediones do not cause hemolysis or affect red cell mass or erythropoiesis [68,69].

Hypoglycemia

Since the thiazolidinediones work independently of the pancreas, and typically reduce insulin levels in patients with type 2 diabetes, there is very little, if any, clinical risk of hypoglycemia with these agents. However, when circulating insulin levels are increased, such as in patients taking a sulfonylurea or insulin, the addition or pioglitazone or rosiglitazone may result in hypoglycemia. This is usually apparent after four or more weeks of therapy, since it takes few months for the full clinical effect of the thiazolidinediones to be manifest in most patients. Under these circumstances, the sulfonylurea or insulin dose should be reduced and therapy with the thiazolidinedione continued.

Pharmacokinetics and Metabolism

Pioglitazone

Pioglitazone is available in 15-, 30-, and 45-mg tablets. When administered in the fasting state, pioglitazone is measurable in serum within 30 min and peak concentrations occur in 2 h [27]. Administration of pioglitazone with food delays the time to peak concentration to 3–4 h but does not diminish the extent of its absorption. Pioglitazone alone has a half-life of 3–7 h; pioglitazone in combination with its active metabolites has a half-life of 16–24 h. Steady-state concentrations are reached within 7 days. Its volume of distribution is 0.63 L/kg and it is more than 99% protein-bound, principally to albumin. Pioglitazone is metabolized by hydroxylation, oxidation, and conjugation into active and inactive metabolites. M-III (an active keto derivative), and M-IV (an active hydroxy derivative) are the principal metabolites in humans. Hepatic metabolism is extensive and occurs via cytochrome (CYP) P450 isoforms CYP2C8 and CYP3A4 [28]. Urinary excretion is 15–30% and is primarily in the form of metabolites. The primary excretion of pioglitazone and its metabolites appears to be through bile and feces [27].

Rosiglitazone

Rosiglitazone is available in 2-, 4-, and 8-mg tablets and is 99% orally bioavailable [67]. Peak plasma concentrations occur in 1 h. When administered with food, there is a decrease in the time to peak concentration and in the maximum concentration; however, these effects are not felt to be clinically significant [70]. The elimination half-life of rosiglitazone is 3–4 h and independent of the dose [67]. Its volume of distribution is 17.6l. It is 99.8% plasma protein-bound, primarily to albumin. Rosiglitazone is metabolized via hydroxylation, *N*-demethylation, and conjugation. None of its metabolites are considered active. Metabolism of rosiglitazone differs from pioglitazone in that it occurs via hepatic cytochrome P450 (CYP) 2C8 and to a lesser extent by CYP2C9, avoiding the 3A4 system, which is a common route for the metabolism of a variety of drugs used in clinical practice. Urinary excretion of rosiglitazone metabolites is 64%; fecal excretion is 23% [67].

Drug Interactions

Pioglitazone

The concurrent administration of pioglitazone with digoxin, glipizide, metformin, and warfarin, respectively, has been studied in healthy volunteers. Medication pharmacokinetics was not altered with any of these drug combinations [27]. The p450 system CYP3A4 metabolizes pioglitazone and can be associated with drug interactions if this enzyme is induced or inhibited, although pioglitazone itself does not affect the function of CYP3A4 [28]. Since estrogens are also metabolized by CYP3A4, pioglitazone has been studied in combination with oral contraceptives and other hormone replacement therapies. The pharmacokinetics of both agents remained unchanged with administration of pioglitazone, indicating that dosing adjustments are ordinarily not necessary [71].

Rosiglitazone

Rosiglitazone has been studied in combination with acarbose, digoxin, metformin, nifedipine, ranitidine, warfarin, and oral contraceptives [67,72] There have been no clinically significant effects on the pharmacokinetics of any of these agents in combination with rosiglitazone.

Special Populations

No adjustment in the dosage of either pioglitazone or rosiglitazone is required in renal insufficiency or in elderly populations [27,67]. However, there are now few reports of congestive heart failure caused or exacerbated by thiazolidinediones in the setting of chronic renal insufficiency [73], which suggests that in patients with renal insufficiency, a lower dose of a thiazolidinedione may be safer to use. Neither drug should be used in patients who have serum hepatic transaminase levels greater than 2.5 times the upper limit of normal (see adverse effects). Both agents are classified as pregnancy category C and should be avoided in pregnant women. It is not known whether either drug is excreted in breast milk. There are insufficient data supporting the use of either drug in pediatric populations [27,67].

Learning Elements

Key Points

1. Thiazolidinediones act via PPAR-gamma receptors to change the metabolism and distribution of adipose stores in the body, resulting in enhanced insulin sensitivity.
2. Improvement in the insulin resistance that underlies the pathogenesis of type 2 diabetes and the metabolic syndrome leads to pleiotropic effects, including reduced glycemia, enhanced beta cell function, reduction in the inflammatory milieu, improvement in dyslipidemia and blood pressure vascular endothelial function, cardiovascular risk reduction, and in the prevention of diabetes.
3. These agents act independently of the pancreas and reduce circulating insulin levels, enabling them to provide aggressive glycemic control without hypoglycemia.

Pitfalls/Complications

1. In some patients, thiazolidinediones are associated with fluid retention and weight gain, which can be exaggerated when used in combination with insulin secretagogues or insulin. These adverse effects appear to be integral to the insulin-sensitizing effects of these drugs and may be mediated by the PPAR-gamma receptor.

Because of these issues, neither thiazolidinediones is appropriate for use in patients with symptomatic congestive heart failure or severely compromised cardiac function.

References

1. Adams M, Montague CT, Prins JB, et al. Activators of Peroxisome Proliferator-Activated Receptor gamma Have Depot-Specific Effects on Human Preadipocyte Differentiation. J Clin Invest. 1997; 100(12):3149–3153.
2. Vidal-Puig AJ, Considine RV, Jimenez-Liñan M, et al. Peroxisome proliferator-activated receptor gene expression in human tissues: effects of obesity, weight loss, and regulation by insulin and glucocorticoids. J Clin Invest. 1997;99(10): 2416–2422.
3. Roden M, Price TB, Perseghin G, et al. Mechanism of free fatty acid-induced insulin resistance in humans. J Clin Invest. 1996;97:2859–2865.
4. Oakes ND, Thalen PG, Jacinto SM, et al. Thiazolidinediones increase plasma-adipose tissue FFA exchange capacity and enhance insulin-mediated control of systemic FFA availability. Diabetes. 2001;50:1158–1165.
5. Iwata M, Haruta T, Usui I, et al. Pioglitazone ameliorates tumor necrosis factor-alpha-induced insulin resistance by a mechanism independent of adipogenic activity of peroxisome proliferator-activated receptor-gamma. Diabetes. 2001;50:1083–1092.
6. Phillips SA, Ciaraldi TP, Kong AP, et al. Modulation of circulating and adipose tissue adiponectin levels by antidiabetic therapy. Diabetes 2003;52(3): 667–674.
7. Akazawa S, Sun F, Ito M, et al. Efficacy of troglitazone on body fat distribution in type 2 diabetes. Diabetes Care 2000;23:1067–1071.
8. Inzucchi SE, Maggs DG, Spollett GR, et al. Efficacy and metabolic effects of metformin and troglitazone in type II diabetes. New Engl J Med. 1998;338(13): 867–872.
9. Nolan JJ, Bernhard L, Beerdsen P, et al. Improvement in glucose tolerance and insulin resistance in obese subjects treated with troglitazone. N Engl J Med. 1994;331(18):1188–1193.
10. Petersen KF, Krssak M, Inzucchi S, et al. Mechanism of troglitazone action in type 2 diabetes. Diabetes. 2000;49:827–831.
11. Maggs DG, Buchanan TA, Burant CF, et al. Metabolic effects of troglitazone monotherapy in type 2 diabetes mellitus: a randomized, double-blind, placebo-controlled trial. Ann Intern Med. 1998; 128(3):176–185.
12. Shimabukuro M, Zhou YT, Lee Y, et al. Troglitazone lowers islet fat and restores beta cell function of Zucker diabetic fatty rats. J Biol Chem. 1998;273(6):3547–3550.
13. Unger RH. Lipotoxic diseases. Annual Rev of Medicine 2002;53:319–336.
14. Yang L, An HX, Deng XL, et al. Rosiglitazone reverses insulin secretion altered by chronic exposure to free fatty acid via IRS-2-associated phosphatidylinositol 3-kinase pathway. Acta Pharmacologica Sinica. 2003;24(5):429–434.
15. Finegood DT, McArthur MD, Kojwang D, et al. Beta-cell mass dynamics in Zucker diabetic fatty rats. Rosiglitazone prevents the rise in net cell death. Diabetes 2001;50(5):1021–1029.
16. Buckingham RE, Al-Barazanji KA, Toseland CD, et al. Peroxisome proliferator-activated receptor-gamma agonist, rosiglitazone, protects against nephropathy and pancreatic islet abnormalities in Zucker fatty rats. Diabetes. 1998;47(8): 1326–1334.

17. Aronoff S, Rosenblatt S, Braithwaite S, et al. Pioglitazone hydrochloride improves glycemic control in the treatment of patients with type 2 diabetes. Diabetes Care. 2000;23(11):1605–1611.
18. Kipnes M S, Krosnick A, Rendell MS, et al. Pioglitazone hydrochloride in combination with sulfonylurea therapy improves glycemic control in patients with type 2 diabetes mellitus: a randomized, placebo-controlled study. Am J Med. 2001;111(1): 10–17.
19. Einhorn D, Rendell M, Rosenzweig J, et al. Pioglitazone hydrochloride in combination with metformin in the treatment of type 2 diabetes mellitus: a randomized, placebo-controlled study. Clin Ther. 2000;22(12):1395–1409.
20. Rubin C, Egan J, Schneider R. Combination therapy with pioglitazone and insulin in patients with type 2 diabetes [abstract 0474]. Diabetes. 1999;48(suppl 1):A110.
21. Phillips LS, Grunberger G, Miller E, et al. Once- and twice-daily dosing with rosiglitazone improves glycemic control in patients with type 2 diabetes. Diabetes Care. 2001;24(2):308–315.
22. Lebovitz LE, Dole JF, Patwardhan R, et al. Rosiglitazone monotherapy is effective in patients with type 2 diabetes. J Clin Endocrinol Metab. 2001;86(1):280–288.
23. Wolffenbuttel BHR, Gomist R, Squatrito S, et al. Addition of low-dose rosiglitazone to sulphonylurea therapy improves glycaemic control in type 2 diabetic patients. Diabet Med. 2000;17:40–47.
24. Fonseca V, Rosenstock J, Patwardhan R, et al. Effect of Metformin and rosiglitazone combination therapy in patients with type 2 diabetes mellitus: a randomized controlled trial. JAMA. 2000;283(13):1695–1702.
25. Raskin P, Rendell M, Riddle MC, et al. A randomized trial of rosiglitazone therapy in patients with inadequately controlled insulin-treated type 2 diabetes. Diabetes Care. 2001;24(7):1226–1232.
26. Gerstein H, Yusuf S, Holman R, et al. Effect of rosiglitazone on the frequency of diabetes in patients with impaired glucose tolerance or impaired fasting glucose. Lancet 2006;368:1096–1105.
27. Prescribing information for pioglitazone. Takeda Pharmaceuticals. February, 2000.
28. Aoyama E, Tsujiuchi H, Asahi S, et al. In vitro studies on the metabolic pathways of pioglitazone [abstract 418-P]. Diabetes. 2001;50(suppl 2):A105.
29. Fonseca V, Valiquett TR, Huang SM, et al. Troglitazone monotherapy improves glycemic control in patients with type 2 diabetes mellitus: a randomized, controlled study. J Clin Endocrinol Metab. 1998;83(9):3169–76.
30. Prince MJ, Zagar AJ, Robertson KE. Effect of pioglitazone on HDL-C, a cardiovascular risk factor in type 2 diabetes [abstract 514-P]. Diabetes. 2001; 50(suppl 2):A128.
31. Dormany J, Charbonnel B, Eckland D, et al. Secondary prevention of macrovascular events in patients with type 2 diabetes in the PROactive Study. Lancet. 2005;366:1279–1289.
32. Li AC, Brown KK, Silvestre MJ, et al. Peroxisome proliferator-activated receptor gamma ligands inhibit development of atherosclerosis in LDL receptor-deficient mice. J Clin Invest. 2000;106(4):523–531.
33. Collins AR, Noh G, Hsueh WA, et al. PPARγ ligands attenuate angiotensin-II accelerated atherosclerosis in male low density receptor deficient (LDLR-/-) mice[abstract 292-PP]. Diabetes. 2001;50(suppl 2): A72–A73.
34. Yoshimoto T, Naruse M, Shizume H, et al. Vasculoprotective effects of insulin sensitizing agent pioglitazone in neointimal thickening and hypertensive vascular hypertrophy. Atherosclerosis. 1999; 145:333–340.
35. Minamikawa J, Tanaka S, Yamauchi M, et al. Potent inhibitory effect of troglitazone on carotid arterial wall thickness in type 2 diabetes. J Clin Endocrinol Metab. 1998;83(5):1818–1820.
36. Koshiyama H, Shimono D, Kuwamura N, et al. Inhibitory effect of pioglitazone on carotid arterial wall thickness in type 2 diabetes. J Clin Endocrinol Metab. 2001;86(7):3452–3456.
37. Choi SH, Choi DH, Ko YK, et al. Preventive effects of rosiglitazone on restenosis after coronary stenting in patients with type 2 diabetes. ADA 63rd Scientific Sessions 2003;82-OR.
38. Schneider RL, Shaffer SJ. Long-Term Echocardiographic Assessment in patients with type 2 diabetes mellitus treated with pioglitazone [abstract 504-P]. Diabetes. 2000;49(suppl 1):A124.
39. Sutton MSJ, Dole JF, Rappaport EB. Rosiglitazone does not adversely affect cardiac structure or function in patients with type 2 diabetes [abstract 0438]. Diabetes. 1999;48(suppl 1):A102.
40. Actos (pioglitazone hydrochloride) [package insert]. Lincolnshire, Ill: Takeda Pharmaceuticals America, Inc; 2000.
41. Walker AB, Chattington PD, Buckingham RE, et al. The thiazolidinedione rosiglitazone (BRL-49653) lowers blood pressure and protects against impairment of endothelial function in Zucker fatty rats. Diabetes. 1999;48(7):1448–1453.
42. Buchanan TA, Meehan WP, Jeng YY, et al. Blood pressure lowering by pioglitazone: evidence for a direct vascular effect. J Clin Invest. 1995;96:354–360.
43. Yang T, Michele DE, Park J, et al. Expression of peroxisomal proliferator-activated receptors and retinoid X receptors in the kidney. Am J Physiol. 1999;277(6):F966–F973.

44. Guan YF, Breyer MD. Peroxisome proliferator-activated receptors (PPARs): novel therapeutic targets in renal disease. Kidney Int. 2001;60: 14–30.
45. Asano T, Wakisaka M, Yoshinari M, et al. Peroxisome proliferator-activated receptor gamma1 (PPARgamma1) expresses in rat mesangial cells and PPARgamma agonists modulate its differentiation. Biochim Biophys Acta. 2000;1497(1): 148–154.
46. Nicholas SB, Kawano Y, Wakino S, et al. Expression and function of peroxisome proliferator-activated receptor-gamma in mesangial cells. Hypertension. 2001;37(2 part 2):722–727.
47. Yoshimoto T, Naruse M, Nishikawa M, et al. Antihypertensive and vasculo- and renoprotective effects of pioglitazone in genetically obese diabetic rats. Am J Physiol. 1997;272(6):E989–E996.
48. Nakamura T, Ushiyama C, Shimada N, et al. Comparative effects of pioglitazone, glibenclamide, and voglibose on urinary endothelin-1 and albumin excretion in diabetes patients. J Diabetes Complications. 2000;14(5):250–254.
49. Murata T, Hata Y, Ishibashi T, et al. Response of experimental retinal neovascularization to thiazolidinediones. Arch Ophthalmol. 2001;119(5): 709–717.
50. Neuschwander-Tetri BA, Brunt EM, Wehmeier KR, et al. Improved nonalcoholic steatohepatitis after 48 weeks of treatment with the PPAR-gamma ligand rosiglitazone. Hepatology 2003;38(4):1008–1017.
51. Sanyal AJ, Contos MJ, Sargeant C, et al. A randomized controlled pilot study of pioglitazone and vitamin E versus vitamin E for nonalcoholic steatohepatitis (abstract). Hepatology 2002;382A.
52. Promrat K, Lutchman G, Kleiner DE, et al. Pilot study of pioglitazone in nonalcoholic steatohepatitis (abstract). Gastroenterology, 2003;124(4) (Suppl 1):A708.
53. Ghazeeri G, Kutteh WH, Bryer-Ash M, et al. Effect of rosiglitazone on spontaneous and clomiphene-induced ovulation in women with polycystic ovary syndrome. Fertil Steril 2003;79(3):562–566.
54. Brettenthaler N, De Geyter C, Huber P, et al. Effect of Insulin Sensitizer Pioglitazone on Insulin resistance, Hyperadrongenism, and Ovulatory Dysfunction in Women with Polycystic Ovary Syndrome. J of Clin Endocrinol Metabolism. 2004; 89(8):3835–3840.
55. Watkins PB, Whitcomb RW. Hepatic dysfunction associated with troglitazone. N Engl J Med. 1998;338(13):916–917.
56. Misbin, RI. Troglitazone-associated hepatic failure. Am J Med. 1999;130(4):330.
57. Forman LM, Simmons DA, Diamond RH. Hepatic failure in a patient taking rosiglitazone. Ann Intern Med. 2000;132(2):118–121.
58. Maeda K. Hepatocellular injury in a patient receiving pioglitazone. Ann Inten Med 2001;135(4):306.
59. Al-Salman J, Arjomand H, Kemp DG, et al. Hepatocellular injury in a patient receiving rosiglitazone: a case report. Ann Intern Med. 2000;132(2): 121–124.
60. Ravinuthala RS, Nori U. Rosiglitazone toxicity. Ann Intern Med. 2000;133(8):658.
61. Donnelly R, Gray S, Idris I. Rosiglitazone and ankle swelling: an acute dose-dependent effect on endothelial permeability [abstract 275-OR]. Diabetes. 2001;50(suppl 1):A68.
62. Niemeyer NV, Janney LM. Thiazolidinedione-induced edema. Pharmacotherapy 2002;22(7): 924–929.
63. Gorson DM. Significant weight gain with rezulin therapy. Arch Intern Med. 1999;159:199.
64. Thomas ML, Lloyd SJ. Pulmonary edema associated with rosiglitazone and troglitazone. Ann Pharmacother. 2001;35:123–124.
65. Shimizu H, Tsuchiya T, Sato N, et al. Troglitazone reduces plasma leptin concentration but increases hunger in NIDDM patients. Diabetes Care. 1998;21:1470–1474.
66. King AB, Armstrong D. Characteristics of the patients who gain weight while on pioglitazone treatment [abstract 481-P]. Diabetes. 2001;50(suppl 1): A120.
67. Prescribing information for rosiglitazone. SmithKline Beecham Pharmaceuticals. February 2001.
68. Young MM, Squassante L, Wemer J, et al. Troglitazone has no effect on red cell mass or other erythropoietic parameters. Eur J Clin Pharmacol. 1999;55:101–104.
69. Dogterom P, Jonkman JHG, Vallance SE. Rosiglitazone: no effect on erythropoiesis or premature red cell destruction [abstract 0424]. Diabetes. 1999;48(suppl 1):A98.
70. Freed MI, Allen A, Jorkasky DK, et al. Systemic exposure to rosiglitazone is unaltered by food. Eur J Clin Pharmacol. 1999;55(1):53–56.
71. Carey RA, Liu Y. Pioglitazone does not markedly alter oral contraceptive or hormone replacement therapy pharmacokinetics [abstract 405-P]. Diabetes. 2000;49(suppl 1):A100.
72. Inglis AML, Miller AK, Culkin KT, et al. Rosiglitazone, a PPARγ agonist, does not alter the pharmacokinetics of oral contraceptives [abstract 0443]. Diabetes. 2000;48(suppl1):A103.
73. Kermani A, Garg A. Thiazolidinedione-associated congestive heart failure and pulmonary edema. Mayo Clin Proc 2003;78(9):1088–1091.

11
Antidiabetic Combination Therapy

Henning Beck-Nielsen and Jan Erik Henriksen

Keywords: Type 2 diabetes, treatment, insulin, Metformin, sulfonylurea, glitazones, triple therapy, glycaemic control.

Introduction

Type 2 diabetes (T2D) is a fast-growing disease with an increase in prevalence of some 5% per year. This increase may, however, in part, be explained by a reduction in mortality indicating that the investment in better treatment has been fruitful [1]. Especially, treatment of arterial hypertension and dyslipidaemia may have had an impact, whereas severe hyperglycaemia still seems to present a serious problem in T2D subjects and therefore needs more attention. The UKPDS clearly showed the existence of a close correlation between blood glucose values and diabetic complications, as also seen in type 1 diabetes [2] (Fig. 1). In fact, the epidemiological calculation based on the UKPDS data showed a reduction of about 20% in both mortality rate and in the risk of developing myocardial infarct per 1% reduction in HbA1c [2]. Consequently, we must aim to normalise HbA1c values in these subjects.

In most countries today, the recommendation is therefore to reduce HbA1c values to a level below 7.0% (normal range: 4.4–6.4%). Several surveys, however, indicate HbA1c levels in most diabetic populations to be above 8–9%, and a clinical experience of values of 10% or higher is not unusual [3]. Therefore, new treatment modalities seem to be needed. In this review, we will discuss the pathophysiology of T2D, the treatment of the pathophysiological defects and thereby end up with a recommendation for a combination of antidiabetic drugs.

Pathophysiology

Until now treatment of hyperglycaemia in T2D subjects has mainly been of empirical origin, and for many years it was based on the experiences gained from type 1 diabetes. However, T2D is not just an insulin deficient disease, but rather an insulin resistant condition. Therefore, insulin action must be improved as part of the treatment as well. The pathophysiology is very complex, but recent years have revealed many details, and today we know that several organs and cellular defects are involved [4]. One defect cannot explain the cascade of events leading to frank hyperglycaemia, and due to the multifactorial aetiology, T2D cannot be treated by a single drug or change in lifestyle alone. This has, however, been the approach until recently, as clearly indicated by UKDPS [5]. The authors of that landmark study also concluded that multifactorial intervention including polypharmacia is necessary [6].

Why is Blood Glucose Elevated in T2D Subjects?

The main reason for the elevation of blood glucose in diabetes is reduced insulin-mediated glucose metabolism due to reduced insulin secretion and insulin resistance. Due to these defects in insulin-mediated

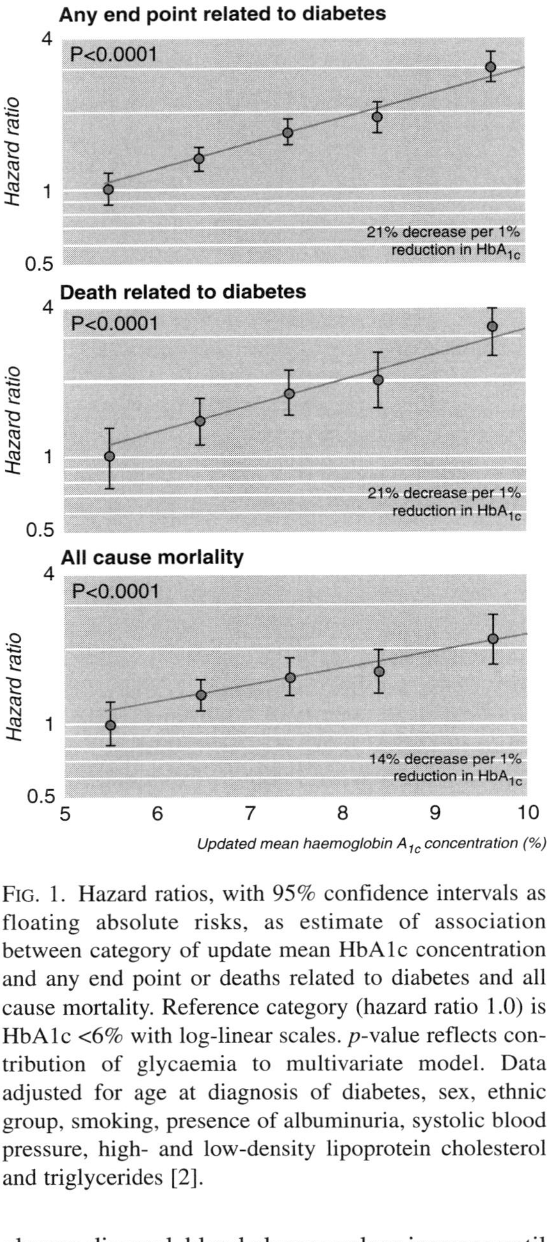

FIG. 1. Hazard ratios, with 95% confidence intervals as floating absolute risks, as estimate of association between category of update mean HbA1c concentration and any end point or deaths related to diabetes and all cause mortality. Reference category (hazard ratio 1.0) is HbA1c <6% with log-linear scales. *p*-value reflects contribution of glycaemia to multivariate model. Data adjusted for age at diagnosis of diabetes, sex, ethnic group, smoking, presence of albuminuria, systolic blood pressure, high- and low-density lipoprotein cholesterol and triglycerides [2].

glucose disposal, blood glucose values increase until reaching a level where glucose itself – glucose-mediated glucose disposal – is able to compensate for the reduced insulin-mediated glucose metabolism, resulting in normal glucose disposal. In other words, the increase in blood glucose in T2D is a compensation for the reduced insulin-mediated glucose disposal. Thus, the degree of hyperglycaemia depends on the degree of impairment of insulin secretion and action. Due to this compensation, diabetic subjects do survive (which is often forgotten), but they pay the price of chronic hyperglycaemia (which may lead to severe diabetic complications). Therefore, we must try to correct this devastating situation by improving the insulin-mediated glucose metabolism. This can be done by improving insulin secretion and action or both.

The Role of the Liver in Fasting and Postprandial Glycaemia

Blood glucose is determined by the rate of glucose appearance (R_a) and the rate of glucose disappearance (R_d). An increase in R_a or a decrease in R_d (or both) may result in hyperglycaemia. Glucose appearing in blood can derive from both ingested carbohydrates and the endogenously produced glucose from liver and kidneys. Most focus has been on the basal hepatic glucose production (HGP), as for several years HGP, alone, was claimed to determine fasting blood glucose values in the morning. This conclusion was based on the finding of a strongly positive correlation between the two variables – a correlation explained partly by the fact that HGP and fasting glucose are mathematically dependent and partly by the fact that the methods used for estimating HGP over-estimated HGP in parallel with the increase in blood glucose, strengthening the positive correlation [7]. Therefore, the importance of this correlation has been weakened, as the methodology was improved [8]. The improved methodology has also led to the conclusion that HGP in the postabsorptive state is normal or only slightly increased (up to 20%) [9]. It therefore seems illogical aiming for a major HGP reduction overnight, for example, by giving long-acting insulin at night, as suppression of glucogenolysis may induce hypoglycaemia at night. Therefore, the concept must be reconsidered.

If fasting hyperglycaemia is not alone caused by an increase in HGP overnight, what could then add to fasting hyperglycaemia? Naturally, the reduced insulin-mediated glucose disposal (R_d) may play a role, but it is well known that glucose uptake in skeletal muscle during the fasting state is trivial, and therefore defects here may only play a minor role. Another possibility is that a spillover is created from the daytime when postprandial blood glucose values are severely increased. Reduced glucose disposal after the meal may result in glucose accumulation in blood, which is not metabolised before bedtime, and this may add to fasting hyperglycaemia through overnight hyperglycaemia. This hypothesis is supported by the finding that reduction of postprandial glycaemia by diet (low carbohydrate) alone also results in reduction of fasting blood glucose. As a consequence, treatment of fasting hyperglycaemia may not primarily aim to reduce HGP overnight, but rather aim to improve the insulin-mediated glucose disposal postprandially.

Postprandial hyperglycaemia can be addressed using pharmacological treatment, and also by changing the diet, since the major part of glucose appearance in the body during a 24-h period is due to intake of carbohydrates. T2D subjects overeat and this can therefore explain postprandial hyperglycaemia as the values decline immediately after reducing the carbohydrate intake [10]. Several studies have shown a dramatic effect when reducing energy intake for a few days only [10]. Therefore, diet treatment must be part of the hyperglycaemic treatment in T2D subjects. However, despite the significant effect obtained immediately, hypocalory diet treatment is disappointing in the long term as indicated by the UKPDS study, probably due to a decline in compliance [6]. Pharmaceutical compounds are therefore needed in most diabetic subjects in order to normalise postprandial blood glucose values. The only drug known to improve hepatic insulin sensitivity is Metformin, but reconstruction of the first-phase insulin response is another and more promising possibility for reduction of postprandial hypoglycaemia.

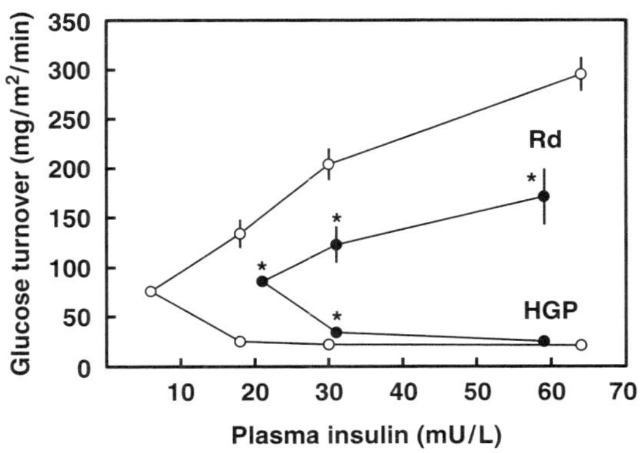

FIG. 2. Dose–response effects of insulin on glucose disposal (Rd) and HGP in T2D patients with fasting hyperinsulinaemia (closed symbols) and in age- and weight-matched control subjects (open symbols). $^*p < 0.05$ [9].

Is the Glucose Disappearance Rate Reduced in T2D?

Glucose disappears into skeletal muscle, fat tissue and liver, mediated by insulin, and into the central nervous system, blood cells and several other tissues mediated by the mass action of glucose itself. The insulin-mediated glucose uptake in skeletal muscle is significantly reduced in T2D subjects due to a reduced glycogen synthesis and glucose oxidation (Fig. 2) [11]. Since most glucose after a meal is taken up in skeletal muscle, the defect in insulin action adds to the degree of postprandial hyperglycaemia. Thus, insulin resistance plays an important role in postprandial blood glucose values [12]. Improvement of insulin action in T2D subjects must therefore be a primary aim for the normalisation of blood glucose values, mainly in the postprandial state. Normalisation of insulin sensitivity in peripheral tissues in T2D has, however, never been the main objective, as we possessed no tools carrying the potential for reaching this objective. However, the recently discovered PPAR (peroxisome proliferator-activated receptor) gamma agonists, namely glitazones, carry this potential.

Lack of First-Phase Insulin Response in T2D Subjects

Besides the reduced insulin-mediated glucose uptake in skeletal muscle (and in liver and fat tissue), the abnormal insulin secretion pattern characterised by a lack of first-phase insulin release may also play a pathophysiological role, since the postprandial insulin peaks disappear in T2D subjects (Fig. 3). A recent publication has shown that the reduction of the first-phase insulin response to meals is already present at normal fasting glucose values in T2D subjects [13]. This indicates a need for an earlier insulin treatment than what has been the routine for several years. Furthermore, these findings indicate that it is unphysiological to treat

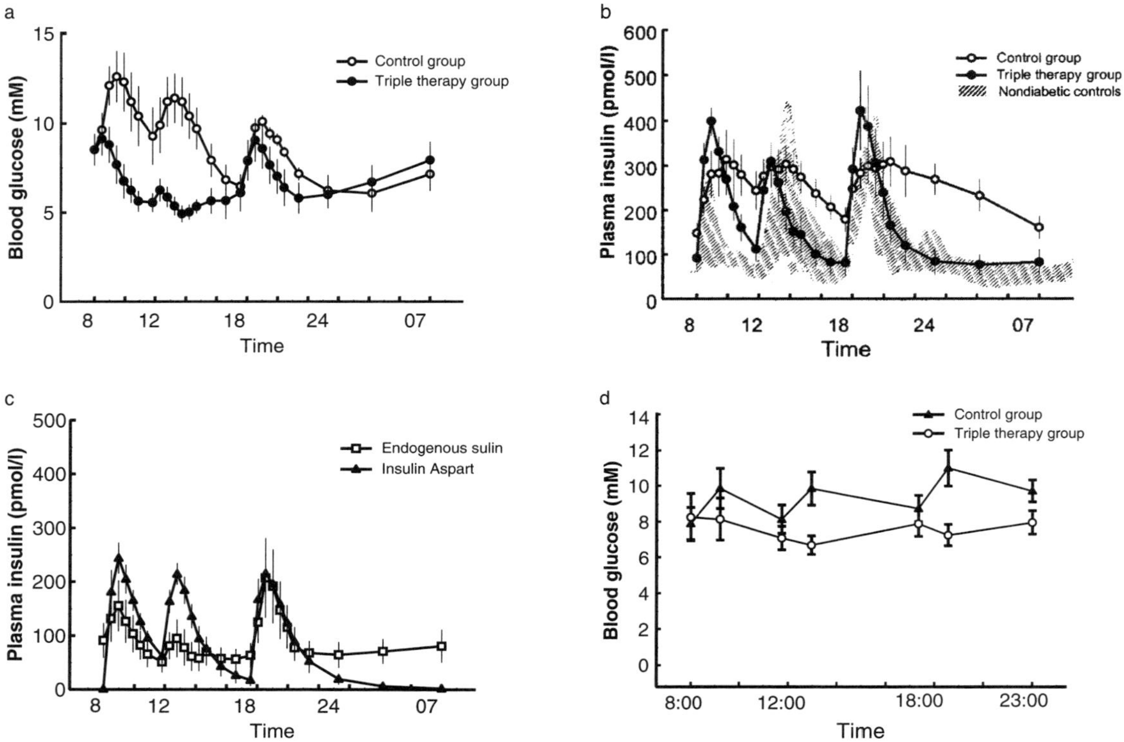

FIG. 3. Twenty-four-hour blood glucose (a) and insulin (b) values together with insulin aspart values (c) after 6 months of treatment with either NPH insulin (control group) or triple therapy. (d) The scattered area represents the 24-h insulin profile in healthy non-diabetic subjects in hospital. Eight-point home-measured blood glucose profiles in all subjects studied (mean values) [17].

T2D subjects with NPH (Neutral Protamine Hagedorn) insulin once or twice daily, as it only increases the 24-h plasma insulin values without reconstructing the physiological insulin profile. However, the insulin response to meals can be reconstructed using rapid-acting insulin analogues. Therefore, based on this pathophysiological consideration, it is difficult to find the arguments for the present routine with NPH insulin or long-acting insulin analogues once or twice daily, without treating postprandial hyperglycaemia.

Conclusion on Pathophysiological Considerations

Obese T2D subjects suffer from insulin resistance in both liver, skeletal muscle and adipocytes. Furthermore, the secretory capacity of insulin in beta cells is reduced compared with the degree of insulin resistance. Due to hyperglycaemia itself, the 24-h insulin profile is elevated compared with controls without diabetes, but the secretion pattern is characterised by reduced, delayed and often absent insulin peaks in the postprandial state compared with normal controls (Fig. 3). The reason for the increase in fasting glucose values has been discussed above, and it was concluded that postprandial glucose excursions also play a role in the post-absorptive values. Thus, it seems very important to treat postprandial hyperglycaemia, and if this is done properly, T2D subjects may go to bed with normal blood glucose values. However, if insulin values during the night are too low or the degree of insulin resistance remains present, HGP will increase and a reduction in HGP may be necessary.

Based on our theories of the pathophysiology of T2D, the obvious question is therefore whether a correction of these three major pathophysiological defects – insulin resistance in the liver, reduced insulin-mediated glucose uptake, specifically in skeletal muscle, and reduced first-phase insulin secretion – will result in normo-glycaemia. Until now, no treatment modalities have been able to normalise these three defects at the same time. However, the recent development in pharmacological treatment has made it possible.

Triple Therapy

Our triple-therapy model combines three antidiabetic drugs in addition to lifestyle changes aiming to treat the three major defects in the pathophysiology of T2D, as mentioned above. To correct these three defects, we chose a rapid-acting insulin analogue, insulin aspart, since it has been shown to be able to reconstruct the insulin peaks after meals [14]; a glitazone, in this case rosiglitazone, since these drugs are the most potent insulin synthesizers on the market improving R_d by 50–75% and furthermore reducing lipid accumulation in skeletal muscle and liver [15]; and finally Metformin, thanks to its effect on gluconeogenesis in the liver resulting in improved insulin sensitivity [16]. Metformin furthermore reduces appetite and thereby theoretically may reduce the glucose intake, and it is also the only drug shown to be able to reduce mortality in T2D subjects [6]. These pharmaceutical compounds are of course supplements to diet treatment, which must always be the basis.

To test this new antidiabetic combination therapy – named triple therapy – we used T2D subjects already treated with insulin after failed peroral treatment. These types of diabetic subjects suffer from severe metabolic disturbances and are the most difficult subjects to control. In this study, subjects were allocated to continue NPH treatment once or twice daily or shifted to triple therapy [17]. In both groups, our aim was to normalise HbA1c values and blood glucose values without inducing severe hypoglycaemia. The subjects measured blood glucose pre- and postprandially daily and at night. Based on these values, subjects were instructed in adjusting the insulin dose in accordance with an algorithm depending on the use of insulin aspart or NPH insulin. In the triple-therapy group, only insulin aspart was given at meals and no insulin was given at night (in accordance with the hypothesis discussed above). Metformin and rosiglitazone were increased up to full dose, meaning Metformin 1 g twice daily and rosiglitazone 8 mg daily during the first 2 months.

After half a year of triple therapy, Hb1Ac was reduced by 2% from 8.8 to 6.8 in the triple-therapy group, whereas it remained unchanged in the NPH group despite an increase in insulin dose of 50% [17]. The diurnal profile of blood glucose measured at the hospital and at home (Fig. 3) clearly indicated that triple therapy resulted in normalisation of blood glucose values during most of the 24-h period (Fig. 3). At home, no postprandial increase in blood glucose was seen, whereas an increase was seen after supper during hospitalisation only. Fasting blood glucose values were identical in the two groups after 6 months of treatment and blood glucose values increased slightly during the night in both groups. No nocturnal hypoglycaemia was seen at all in the triple-therapy group in spite of the near-normalisation of Hb1Ac values. However, during the day, more mild (but no severe) hypoglycaemic attacks were seen in a few subjects. Thus, triple therapy, which affects the three major pathophysiological defects in T2D, was able to eliminate postprandial hyperglycaemia and keep nightly blood glucose values stable without inducing severe hypoglycaemia. This clearly supports our hypothesis indicating that the three defects described are essential to the development of hyperglycaemia and that focusing on postprandial hyperglycaemia using a specific treatment is important. It furthermore seems to be less important trying to treat basal HGP values during the night by night time basal insulin if postprandial elevation is eliminated.

How Does Triple Therapy Improve Glucose Metabolism?

First of all, insulin aspart given at the initiation of the meal was in fact able to reconstruct the necessary fast and high insulin peaks compared with non-diabetic subjects (Fig. 3). This seems to be important since the insulin concentration obtained (24-h area under the curve) is much lower in triple therapy despite much lower blood glucose values. This indicates that the insulin profile is more important than the absolute amount of insulin given. We were able to measure insulin aspart with a specific antibody and thereby, for the first time in insulin-treated subjects, measure the amount of endogenous insulin produced together with exogenous insulin. Endogenous insulin secretion is still seen to continue with relatively low peaks at meals and with an overnight concentration of about 50 pmol/L, which is interestingly close to the values seen in non-diabetic controls (Fig. 3). However, the exogenous insulin aspart gives rise to significant peaks after meals, with a steep rise just after injection and an appropriately declining rate following the peak. Interestingly, all exogenous insulin was metabolised around midnight and therefore the T2D subjects rely on endogenous insulin only during the night. To our knowledge this is very important since it protects against nightly hypoglycaemia, as a fall in blood glucose during the night will immediately result in reduced insulin secretion. This can explain why no hypoglycaemic attacks were seen in the triple-therapy group during the night, and this is one of the greatest fortunes when using this new approach.

Blood glucose values increased during the night in the triple-therapy group despite "normal" serum-insulin values. The reason for this must of course be that both the liver and peripheral tissue are insulin resistant. However, during home blood glucose measurements, the mean value reached in the morning was between 7 and 8 mmol/L (based on measurements every morning during 6 months), which is an acceptable value.

As seen in Fig. 3, blood glucose values during triple therapy were not completely normalised during the 24-h period. This may be explained by insulin resistance, since our euglycaemic hyperinsulinaemic clamp studies showed an improvement only in peripheral insulin sensitivity of about 60%. Therefore, to completely normalise blood glucose values, a more potent insulin synthesizer than rosiglitazone is needed.

Drawbacks of the Proposed Triple-Therapy Regime

First of all, triple therapy is an expensive treatment, but several studies of intensive therapy in T2D, including UKDPS, have shown it to be cost-effective because of the heavy expenses related to the treatment of diabetic complications [18]. Secondly, subjects may gain weight. During this half-a-year study, it was, however, only about 2 kg and this may be explained by the 2% reduction in HbA1c.

Comparative Studies to Triple Therapy

The combination of three oral antidiabetics can be compared with our approach, but the small number of trials published has not been able to bring HbA1c levels below 7.8% [19]. In three other published studies, Metformin and a sulfonylurea (SU) preparation have been combined with NPH insulin with only a modest effect on HbA1c values (probably due to a modest improvement of peripheral insulin resistance).

In a recent study (more alike ours), in which Metformin, troglitazone and NPH insulin were given in combination, a near-normalisation of HbA1c was described, too. These two triple-therapy models including glitazones (reducing peripheral insulin resistance) are both very effective, probably due to treatment of peripheral insulin resistance [20].

Both insulin aspart and insulin lispro have been tested as a part of the classical basal bolus insulin regime in type 1 diabetes and were tested in T2D as a part of that regime. However, for several reasons none of these studies turned out to be successful when compared with the combination of NPH insulin and SU or with treatment with regular insulin three times a day and NPH at night [19]. An obvious conclusion is that the insulin sensitivity must be improved in accordance with the application of the analogues in order to obtain the full effect of these short-acting analogues. However, it is difficult to compare insulin regimes if they are not administered in the same trials and in comparable groups of diabetic subjects, since T2D is very heterogeneous.

What Have We Learned from these Studies?

We conclude that treatment of the three major pathophysiological defects in T2D using drugs affecting specifically theses abnormalities results in proper insulin peaks at meals and improved insulin sensitivity in both the periphery and in the liver. These interventions induced near-normalisation of the 24-h glucose profile and HbA1c values. Therefore, a normalisation of the physiological glucose homeostatis must be the goal for the treatment of T2D. This does not always imply initiation of triple therapy since dual therapy may also be effective in many subjects, whereas monotherapy only works in fewer subjects and for a shorter period.

Which Drugs Should be Considered for Combination in T2D?

Most T2D patients without contraindications for Metformin should start with that drug – but not until lifestyle intervention has failed [21]. In most patients, monotherapy by Metformin is not sufficient in time due to a decline in beta-cell function and/or weight gain or non-adherence to the lifestyle guidelines. Therefore, a secondary drug must be added. Here, we have three choices: SU (gliclazide, glimepiride, glipizide), glitazones (pioglitazone and rosiglitazone) and insulin. Despite these choices, dual therapy may also fail in time and a third drug must be added in order to reach the goal for HbA1c, namely ≤7.0% (in Europe ≤6.5%). Thus, a combination of 2–3 antidiabetic drugs, including insulin when necessary, has now become more usual. In this review, acarbose, which may have a minimal effect as well as severe side-effects, will not be discussed. Furthermore, the new GLP-1 analogues and the DPPIV inhibitors are too new to be put into perspective in this review.

Advantages and Disadvantages of the Antidiabetic Drugs Metformin, Su, Glitazones and Insulin and a Combination of those

Metformin

The unique advantage of Metformin is that it has been shown to reduce the risk of myocardial infarction and the mortality rate in T2D subjects (UKPDS) [21]. Therefore, it is today the first drug of choice. It may induce lactacidosis in very few subjects and therefore it should not be used in subjects with increased serum creatinine. In that case, SU or a glitazone will be the first drug of choice. In about 5% of subjects, Metformin may induce severe gastrointestinal discomfort. An advantage is that the drug does not induce weight gain and hypoglycaemia. In lean subjects, Metformin is not the first choice.

SU

SU is the most used antidiabetic drug in T2D today, as mentioned above. The difference in potency of the preparations mentioned above is minimal and no major differences in side-effects are seen either. The tendency is to use either glimepiride, since it may not impair cardiac function after a myocardial infarction, or gliclazides, which may have a beneficial effect on endothelial function. The drawback of SU preparations is that they can result in prolonged hypoglycaemic events [22].

Glitazones

Two drugs exist on the market, as mentioned above. They are identical in potency on glucose metabolism. They reduce blood pressure and improve lipid profile [23]. Pioglitazone may have an advantage compared with rosiglitazone when triglycerides are taken into account. They are not recommended as the first drug of choice, but they can be used in specifically obese subjects, where Metformin is contraindicated or not tolerated. The side-effects are weight gain and oedema (fluid retention) [23]. The weight gain is a few kilograms more than the weight gain seen in patients treated with SU or insulin. However, glitazones may change the body composition in a more beneficial way. More important is that glitazones reduce fat in the liver, which turns out to be of clinical importance. Fluid retention is seen in about 5% of T2D subjects and, in patients with reduced ejection fraction, this may result in heart failure. T2D subjects should therefore not be prescribed glitazones if they suffer from congestive heart failure. A combination with insulin may further increase this risk.

Insulin

In combination with oral antidiabetic drugs both NPH insulin and short-acting insulin can be used. The most successful combination until now has been Metformin and NPH insulin given at night, where the insulin doses have been titrated up based on measurements of fasting blood glucose values. This combination is powerful and fairly weight neutral, meaning a slight increase in body weight in most subjects. It is safe to use and can be handled by the patients themselves based on an algorithm [24].

Only a few studies on the combination of Metformin with long-acting insulin analogues, such as glargine and determir, have been published. In a treat-to-target study, NPH insulin was compared with glargine and no difference was shown in antidiabetic potential, but glargine may induce fewer hypoglycaemic attacks during the night [25]. However, more studies are needed, especially investigating the combination of determir and Metformin.

Based on a Cochrane analysis, insulin in combination with SU has no beneficial effect compared with insulin alone. Moreover, this combination will increase the body weight [26].

Trials investigating the combination of Metformin with rapid-acting insulin or insulin analogues, such as lispro and insulin aspart, are few, but indicate that the effect on HbA1c is identical to what is seen when combining Metformin with long-acting insulin, but postprandial blood glucose values are of course lower. This combination has been discussed previously under the heading "Triple therapy" [17].

From a theoretical point of view the choice between long-acting or intermediate-acting insulin and rapid-acting insulin and insulin analogues may of course also depend on the patient's phenotype and preference.

A combination of more than three antidiabetic drugs seems hazardous and has not been justified by the literature so far.

What Shall We Aim for?

It is obvious that the aim must be to use as few drugs as possible – this is an old lesson. On the other hand, we should aim for near-normalisation of blood glucose values, since a normalisation of HbA1c seems to reduce the risk of diabetic complications tremendously (Fig. 1). In that respect, the economy may be taken into account, since combination therapy may be expensive. It is, however, much more expensive to treat diabetic complications.

Therefore, it seems obvious to attack the three major pathophysiological defects in T2D, peripheral insulin resistance, increased HGP in the liver and the loss of first-phase insulin response related to a meal, using lifestyle changes and at least three pharmaceutical drugs. This suggestion is based on a few short-time studies, but longer studies are on their way.

Algorithm for Combination Treatment of T2D Subjects

The algorithm proposed by us is based on the statement paper by the American Diabetes Association (ADA) and the European Association for the Study of Diabetes (EASD) [27] and our own experience based on current pathophysiological knowledge. The algorithm will be changed in time in accordance with the new literature, but until then the following proposal will be useful. This algorithm takes into account the specific characteristics of the drugs used, their synergies, expenses and side-effects. The goal is – based on the recent literature – to maintain HbA1c values as close as possible to the non-diabetic range and to change medication as rapidly as necessary based on the effect obtained and the side-effects. The algorithm is based on the most used and best documented drugs in the field: Metformin, SU (glimiperide, gliclazide or glipizide), glitazones (pioglitazone or rosiglitazone) and insulin (mainly NPH insulin, but analogues when indicated – see above).

Algorithm

Lifestyle intervention is the basis for all treatment of T2D [27]. The improvements of glucose metabolism obtained initially, specifically on body weight, may influence the results of the drug added later on (Fig. 4). Specifically, a change of diet is important as it has an immediate effect. The amount of calories should be reduced by reducing intake of not only fat, but also rapidly absorbed carbohydrates. The patient should remain on non-pharmacological treatment for a couple of months before starting drug treatment in order to obtain the full beneficial effect of lifestyle changes. The time spent on lifestyle changes alone of course depends on the achieved blood glucose values and the clinical situation.

The first drug of choice is Metformin, which should be titrated up to the highest dose tolerated. To start with a low dose is recommendable to avoid side-effects. However, most patients suffer some gastrointestinal side-effects, but these side-effects disappear in most subjects in time. If the goal for HbA1c – either the international goal or the individually decided goal – is not reached within 2–3 months, another group of drugs may be added. As mentioned in Fig. 4,

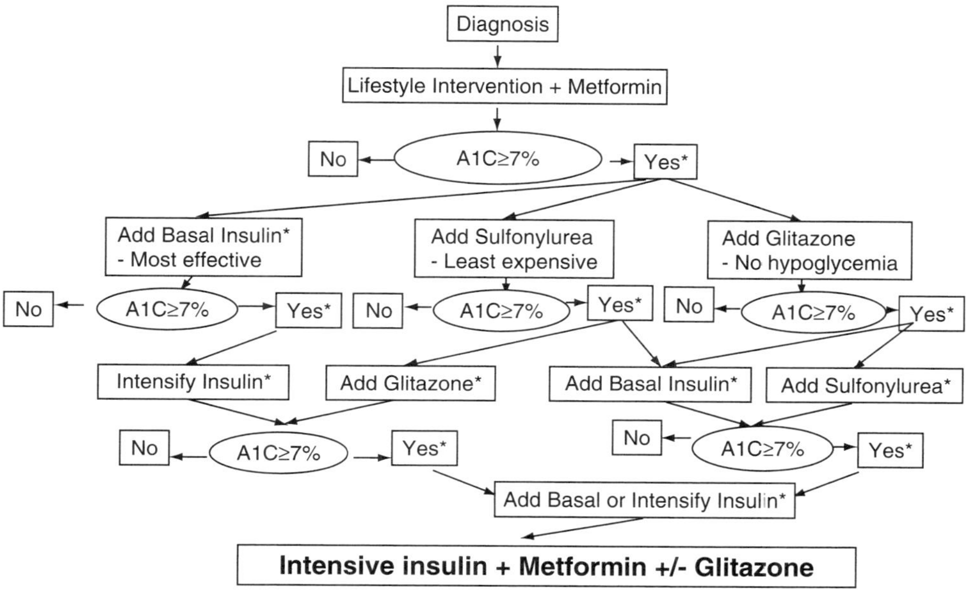

FIG. 4. Algorithm for the metabolic management of type 2 diabetes [27].

three possibilities exist: insulin, SU or glitazones. The choice depends on several factors: the level of HbA1c, body weight, age and phenotype. Furthermore, some drugs may be contraindicated. The patient's preference must also be taken into account, as the patient's compliance has immediate impact on the results obtained. Since T2D subjects need many drugs for treatment, individual education and motivation are important.

Insulin

Insulin treatment may be initiated earlier in young subjects, in lean subjects and in subjects with high HbA1c levels (>8.5%). Today, in addition to Metformin, intermediate-acting insulin once daily – often given at night – will be the regime to choose [24]. This regime is easy to handle, as the patients themselves can titrate the dose of insulin based on the fasting blood glucose values. The goal is a fasting blood glucose of <6 mmol/L. The patients may start with NPH insulin at night and titrate according to the individually given algorithm. The long-acting insulin analogues may be used instead of NPH insulin, since they have demonstrated the same potency as NPH [25], but with fewer hypoglycaemic attacks. However, more studies are needed before recommending the new insulins in general, but in subjects showing a tendency of hypoglycaemia or poor control, glargine or determir must be considered.

A few studies used rapid-acting insulin or rapid-acting insulin analogues at meal time instead of intermediate- or long-acting insulin at night, since it is important to treat postprandial blood glucose values as stated above (triple therapy). Only a few studies have been published until now investigating the combination of these fast-acting insulins with Metformin. The concept of treating postprandial blood glucose alone seems as effective as treating with long-acting or intermediate-acting insulin at night. The advantage is that the postprandial values will be lower. However, fasting blood glucose values may be higher, and therefore more long-term studies are needed before this change of concept can be recommended. The only obvious situation is lean, young T2D subjects with reduced beta-cell function indicated by C-peptide values fasting lower than 300 pmol/L. In this case the classical basal bolus regimes should be considered.

SU

SU is another possibility as add-on medication to Metformin in cases where the metabolic goal is not obtained. These drugs may be considered in young and lean subjects and in T2D subjects with a HbA1c value lower than 8.5% after 2–3 months of monotherapy with Metformin. These drugs can induce severe hypoglycaemia and are therefore relatively contraindicated in subjects prone to hypoglycaemia, that is, elderly subjects and subjects suffering from liver diseases [22]. It has been claimed that SU should not be given to T2D subjects with coronary arteriosclerosis, but data supporting this are not very solid. The three different SUs mentioned above have the same potency and, for the moment, no scientific evidence exists to choose one for the other, but the patient's individual phenotype must naturally be taken into account.

Glitazones

Glitazones are the newest antidiabetic drugs on the market, and we therefore have less experience with these drugs. Both pioglitazone and rosiglitazone can reduce HbA1c levels by 1–2% in combination with Metformin. They seem to work best in obese subjects with preserved beta-cell function indicated by a C-peptide level higher than 300 pmol/L in the fasting state. They should not be used in subjects showing signs of reduced cardiac function due to fluid retention and oedema, as stated above. A combination of Metformin and glitazones seems to be equal to the combination of Metformin and SU in their blood glucose reducing effect. Glitazones should be considered as add-on medications in subjects not tolerating SU, specifically obese subjects, and in subjects where Metformin is contraindicated or not tolerated, glitazones could be the first drug of choice.

Triple Therapy

In some diabetic subjects, the goal is not reached by dual therapy, and add-on of the third antidiabetic drug must be considered. The combination of insulin and glitazones has been shown to be powerful and must be considered if the goals are not reached, as stated above. Now, this combination has also been approved in Europe. Another possibility is to combine the three oral antidiabetic drugs: SU, Metformin and glitazones [28].

The algorithm given in Fig. 4 based on the ADA and the EASD criteria can be recommended as the basis for the individual treatment.

Conclusion

It is obvious both from the literature and the daily clinical experience that most T2D subjects need combination therapy consisting of two or three antidiabetic drugs. The long-term effect on complications (hard end-points) and the potential side-effects (of combinations) have still not been demonstrated in the literature, but from the UKPDS study we learned the importance of normalisation of blood glucose values.

References

1. Stovring H, Andersen M, Beck-Nielsen H, et al. Rising prevalence of diabetes: evidence from a Danish pharmaco-epidemiological database. Lancet 2003;362(9383):537–538.
2. Stratton IM, Adler AI, Neil HA, et al. Association of glycaemia with macrovascular and microvascular complications of type 2 diabetes (UKPDS 35): prospective observational study. BMJ 2000;321(7258):405–412.
3. Liebl A, Mata M, Eschwege E. Evaluation of risk factors for development of complications in Type II diabetes in Europe. Diabetologia 2002; 45(7):S23–S28.
4. Beck-Nielsen H, Groop LC. Metabolic and genetic characterization of prediabetic states. Sequence of events leading to non-insulin-dependent diabetes mellitus. J Clin Invest 1994;94(5):1714–1721.
5. Turner RC, Holman RR, Cull CA, et al. Intensive blood-glucose control with sulphonylureas or insulin compared with conventional treatment and risk of complications in patients with type 2 diabetes (UKPDS 33). Lancet 1998;352(9131):837–853.
6. Turner RC, Cull CA, Frighi V, et al. Glycemic control with diet, sulfonylurea, metformin, or insulin in patients with type 2 diabetes mellitus: progressive requirement for multiple therapies (UKPDS 49). UK Prospective Diabetes Study (UKPDS) Group. JAMA 1999;281(21):2005–2012.
7. Hother-Nielsen O, Beck-Nielsen H. On the determination of basal glucose production rate in patients with type 2 (non-insulin-dependent) diabetes mellitus using primed-continuous 3-3H-glucose infusion. Diabetologia 1990;33(10):603–610.
8. Beck-Nielsen H, Hother-Nielsen O, Staehr P. Is hepatic glucose production increased in type 2 diabetes mellitus? Curr Diab Rep 2002; 2(3):231–236.
9. Staehr P, Hother-Nielsen O, Beck-Nielsen H. The role of the liver in type 2 diabetes. Rev Endocr Metab Disord 2004;5(2):105–110.

10. Beck-Nielsen H, Pedersen O, Sorensen NS. Effects of diet on the cellular insulin binding and the insulin sensitivity in young healthy subjects. Diabetologia 1978;15(4):289–296.
11. Damsbo P, Vaag A, Hother-Nielsen O, et al. Reduced glycogen synthase activity in skeletal muscle from obese patients with and without type 2 (non-insulin-dependent) diabetes mellitus. Diabetologia 1991; 34(4):239–245.
12. DeFronzo RA. Pathogenesis of type 2 (non-insulin-dependent) diabetes mellitus: a balanced overview. Diabetologia 1992;35(4):389–397.
13. Ferrannini E, Gastaldelli A, Miyazaki Y, et al. Predominant role of reduced beta-cell sensitivity to glucose over insulin resistance in impaired glucose tolerance. Diabetologia 2003;46(9):1211–1219.
14. Raskin P, Guthrie RA, Leiter L, et al. Use of insulin aspart, a fast-acting insulin analog, as the mealtime insulin in the management of patients with type 1 diabetes. Diabetes Care 2000;23(5):583–588.
15. Carey DG, Cowin GJ, Galloway GJ, et al. Effect of rosiglitazone on insulin sensitivity and body composition in type 2 diabetic patients [corrected]. Obes Res 2002;10(10):1008–1015.
16. DeFronzo RA, Goodman AM. Efficacy of metformin in patients with non-insulin-dependent diabetes mellitus. The Multicenter Metformin Study Group. N Engl J Med 1995;333(9):541–549.
17. Poulsen MK, Henriksen JE, Hother-Nielsen O, et al. The combined effect of triple therapy with rosiglitazone, metformin, and insulin aspart in type 2 diabetic patients. Diabetes Care 2003; 26(12):3273–3279.
18. Gray A, Raikou M, McGuire A, et al. Cost effectiveness of an intensive blood glucose control policy in patients with type 2 diabetes: economic analysis alongside randomised controlled trial (UKPDS 41). United Kingdom Prospective Diabetes Study Group. BMJ 2000;320(7246):1373–1378.
19. Yki-Jarvinen H, Kauppila M, Kujansuu E, et al. Comparison of insulin regimens in patients with non-insulin-dependent diabetes mellitus. N Engl J Med 1992;327(20):1426–1433.
20. Strowig SM, Aviles-Santa ML, Raskin P. Improved glycemic weight control without gain using triple therapy in type 2 diabetes. Diabetes Care 2004; 27(7):1577–1583.
21. Turner RC, Holman RR, Stratton IM, et al. Effect of intensive blood glucose control with metformin on complications in overweight patients with type 2 diabetes (UKPDS 34). The UK Prospective Diabetes Study Group. Lancet 1998;352(9139):854.
22. Holstein A, Plaschke A, Egberts EH. Lower incidence of severe hypoglycaemia in patients with type 2 diabetes treated with glimepiride versus glibenclamide. Diabetes Metab Res Rev 2001;17(6):467–473.
23. Yki-Jarvinen H. Drug therapy: Thiazolidinediones. N Engl J Med 2004;351(11):1106–1118.
24. Yki-Jarvinen H, Dressler A, Ziemen M. Less nocturnal hypoglycemia and better post-dinner glucose control with bedtime insulin glargine compared with bedtime NPH insulin during insulin combination therapy in type 2 diabetes. HOE 901/3002 Study Group. Diabetes Care 2000;23(8):1130–1136.
25. Riddle MC, Rosenstock J, Gerich J. The treat-to-target trial: randomized addition of glargine or human NPH insulin to oral therapy of type 2 diabetic patients. Diabetes Care 2003;26(11):3080–3086.
26. Goudswaard AN, Furlong NJ, Rutten GE, et al. Insulin monotherapy versus combinations of insulin with oral hypoglycaemic agents in patients with type 2 diabetes mellitus. Cochrane Database Syst Rev 2004;(4):CD003418.
27. Nathan DM, Buse JB, Davidson MB, et al. Management of hyperglycemia in type 2 diabetes: A consensus algorithm for the initiation and adjustment of therapy: a consensus statement from the American Diabetes Association and the European Association for the Study of Diabetes. Diabetes Care 2006; 29(8):1963–1972.
28. Roberts VL, Stewart J, Issa M, et al. Triple therapy with glimepiride in patients with type 2 diabetes mellitus inadequately controlled by metformin and a thiazolidinedione: results of a 30-week, randomized, double-blind, placebo-controlled, parallel-group study. Clin Ther 2005;27(10):1535–1547.

12
The Incretin Modulators – Incretin Mimetics (GLP-1 Receptor Agonists) and Incretin Enhancers (DPP-4 Inhibitors)

Michael A. Nauck, Wolfgang E. Schmidt, and Juris J. Meier

Keywords: Incretin, glucagon-like peptide-1 (GLP-1), gastric inhibitory polypeptide (GIP), entero-insular axis, exenatide, liraglutide, vildagliptin, sitagliptin, saxagliptin, DPP-4.

Introduction

The stimulation of insulin secretion has been a therapeutic principle since the introduction of sulfonylureas in the 1950s, when tolbutamide and carbutamide were introduced. Second- and third-generation sulfonylureas like glibenclamide and glimeperide remain to be among the most commonly used antidiabetic agents, attesting to the fact that promoting β-cell secretory function is a feasible way of controlling plasma glucose in patients with type 2 diabetes. Nevertheless, sulfonylureas are far from ideal as antidiabetic agents, since their use is associated with weight gain and with the provocation of hypoglycemia [1]. The latter is caused by the absence of a strict glucose dependency of the ability to promote insulin secretion, since sulfonylureas per se are able to close the ATP-dependent K^+ channel, even at rather low glucose concentrations [2].

The incretin concept was developed when it had become obvious that the oral ingestion of nutrients, especially carbohydrates (glucose, starch, etc.) releases insulinotropic hormones from the gut mucosa, which in turn augment the insulin secretory response induced by meal-related glycemic excursions [3,4]. When the first incretin hormone to be described in detail, Glucose-dependent *I*nsulinotropic *P*olypeptide (*G*astric *I*nhibitory *P*olypeptide, GIP) was characterized [5–7], one of the remarkable properties was the strict glucose dependency of its insulinotropic actions, both in perfused rat pancreas [8] and in human subjects in vivo [9]. Werner Creutzfeldt, in his 1978 Claude–Bernard lecture to the European Association for the Study of Diabetes [3], made this characteristic of GIP a core component of the definition of incretin hormones in general. Obviously, with a peptide like GIP, it was impossible to provoke hypoglycemic episodes, even when it was administered at high doses. A natural compound that potently stimulates insulin secretion, however, without a risk of provoking hypoglycemia, attracted attention as a potential candidate parent compound for the development of antidiabetic drugs. Because GIP has lost most of its insulinotropic activity in patients with type 2 diabetes [10–13], it was not until the identification of glucagon-like peptide-1 (GLP-1) [14–18] and the demonstration that GLP-1 had preserved insulinotropic (and additional) activities in patients with type 2 diabetes [11,19,20] that the idea of using incretin hormones as the basis for novel antidiabetic drugs could be actively persued.

Definition of the Problem and Basic Pathophysiology

Secretion and Action of Incretin Hormones in Physiology

Physiological Roles of Gastrointestinal Peptide Hormones

The ingestion of nutrients elicits the secretion of gastrointestinal hormones intimately involved in the regulation of gut and gallbladder motility, digestive juice secretion, and postprandial carbohydrate metabolism. In particular, incretin hormones stimulate insulin secretion from the endocrine pancreas. Through the action of incretin hormones, enteral nutrition provides a more potent insulinotropic stimulus relative to an isoglycemic intravenous challenge. This phenomenon is named the "incretin effect" [3,21–23].

GIP

The first incretin to be identified, GIP, was purified from porcine intestine extracts by virtue of its ability to inhibit gastric acid secretion (therefore, the original name was *gastric inhibitory polypeptide*) [7,24]. Soon, it was discovered that GIP displayed potent insulinotropic actions in animals [8,25] and in human subjects [9]. GIP was shown to be a 42 amino acid peptide hormone [7,24] synthesized in duodenal and jejunal enteroendocrine K cells [26] in the proximal small bowel (duodenum and jejunum) (Fig. 1).

GLP-1

Much later, the second incretin hormone, glucagon-like peptide-1 (GLP-1), was identified as a partial sequence of the cDNAs and genes encoding proglucagon [14,27]. After posttranslational processing of proglucagon in gut endocrine L-cells [16,28–30], GLP-1 exists in two circulating equipotent molecular forms, GLP-1 ("glycine-extended GLP-1") and GLP-1 [7–36] amide ("amidated GLP-1") [31,32] (Fig. 1). The amidated form is more abundant in the circulation following meal ingestion in humans [32]. Although the majority of GLP-1 is synthesized in the distal ileum and colon, plasma levels of GLP-1, like GIP, increase shortly after starting meals. This leaves two possibilities: Either there is an upper gut signal mediating GLP-1 release from more distal stores [33] (i.e. the locations where GLP-1 is most abundant [28]). Alternatively, GLP-1 is predominantly released from the sparse L-cells that are present in the upper gut [28,34]. Quantitative considerations make it appear feasible that GLP-1 from gut segments coming into direct contact with chyme is the source of postprandial increments in GLP-1 concentrations [35].

Proteolytic Degradation of Incretin Hormones by Dipeptidyl Peptidase-4

Plasma levels of total GLP-1 (including proteolytic degradation products) are low ("basal") in the fasted state (approximately 5 pmol/L) and increase rapidly following meal ingestion, reaching levels in plasma

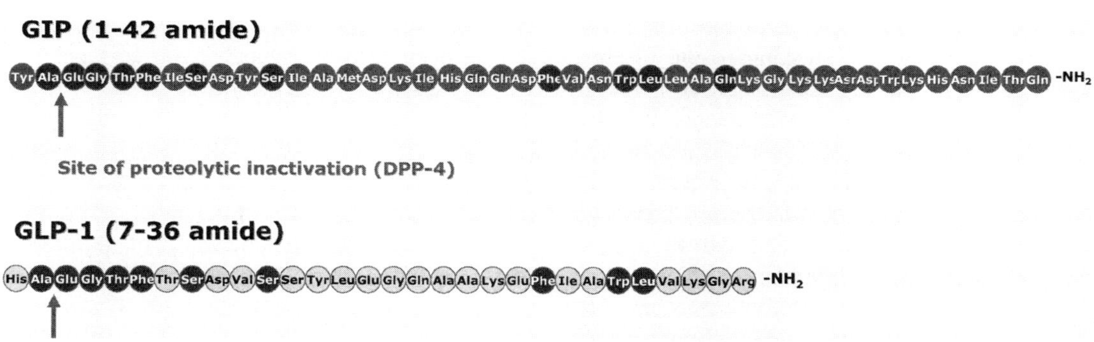

FIG. 1. Peptide structures of the two main incretin hormones, glucose-dependent insulinotropic polypeptide (gastric inhibitory polypeptide, GIP), and glucagon-like peptide 1 (GLP-1). Amino acids shared between both peptides are shown in dark blue, and amino acids unique to GIP and GLP-1 are shown in light and dark green, respectively. The red arrow indicates the position of cleavage by dipeptidyl peptidase-4 (DPP-4), the alanine residue in position 2, which is recognized by DPP-4, is highlighted by a red margin.

of 15–50 pmol/L [32]. Only a minor proportion of circulating GLP-1 (approximately 10–20%) is intact, biologically active GLP-1. This is true after endogenous secretion [36] as well as during exogenous administration, for example, during continuous intravenous infusion or after subcutaneous injection [37]. The major reason is the rapid proteolytic degradation and inactivation by dipeptidyl peptidase-4 (DPP-4) [38], an aminopeptidase recognizing peptides with a proline or alanine in the second aminoterminal position [39]. It removes the first two aminoterminal amino acids, rendering the breakdown products (GLP-1 [9–36] amide or GLP-1 [9–37]) biologically inactive or even weakly antagonistic [40–44]. The circulating levels of intact GLP-1 and GIP are further kept low by rapid renal clearance [45,46]. Whether additional proteases such as human neutral endopeptidase 24.11 are also essential determinants of GLP-1 inactivation remains under active investigation [47,48]. Mice with targeted inactivation of the DPP-4 gene exhibit increased levels of plasma GIP and GLP-1, increased insulin secretion, and reduced glucose excursion following a glucose challenge [49].

GIP and GLP-1 Receptors

GIP and GLP-1 exert their actions via engagement of structurally distinct G protein-coupled receptors. GIP receptors are predominantly expressed on islet β-cells, and to a lesser extent, in adipose tissue and in the central nervous system [50–53]. In contrast, GLP-1 receptors are expressed in pancreatic endocrine β-cells [54,55] and in several peripheral tissues including the central and peripheral nervous system, heart, kidney, lung, and the gastrointestinal tract [56,57]. Activation of both incretin receptors on β-cells leads to rapid increases in levels of cyclic AMP and intracellular calcium, followed by insulin exocytosis, in a glucose-dependent manner [58]. Incretin receptor signaling is associated with protein kinase A activation, induction of gene transcription, enhanced levels of (pro-)insulin biosynthesis [59], and the stimulation of β-cell proliferation [60,61]. GLP-1 and GIP receptor activation protect β-cells against toxin-induced apoptosis (elicited by glucotoxicity – hyperglycemia, lipotoxicity – high concentrations of free fatty acids, streptozotocin, or hydrogen peroxide) and enhanced β-cell survival, findings observed in studies of both rodent [62–64] and human islets [65].

Biological activity of GIP and GLP-1

The main functions of GIP are the glucose-dependent augmentation of insulin secretion during periods characterized by physiological hyperglycemia, the incretin function *sensu strictu* [8,9,18,66,67]. Animal experiments suggest that GIP receptors on adipose tissue are essential for adipocyte triglyceride storage after meal ingestion: GIP receptor knock-out mice do not become obese when fed a high-fat diet [53].

GLP-1 does not only display glucose-dependent insulinotropic ("incretin") activity [15,17,18,68], but also inhibits glucagon secretion [11,69], decelerates gastric emptying [70–73] and reduces food ingestion [74–78], and promotes enhanced glucose disposal via neural mechanisms involving receptors in the "hepatoportal" region [79]. All these actions, which are summarized in Fig. 2 and Table 1, potentially contribute to glucoregulation. It is of interest that GLP-1 effects on glucagon secretion, like those on insulin secretory responses, are glucose-dependent, whereas counter-regulatory release of glucagon in response to hypoglycemia remains undisturbed even in the presence of pharmacological concentrations of GLP-1 [68].

Effect of Incretin Receptor Knock-out in Mice

The physiological importance of endogenous GIP and GLP-1 for glucose homeostasis can be examined using specific receptor antagonists or knock-out mice. Acute antagonism of either GIP or GLP-1 action lowers insulin secretion and increases plasma glucose following oral glucose ingestion in rodents [80,81]. Similarly, mice with inactivating mutations in the GIP or GLP-1 receptors exhibit reduced glucose-stimulated insulin secretion and impaired glucose tolerance [66,82]. GLP-1, but probably not GIP, is essential also for the control of fasting glucose concentrations, as acute antagonism or genetic disruption of GLP-1 action leads to increased levels of fasting glucose in rodents [82].

Effects of GLP-1 Receptor Antagonists in Human Subjects

The GLP-1 receptor antagonist exendin [9–39] has been used to elucidate the role of endogenously secreted GLP-1 in human volunteers. Administration of exendin [9–39] leads to a

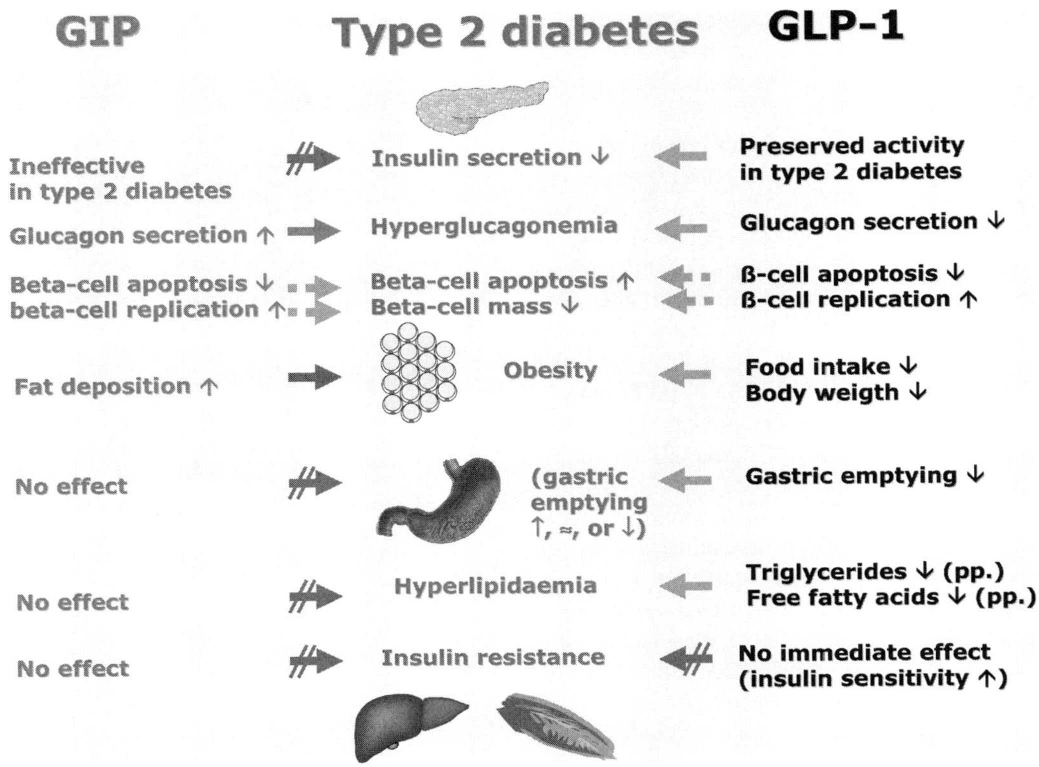

FIG. 2. Biological actions of GIP and GLP-1 on various target organs/cells in relation to pathophysiologically important facets of type 2 diabetes. See Table 1 for related literature.

reduction in glucose-stimulated insulin secretion, diminished glucose clearance, and increased glucagon secretion [83,84]. Indirect evidence suggests more rapid gastric emptying following disruption of GLP-1 action in humans as expected from the activity profile of GLP-1 (Fig. 2) [85].

Activity of the Entero-Insular Axis and Incretin Hormones in Type 2-Diabetic Patients

Reduced Incretin Effect in Patients with Type 2 Diabetes

In healthy human subjects oral glucose elicits a considerably higher insulin secretory response than does intravenous glucose (even if leading to the same glycemic increments). This incretin effect is substantially reduced or even completely lost in patients with type 2 diabetes [86]. The reduction in the incretin effect probably is an acquired defect, since it is also found in patients with diabetes secondary to chronic pancreatitis, whereas chronic pancreatitis without diabetes is characterized by a normal incretin effect [87].

Secretion of Incretin Hormones in Patients with Type 2 Diabetes

Cross-sectional analyses of larger cohorts suggest that there is a slight reduction in postprandial GLP-1 secretion following the ingestion of a mixed meal in patients with type 2 diabetes. Subjects with impaired glucose tolerance display intermediate results between healthy controls (normal response) and type 2-diabetic patients (reduced response) [88]. This is true for both total and intact GLP-1 [36]. However, the overall difference is small, and concerns the second and third hour after starting meal ingestion, whereas the characteristic differences in insulin secretory pattern are found in the early period after glucose or meal ingestion [89].

TABLE 1. Typical features of the type 2 diabetic phenotype and the complementary activity profile of GLP-1, incretin mimetics, and DPP-4 inhibitors. (Modified from Drucker and Nauck 2006 [145]).

			Incretin mimetics		DPP-4 inhibitors	
Characteristics of type 2 diabetes	Biological actions of incretin-related hormones/medications	Native GLP-1[a]	Exenatide	Liraglutide	Sitagliptin	Vildagliptin
Defective insulin secretion	Stimulation of insulin secretion (glucose-dependent)	Yes [11]	Yes [221]	Yes [222]	Yes	Yes [150]
Lack of early phase[b]	Restoration of early phase	Yes [223]	Yes [224]	Not tested	Not tested	Not tested
Delayed insulin secretion after meals [225]	More rapid insulin secretion after meals[c]	Yes [113, 226]	Yes [221]	Yes [222]	Yes	Yes [150]
Reduction in the incretin effect [86]	Replacement of incretin activity/enhanced incretin effect	Yes[c]	Yes[c]	Yes[c]	Not tested, but probable	Not tested, but probable
Hyperglucagonemia [227]	Suppression of glucagon	Yes [11]	Yes [221]	Yes [222]	Yes	Yes [150]
Hypoglycemia counter-regulation	Glucagon secretion, when plasma glucose is low	Yes [68]	Yes [228]	Yes [229]	Not tested	Not tested
Reduced β-cell insulin content	Stimulated synthesis of proinsulin	Yes [230]	Yes	Yes	Yes (?)	Yes (?)
Reduced β cell mass [193, 231]	Increase in β-cell mass[e]	Yes [232]	Yes [199]	Yes [205]	Yes [208]	Yes [216]
	Differentiation of islet precursor cells into β-cells[e]	Yes [214]	Yes	Yes	Unknown	Unknown
Enhanced β-cell apoptosis [193]	Inhibition of β-cell apoptosis[e]	Yes [63, 213]	Yes [233]	Yes [234]	Probable [207]	Probable
Normal, slowed, or accelerated [235] gastric emptying	Deceleration in gastric emptying	Yes [70]	Yes [175]	Yes [222]	Not tested	Marginal [165,182]
High energy intake/obesity [236]	Suppression of appetite/induction of satiety	Yes [74]	Probable	Yes [157]	No obvious effect	No obvious effect
	Weight loss	Yes [114]	Yes [119–121]	Yes [158]	No weight change	No weight change [153]

[a]GLP-1 may be in a "glycine-extended" form [7–37] or the predominant "amidated" form, [7–36] amide; both forms have similar biological activities.

[b]A separate early-phase insulin response is only seen under artificial conditions leading to a rapid rise in glucose concentrations (glucose bolus injection, "squarewave stimulus" when starting a hyperglycemic clamp).

[c]Shown by an improvement (normalization) of postprandial glucose excursions.

[d]By definition, GLP-1 and incretin mimetics replace incretin activity.

[e]These actions have only been reported from animal or in vitro (e.g., islet) studies. Methods to assess human β-cell mass in vivo are not available.

Therefore, it cannot be considered likely that the slight reduction in postprandial GLP-1 secretion in patients with type 2 diabetes has any immediate impact on glycemic control. Along the same lines, any administration of GLP-1 receptor agonists should not be simply considered a replacement of an essential hormone (e.g. GLP-1) that is lacking in patients with type 2 diabetes.

GIP secretion in patients with type 2 diabetes has been reported as exaggerated [90], normal (on average) [91], or reduced [88]. In all cases, the differences were small in comparison with appropriate control subjects and are not likely to indicate any importance for the pathophysiology of the entero-insular axis in type 2 diabetes. Certainly, there is no complete lack in GIP in patients with type 2 diabetes.

Insulinotropic Activity of GIP and GLP-1 in Patients with Type 2 Diabetes

While the interaction of both GIP and GLP-1 with their respective receptors on healthy pancreatic endocrine β-cells leads to cAMP production and the augmentation of glucose-stimulated insulin release in a very similar manner [92], the insulinotropic activity of GIP is almost completely lost in patients with type 2 diabetes [10–13,93]. This does not appear to indicate a lack of expression of GIP receptors on type 2-diabetic β-cells, since a bolus injection of GIP still elicits some insulin secretory response [13]. However, prolonged infusion, even of highly pharmacological doses of GIP, is unable to meaningfully stimulate insulin secretion. This certainly is the fundamental defect underlying the reduced incretin effect in patients with type 2 diabetes. The pathophysiology of the entero-insular axis in type 2 diabetes is outlined elsewhere in more detail [94,95].

On the other hand, a considerable proportion of the insulinotropic activity of GLP-1 as found in healthy subjects is preserved in patients with type 2 diabetes (Table 1). Physiological concentrations of GLP-1 (as found after meal ingestion), however, have little if any effect on insulin secretion in patients with type 2 diabetes [11].

Upon a closer look, the insulinotropic activity of GLP-1 is also somewhat reduced in patients with type 2 diabetes compared with healthy control subjects [96]. However, even a relatively low dose of GLP-1 can acutely restore the ability of β-cells to respond to increasing glucose concentrations with an insulin secretory response similar to healthy subjects. Nevertheless, the insulin response remains at approximately 20–25% relative to the effect in healthy subjects exposed to the same GLP-1 doses and concentrations [96]. This partial preservation of insulin secretory effects is sufficient to make GLP-1 a potent insulinotropic agent in patients with type 2 diabetes.

Pharmacological doses of GLP-1 display the full spectrum of activities also in patients with type 2 diabetes (Fig. 2, Table 1). This includes effects on insulin [11,97] and glucagon [11] secretion, gastric emptying [20,97], appetite, and meal size [76]. As a consequence, antidiabetic properties of pharmacological doses of GLP-1 have been examined in patients with type 2 diabetes.

Therapeutic Potential of Incretin Hormones

Owing to their pivotal role in the postprandial regulation of insulin secretion, both GIP and GLP-1 have been suggested as potential antidiabetic drug candidates [4,98]. However, no significant reduction in glycemia could be achieved in studies with intravenous infusions of the GIP in hyperglycemic patients with type 2 diabetes [99]. Indeed, while GIP exhibits potent insulinotropic properties in healthy subjects and probably mediates the major proportion of the incretin effect under physiological circumstances [9,10,18,100,101], its insulinotropic effect is markedly diminished in patients with type 2 diabetes [11–13]. It is a current matter of debate whether this loss of incretin activity in type 2 diabetes is due to a specific defect, for example, in GIP signaling on pancreatic β-cells, or whether it goes along with a general decline in β-cell mass and function in such patients [102,103]. In support of the latter hypothesis, the insuliotropic effect of GIP is not only reduced in patients with type 2 diabetes, but also in individuals with other forms of diabetes, such as MODY or type 1 diabetes [104]. A number of GIP analogues exhibiting prolonged biological half-lives due to the chemical modifications, mostly at the N-terminal end of the peptide chain, have been proposed as potential drug candidates for the pharmacotherapy of type 2 diabetes [105–107], but as yet none of these compounds has been tested in patients with diabetes. Given the obvious inefficacy of native GIP in such patients, it is questionable whether GIP analogues will indeed exhibit a significant antihyperglycemic potential. Furthermore, unlike GLP-1, GIP even stimulates glucagon secretion [108,109], thereby potentially counteracting its insulinotropic effect.

Antidiabetic Actions of GLP-1

Short-term intravenous infusions of GLP-1 (approximately 1.2 pmol/kg/min, leading to pharmacological plasma concentrations of total GLP-1 of approximately 100 pmol/L, and intact biologically active GLP-1 of approximately 15 pmol/L) lower blood glucose in human subjects with type 2 diabetes through a transient glucose-dependent stimulation of insulin and suppression of glucagon secretion and gastric emptying [110–113]. A 6-week subcutaneous infusion of GLP-1 in patients with type 2 diabetes achieving plasma levels of total GLP-1 of around 65 pmol/L [114] was followed by a substantial improvement in insulin secretory capacity, insulin sensitivity, a reduction in HbA_{1c} by 1.2%, and weight loss [114]. Although intravenous or subcutaneous GLP-1 infusions may be useful for the short-term control of hyperglycemia under a variety of clinical conditions [115,116], the long-term treatment of type 2 diabetes requires a more feasible approach for achieving sustained GLP-1 receptor activation. The proof-of-principle that GLP-1 can help lower, even normalize plasma glucose in a substantial number of patients with type 2 diabetes [112], has paved the way to explore the clinical efficacy of (i) peptides that act as GLP-1 receptor agonists, but have more suitable pharmacokinetic properties than are characteristic for the parent compound, GLP-1, and (ii) DPP-4 inhibitors (small molecules with substantial oral bioavailability) (Figs. 3 and 4, Table 2).

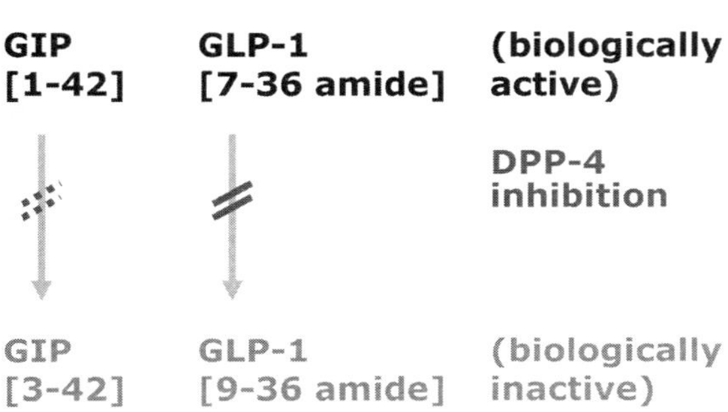

FIG. 3. Schematic diagram illustrating the action of dipeptidyl peptidase-4 (DPP-4) on the incretin hormones GIP and GLP-1.

Therapeutical Approach of Relevant Drugs, Understanding and Pinpointing Clinical Pharmacology. Critical Evaluation of Drugs

GLP-1 Receptor Agonists

Exenatide (synthetic exendin-4)

Exenatide (synthetic exendin-4) was isolated from the salivary gland of the gila monster, a lizard found in the deserts of Arizona [117]. Due to an ~50% amino acid homology with native human GLP-1 (Figs. 1 and 4), this peptide acts as a potent agonist at the mammalian GLP-1 receptor, but is not substrate to proteolytic cleavage by DPP-4 [117]. This leads to a circulating plasma half-life of 2–4 h, with exenatide levels being raised for ~6 h after a single subcutaneous injection [118].

The clinical effects of exenatide in the treatment of type 2 diabetes have been examined in phase 3 trials (Fig. 5). In these studies, exenatide (5 or 10 μg s.c. twice daily) was added to an existing therapy with metformin [119], sulfonylureas [120], a combination of both [121], or thiazolidinediones [122]. HbA_{1c}-reductions achieved after exenatide treatment over 30 weeks ranged from 0.8% to 1.0%, with HbA_{1c}-levels at baseline ranging between 8.2% and 8.6%. In addition, body weight was reduced by ~1–3 kg after 30 weeks (baseline weight: ~100 kg), and patients continuing in an open-label extension study for 80 weeks exhibited a total weight loss averaging ~4.5 kg [123]. The latter effect is remarkable in that all other insulinotropic drugs (sulfonylureas and glinides) as well as insulin itself typically cause weight gain during long-term administration [1].

In an open-label comparison of exenatide with insulin glargine in diabetic patients suboptimally controlled with metformin and sulfonylurea, both treatment regimens led to a reduction in HbA_{1c} levels by ~1.1% after 26 weeks (baseline: 8.2%)

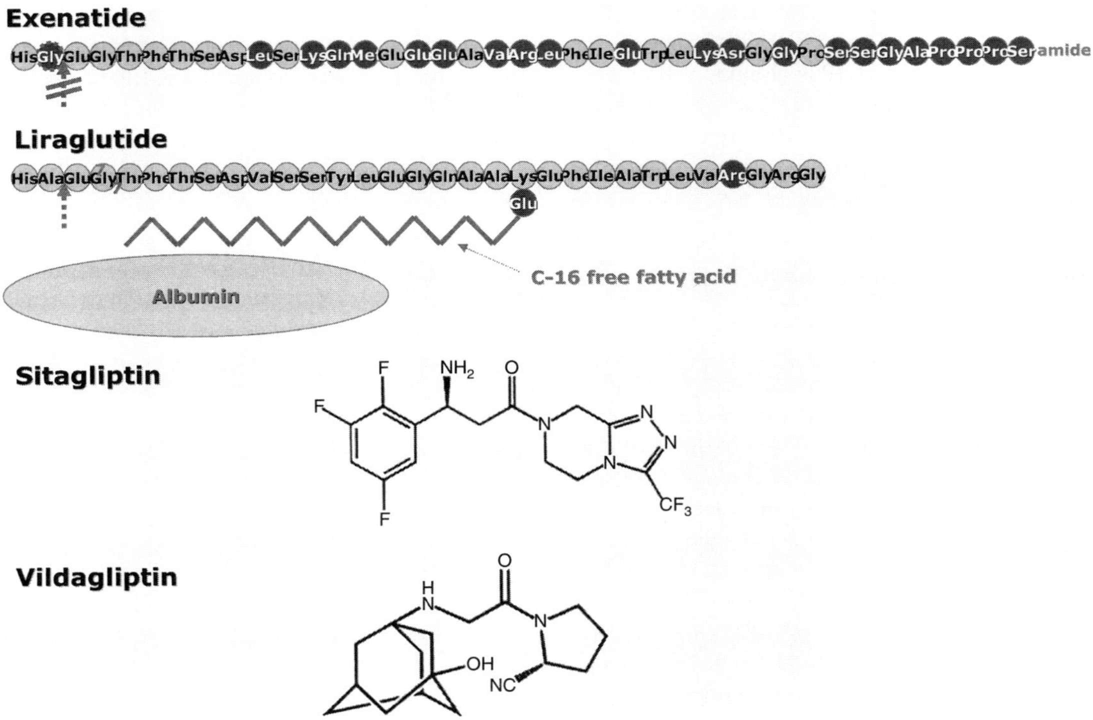

FIG. 4. Peptide and chemical structure, respectively, of the incretin mimetics exenatide and liraglutide and the DPP-4 inhibitors sitagliptin ((2R)-4-oxo-4-[3-(trifluoromethyl)-5,6-dihydro[1,2,4]triazolo[4,3-α]pyrazin-7(8*H*)-yl]-1-(2,4,5-trifluorophenyl)butan-2-amine) and vildagliptin (1-[[(3-hydroxy-1-adamantyl)amino]acetyl]-2-cyano-(S)-pyrrolidine). (Modified from Drucker and Nauck 2006 [145]).

TABLE 2. Comparison of the incretin mimetics exenatide, exenatide LAR and liraglutide.

	Exenatide	Exenatide LAR[a]	Liraglutide
Administration	s.c. injection	s.c. injection	s.c. injection
Half-life (h)	≈2–4	>1 week[b]	≈12–14
Frequency of injections	Twice daily	Once weekly	once daily
Dose per injection	5–10 μg	Up to 2 mg[c]	Up to 2 mg
DPP-4 substrate?	No	No	No
Insulin secretion[d]	↑	↑[e]	↑
Glucagon secretion[d]	↓	↓[e]	↓
Fasting glucose	↓	↓↓↓	↓↓↓
Postprandial glucose excursions	↓↓↓	↓↓↓	↓↓
Weight reduction	Yes	Yes	Yes
Gastric empting	↓	?	(↓)
Hypoglycemia	No[f]	No	No
Nausea	Yes (≈50%)	Yes (≈25%)	Yes (≈10%)
Antibody production	Yes (≈45%)	Probably yes	No

[a]LAR = long-acting release preparation (biodegradable polymeric microspheres).
[b]Estimate, since no pharmacokinetic characteristics have been published.
[c]Since liraglutide strongly binds albumin, only 1–2% are non-albumin bound, free liraglutide able to interact with GLP-1 receptors.
[d]The influence on insulin and glucagon secretion is glucose-dependent.
[e]The active ingredient of exenatide LAR is identical to unretarded exenatide; no studies have reported the action profile of exenatide LAR with respect to insulin and glucagon secretion.
[f]Only if combined with other agents which can cause hypoglycemic episodes (e.g., sulfonylureas).

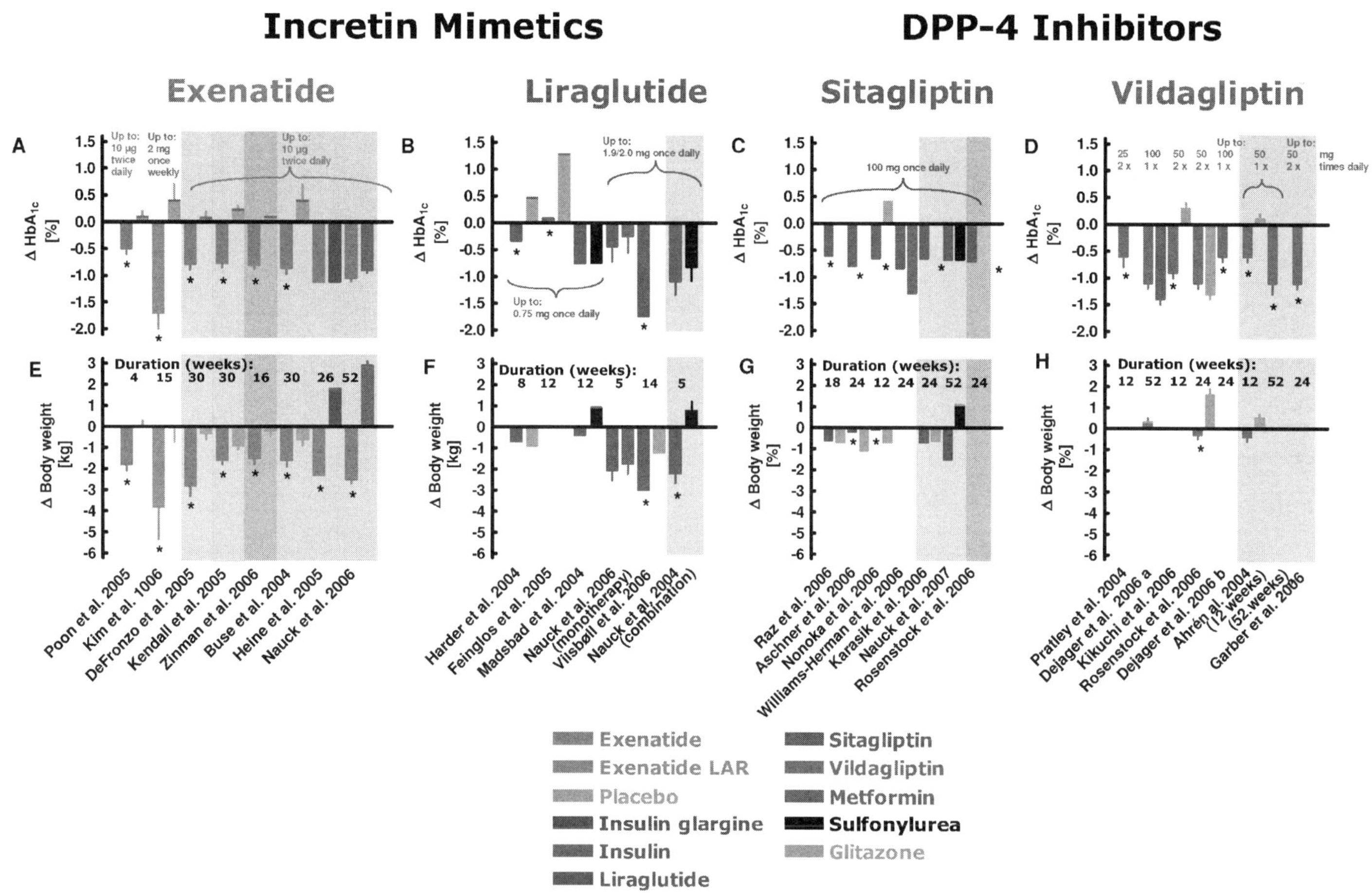

FIG. 5. Results from clinical trials of using incretin mimetics like exenatide injected subcutaneously twice daily, a long-acting release form of exenatide injected subcutaneously once weekly (*left panels*) and liraglutide injected once daily (second column of panels) and DPP-4 inhibitors like sitagliptin (third column of panels) and vildagliptin (*right panels*) on HbA_{1c} (*upper panels*) and body weight (*lower panels*). Background colors indicate concomitant antidiabetic treatment (pink: metformin, light green: sulfonylurea; orange: thiazolidinediones; gray: combinations of oral antidiabetic agents). Columns and bars represent mean change from baseline ± SEM. If no comparator is shown, the results are placebo-corrected. Asterisks indicate significant differences to placebo or the respective comparator. Doses are indicated in the top panels; duration of trials is presented in the lower panels. Results are from the following studies: exenatide [119,121,122,124,125,185,237]; exenatide LAR [135]; liraglutide [130–133,238]; sitagliptin [148,170,239–243]); vildagliptin [153,155,156,244–247]. (Extensively modified from Drucker and Nauck 2006 [145]).

[124]. However, while fasting glucose concentrations were reduced to a greater extent with insulin glargine, exenatide treatment elicited greater reductions in postprandial glycemia. The most striking differences between both treatment regimens were observed in body weight. Thus, patients treated with insulin glargine experienced a weight gain of 1.8 kg, whereas patients on exenatide lost on average 2.3 kg over the treatment period [124]. Similar findings have been reported for the comparison of exenatide and premixed insulin aspart, both injected subcutaneously twice daily [125] (Fig. 5).

In April 2005, exenatide (trade name, Byetta) was approved by the FDA for the treatment of type 2 diabetic patients who have not achieved adequate glycemic control on maximally tolerated doses of metformin and/or a sulfonylurea. In Europe, exenatide was approved in November 2006.

Liraglutide

Liraglutide (NN2211; Arg34, Lys26-[*N*-∈ (γ-Glu[*N*-α-hexadecanoyl])]-GLP-1[7–37]) is a GLP-1 derivative developed by Novo Nordisk, which is currently undergoing phase 3 clinical trials. The plasma half-life of this compound has been extended to ~10–14 h through an amino acid substitution (Arg_{34}→Lys) and the attachment of a glutamic acid and a 16-C-free fatty acid addition to Lys_{26} [126–128]. The acyl moiety induces non-covalent binding to albumin with ~1–2% of Liraglutide circulating as the non-albumin bound, "free" peptide [129]. These modified pharmacokinetic properties make the compound suitable for once-daily s.c. administration. In clinical studies in patients with type 2 diabetes, liraglutide reduced HbA_{1c} levels by up to 1.75% [130]. Liraglutide induced a moderate weight loss during chronic administration [131–133], similar to the effects of native GLP-1 and exenatide.

Long-acting GLP-1 Receptor Agonists

As a single subcutaneous injection of exenatide does not produce effective glucose control for more than 6–8 h, there is considerable interest in the development of longer-acting GLP-1 receptor agonists, which require less frequent parenteral administration. Exenatide LAR ("long-acting release") is a poly-lactide-glycolide microsphere suspension containing 3% exendin-4 peptide, which exhibits sustained dose-dependent glycemic control in diabetic fatty Zucker rats for up to 28 days following a single subcutaneous injection [134]. Preliminary experience with exenatide LAR in 45 subjects with type 2 diabetes mellitus indicates a much greater reduction in fasting glucose concentrations and HbA_{1c} following once-weekly administrations of exenatide LAR for 15 weeks [135]. However, long-term experience with exenatide LAR in larger numbers of patients has not yet been reported. Exenatide LAR is currently being examined in a Phase 3 trial head to head against twice-daily exenatide.

Properties of exenatide, exenatide LAR, and liraglutide are compared systematically in Table 2.

Additional strategies for development of long-acting GLP-1 receptor agonists include the use of chemical linkers to form covalent bonds between GLP-1 (CJC-1131) or exendin-4 (CJC-1134) (ConjuChem Inc.) [136]. Similarly, recombinant albumin-GLP-1 proteins (e.g., "albugon") have been developed, which mimic the full spectrum of GLP-1 actions in preclinical studies [137]. Although these drugs are expected to exhibit a prolonged pharmacokinetic profile suitable for once-weekly dosing in diabetic patients, only limited clinical information is available about the efficacy and safety of these albumin-based drugs in human subjects.

DPP-4 Inhibitors

The therapeutic use of GLP-1 is primarily limited by its rapid in vivo degradation by the enzyme DPP-4 [37,38,138]. DPP-4 is a ubiquitous membrane-spanning cell-surface amino-peptidase widely expressed in many tissues including liver, lung, kidney, intestinal brush-border membranes, lymphocytes, and endothelial cells, which can also be found circulating in plasma [39,139,140]. DPP-4 nonspecifically cleaves peptides displaying a proline or alanine residue in the second amino-terminal position, thereby making a number of gastrointestinal hormones, including GIP [38,138,141], GLP-1 [37,38,138,142], GLP-2, PACAP, Neuropeptide Y, and Peptide YY substrates to DPP-4 degradation [39].

Endogenous GLP-1 plasma levels typically increase by ~2–3-fold after meal ingestion and return to baseline values within ~3–6 h [18,143,144]. Inhibiting DPP-4 activity extents the circulating half-life of the incretin hormone, thereby raising intact GLP-1 levels (Fig. 3) for up to 5 h after meal ingestion. While DPP-4 inhibitors primarily lower postprandial glycemic excursions, there is now evidence that basal concentrations of intact GLP-1 are also raised to some extent by DPP-4 inhibition, which may explain their (modest) effects on fasting glycemia [145].

As a rule, DPP-4 inhibitors mimic many of the actions of native GLP-1, such as the stimulation of insulin and inhibition of glucagon secretion. However, unlike GLP-1 and its analogues, DPP-4 inhibitors do not typically influence body weight or gastric emptying [146]. These discrepancies might be due to the nonspecific mode of action of the DPP-4 inhibitors, which also prevent the degradation of other peptides, especially GIP and NPY, which might exert opposite effects on gastric motility and the central nervous control of appetite. As an alternative explanation, it seems possible that the modest elevations in intact GLP-1 levels (approximately doubled) seen after DPP-4 inhibition are of insufficient magnitude to elicit significant effects on gastric emptying and food intake.

A number of small molecule DPP-4 inhibitors suitable for oral administration are currently undergoing clinical trials. This article focuses on the two major compounds with available reports regarding phase 3 clinical trials. Important results are summarized in Fig. 5.

Sitagliptin

The DPP-4 inhibitor sitagliptin has been developed by Merck Pharmaceuticals and was recently approved for the therapy of type 2 diabetes by the FDA under the name Januvia. The elimination half-life of sitagliptin is 12–14 h [147], thereby allowing for once-daily administration. In phase 3 trials enrolling drug-naïve patients with type 2 diabetes, sitagliptin led to HbA_{1c} reductions of 0.79% and 0.94% a dose of 100 and 200 mg, respectively (baseline: 8.0%) [148]. In diabetic patients inadequately controlled with metformin (baseline HbA_{1c}: 8.0%), HbA_{1c}-levels were reduced by 0.65% after 24 weeks of sitagliptin treatment [149]. Likewise, patients pretreated with pioglitazone (baseline HbA_{1c}: 8.1%) exhibited a 0.7% HbA_{1c}-reduction after 24 weeks of sitaglitin treatment [149]. Regarding the control of glycemia (HbA_{1c}), sitagliptin was equipotent to the sulfonylurea glipizide, when added to metformin pretreatment. Glipizide, however, caused significant weight gain (Fig. 5). Similar to vildaglitin, sitagliptin does not have any systematic effect on body weight (Fig. 5).

Vildagliptin

The DPP-4 inhibitor vildagliptin has been developed by Novartis Pharma and is currently awaiting approval. Vildagliptin has been studied at doses between 50 and 100 mg administered once or twice daily per os [146,150,151]. In a study over 4 weeks, once-daily administration of 100 mg vildagliptin reduced fasting glucose by 0.70 mmol/L, and postprandial glucose excursions by 1.45 mmol/L [150]. This effect was accompanied by a significant reduction glucagon levels, whereas plasma insulin remained rather unchanged [150]. However, similar insulin profiles at lower glucose concentrations indicate an improvement in glucose-stimulated insulin secretion. Consistent with this, indirect evidence from mathematical modeling studies suggested a significant improvement in β-cell function during vildagliptin treatment [152].

In metformin-treated patients with type 2 diabetes, the addition of vildagliptin led to a reduction of HbA_{1c} by ~0.8% (baseline: 7.7%), and this effect was maintained during an open-label extension for 52 weeks [153] (Fig. 5). Recent studies in patients with type 2 diabetes treated with the twice-daily administration of 50 mg vildagliptin also demonstrated a significant improvement in postprandial plasma triglyceride and apolipoprotein B-48-containing triglyceride-rich lipoprotein particle metabolism [154], suggesting that this compound might exert antiatherogenic effects beyond its glucose-lowering actions.

In a direct comparison, vildagliptin did not quite achieve noninferiority in comparison with metformin in terms of lowering HbA_{1c}-levels, but was associated with a lower frequency of GI-side effects [155]. When compared with rosiglitazone, vildagliptin treatment elicited a similar reduction in HbA_{1c}-levels, but did not cause a similar increase in body weight (Fig. 5) [156].

Contrasting Properties of GLP-1 Receptor Agonists and DPP-4 Inhibitors

Properties of incretin mimetics and DPP-4 inhibitors are systematically compared in Table 3.

TABLE 3. Comparison of the classes of incretin mimetics and DPP-4 inhibitors.

Parameter	Incretin mimetics	DPP-4 Inhibitors
Administration	Injection	Tablet
GLP-1/GLP-1 receptor agonist concentration elevated	Up to 24 h/day	Predominantly for 3–6 h after meals, when secretion from endogenous sources is stimulated)
GLP-1 concentration	Pharmacological (> ×5)	Close to physiological (≈ x 2–3)
Action through	GLP-1 receptors	GLP-1 receptors, GIP-receptors (?), other receptors (?)
GLP-1 action via	Circulation > nerves	Nerves > circulation (?)
HbA_{1c} reduction	–0.8–1.8%	–0.5–1.1%
Weight change	–3(–5) kg	±0 kg
β-cell mass effects[a]	Robust	Probable

[a]Animal experiments.

Twice-daily exenatide administered via subcutaneous injection is currently indicated for the treatment of patients with type 2 diabetes mellitus failing one or more oral agents, often as an alternative to institution of insulin therapy. In contrast, once-daily DPP-4 inhibitors may find use as first-line therapy or as add-on therapy to patients failing one or more oral agents. Although there does not appear to be a great difference in the HbA_{1c}-lowering capacity of GLP-1 receptor agonists versus DPP-4 inhibitors, the obvious difference between these classes of drugs is their effect on body weight. Weight loss is a common outcome of therapy with native GLP-1 [114], exenatide [119–121], and liraglutide [157,158], whereas therapy with DPP-4 inhibitors is associated with prevention of weight gain [150,153,159,160] (Fig. 5). In contrast, gastrointestinal side effects, predominantly nausea, are frequently reported following treatment with injectable incretin mimetics, but have not been described with DPP-4 inhibition [150,153,159–162]. These differences may be explained in part by the relatively modest stabilization of postprandial GLP-1 seen after DPP-4 inhibition versus the pharmacological increases in circulating levels of incretin mimetics exemplified by exenatide. Although nausea is a common side effect of exenatide therapy, many patients experience weight loss independent of nausea [163]. Consistent with the above differences in circulating levels of GLP-1, incretin mimetics, but not DPP-4 inhibitors, profoundly decelerate gastric emptying [97,113,164,165] (Table 3).

Practical Outline in the Management

In this chapter, a suggestion will be developed on how incretin mimetics and DPP-4 inhibitors will fit into established treatment algorithms for glycemic control in patients with type 2 diabetes (see Fig. 6A).

FIG. 6. Treatment algorithm for patients with type 2 diabetes. (a) is a simplified version of "a consensus algorithm for the initiation and adjustment of therapy" for the "management of hyperglycemia in type 2 diabetes" recently published by Nathan et al. [166,167]). ?*indicates that a higher than target range HbA_{1c} (e.g., >7.0%) indicates the need for intensification of anti-hyperglycemic therapy. The algorithm is based on the availability of metformin, sulfonylureas, glitazones, and insulin. α-glucosidase inhibitors are not considered. (B) is a development of algorithm (A), but considering the availability of DPP-4 inhibitors (e.g., sitagliptin and vildagliptin) and incretin mimetics (e.g., exenatide). The therapeutic options at each step of intensification considerably increase in number. Dotted lines indicate that progressing through the algorithm this way may require more action than just adding the next antidiabetic drug. In some cases, contraindications need to be addressed (e.g., glitazones in combination with insulin, not approved in Europe).

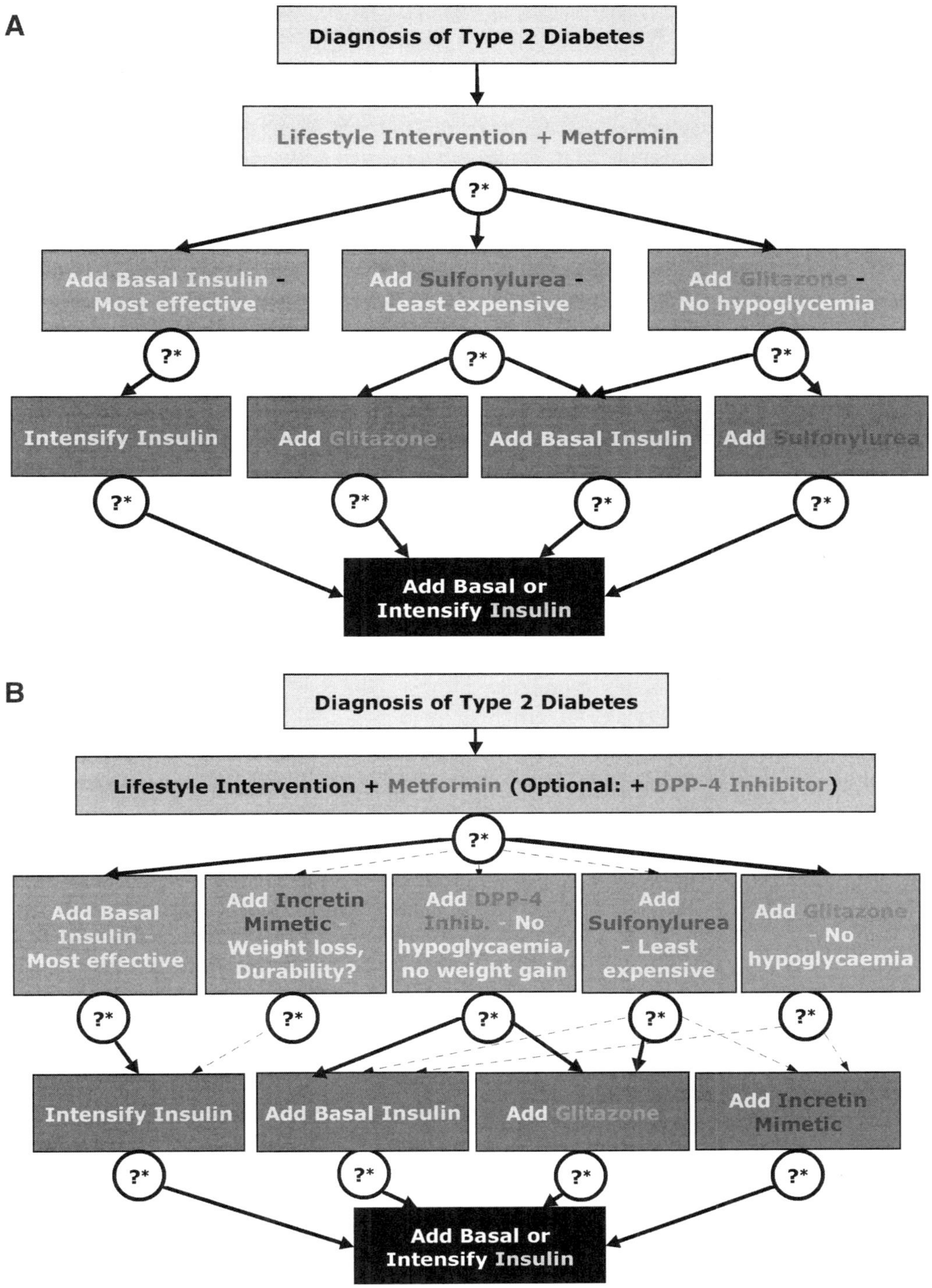

FIG. 6. (*continued*). In other cases, especially if a more potent drug is to be added, which relies on a similar mechanism (e.g., incretin-mediated insulinotropic activity), one of the previously used antidiabetic agents may need to be discontinued (e.g., when adding a sulfonylurea or an incretin mimetic to a patient previously treated with a DPP-4 inhibitor). Note that sufficient study results (see Fig. 5) are not available for all mentioned combinations to provide a sound scientific basis for their use outside clinical studies.

Choice of Patients

Incretin Mimetics

Since incretin mimetics are injectable antidiabetic drugs, their use will most likely be considered, when oral antidiabetic agents in combinations do no longer assure glycemic control of the required quality. This is the moment, when – according to current guidelines – the start of insulin treatment would be considered according to most recommendations [166,167]. However, such guidelines have, until now, not considered the availability of incretin mimetics or DPP-4 inhibitors. An attempt has been made to incorporate these novel antidiabetic treatment choices into a more complex algorithm (Fig. 6B).

Incretin mimetics (e.g. exenatide) would have some advantages over using insulin. In particular, they promote weight loss, whereas the initiation of insulin treatment must be expected to be associated with weight gain [1,168]. This difference has been demonstrated in two head-to-head studies comparing twice-daily exenatide injections either with once-daily insulin *glargine* [124] or twice-daily premixed insulin [125]. It is, however, not known whether the resulting weight difference (approximately 5 kg) represents a significant health benefit in terms of cardiovascular risk or even outcome. Longer-term studies examining cardiovascular endpoints will be necessary to clarify this point. It can, however, be foreseen that for the obese type 2-diabetic patients, who has struggled to lose weight, an agent that will provide a good chance to lose rather than to gain body weight is an attractive choice. Along these lines, for patients in whom insulin therapy had been initiated recently, and in whom this has led to considerable weight gain, switching to incretin mimetics might be a reasonable alternative. However, studies examining the consequences of changing therapy from insulin to incretin mimetics in this particular situation are not yet available.

DPP-4 Inhibitors

Given the fact that metformin is the established first-line drug for the anti-hyperglycemic treatment of obese type 2 diabetes [166,167,169], especially considering the reduction in the incidence of acute myocardial infarction and related mortality demonstrated in the UKPDS (obese cohort) [169], the use of DPP-4 inhibitors may be considered, when metformin alone has failed to maintain adequate glycemic control, or is not likely to achieve treatment goals unless combined with additional agents (Fig. 6 B). An early initiation of anti-hyperglycemic combination treatment is supported by the recent finding that metformin and sitagliptin achieved a higher likelihood of treatment success when given in combination to patients with type 2 diabetes not previously treated with oral agents [170].

As a second oral antidiabetic agent, the use of DPP-4 inhibitors has to be weighed against the alternatives, sulfonylureas, glitazones, α-glucosidase inhibitors, and (basal, "bedtime") insulin (Fig. 6). All other treatment choices (except acarbose or miglitol) will cause weight gain, whereas DPP-4 inhibitors generally can be considered weight-neutral. Sulfonylureas can provoke hypoglycemic episodes [1], and glitazones may precipitate fluid retention and congestive heart failure [171,172]. Given the comparable antidiabetic potency of sitagliptin relative to the sulfonylurea glipizide [125] and of vildagliptine in comparison with the thiazolidindione rosiglitazone [156], their weight-neutrality and unremarkable side-effect profile make DPP-4 inhibitors a serious contender for the second oral antidiabetic agent to be added to metformin treatment.

Given the fact that incretins (both GIP and GLP-1) are eliminated via the kidneys and that patients with impaired renal function have elevated circulating concentrations of GIP and GLP-1, treatment with usual doses of DPP-4 inhibitors might lead to further elevations in incretin plasma levels, potentially causing adverse events. Therefore, lower doses of DPP-4 inhibitors may be appropriate in such patients. Like in the case of renal functional impairment, not much is known on the use of DPP-4 inhibitors in patients with type 2 diabetes and associated diseases leading to severe organ failure (liver cirrhosis, heart failure, pulmonary disorders, etc.).

Initiation of Treatment

Incretin Mimetics

Since starting exenatide injections may be associated with the provocation of nausea, it is better to start treatment at a lower dose (5 μg per injection, twice daily subcutaneously) and to increase the dose to 10 μg twice daily after 4 weeks. This has been shown to make the 10-μg dose more tolerable [173]. Following this regimen has been associated with low withdrawal rates in studies using 10 μg twice daily [124,125].

Initial studies using liraglutide had identified 0.75 mg once daily as a subcutaneous dose close to the maximum tolerated dose upon a single injection into treatment-naïve subjects or patients [127,128,131]. Later, a regimen starting at 0.5 mg once daily, and increasing the dose by 0.5 mg on a weekly basis, was used to extend the final dosage to 2 mg once daily [174] for the majority of patients. Therefore, it appears advisable to start liraglutide at a low dose and titrate the daily dose up to the 2-mg range. The most recent trial has reported the use of 0.65, 1.25, and 1.9 mg once daily [130].

DPP-4 Inhibitors

DPP-4 inhibitors can immediately be started at the target dose, since the initiation of treatment has not been associated with any untoward responses. Since studies examining effects of sitagliptin and vildagliptin at single (100 mg once daily orally) or divided doses (e.g., 50 mg twice daily orally) have not consistently resulted in different efficacy (Fig. 5), once-daily dosing will probably be the standard.

Choice of Dose and Timing

Incretin Mimetics

In studies examining the dose–response relationships for exenatide, 10 μg twice daily has uniformly been more effective than 5 μg twice daily [119–121]. Therefore, for the majority of patients, exploiting the efficacy of 10 μg twice daily will be necessary to reach treatment targets. For those patients achieving their goals already at 5 μg twice daily, continuing at this dosage is an option.

Given the pharmacokinetics of exenatide injected subcutaneously into human subjects [175], a single injection is likely to be clinically effective over a period of 6–8 h. This can be inferred from the fact that the glycemic rise after breakfast and dinner is almost completely abolished when injecting exenatide before breakfast and dinner, whereas there remains a glucose excursion after lunch [124,125].

One consequence of the rather short duration of action of a single injection of exenatide is that timing the injection relative to meals is of some importance. Linnebjerg et al. demonstrated that exenatide should be injected within 60 min before starting meals [176]. This appears plausible, since one important mode of action of exenatide is the deceleration of gastric emptying [177].

Further, the question arises whether more frequent injections of exenatide (three or four per day) would provide even better glycemic control, including a more profound effect on fasting glucose concentrations and lunch-time glycemic control. One study had not found advantages of three over two injections [178]. Rather than increasing the number of injections per day, the development has been in the direction of more extended-acting preparations of exenatide.

Preliminary results of using exenatide LAR indicate that doses of 0.8 and 2.0 mg per week (injected subcutaneously) are effective in reducing HbA_{1c} considerably [135]. Interestingly, only the higher dose significantly reduced body weight, while the effect on HbA_{1c} after 15 weeks was relatively similar. This raises the question whether the dose–response relationship is different for glycemic control and for the reduction in body weight. If this were true, higher doses should be used, if weight reduction is among the treatment goals.

Similarly, liraglutide reduced HbA_{1c} at doses of 0.65, 1.25, and 1.9 mg injected once daily subcutaneously, to a rather similar extent [130], while only the higher dose(s) significantly reduced body weight. Perhaps, the upper end of the dose–response relationship for weight reduction has not been characterized, and doses even higher than 2 mg daily would have more profound effects on body weight. Like with exenatide, the choice of the dose should consider whether or not weight loss is among the individual treatment goals.

DPP-4 Inhibitors

Sitagliptin and vildagliptin exert their antidiabetic activity by inhibiting DPP-4 enzymatic activity. Since a single dose of 100 mg inhibits DPP-4 activity by >90% for most of a 24-h period [150,179], there is no obvious reason why higher doses should be more effective. As a consequence, a dose of 100 mg once daily will most likely be used rather uniformly, both for sitagliptin and vildagliptin, unless they are combined with other antidiabetic agents (like metformin), which are usually administered twice daily [170].

Reduced doses may be necessary for patients with renal functional impairment.

Choice of Antidiabetic Agents to be Used in Combination

Incretin Mimetics

A number of potential combinations are depicted in Fig. 6b. Based on available clinical studies, a combining exenatide with metformin has the most obvious advantages: A substantial reduction in HbA_{1c} is associated with the numerically largest weight loss [119] (compared with combinations including sulfonylureas) [120,121] and no increased risk of hypoglycemia (despite better glycemic control) [119].

Addition to thiazolidinediones is similarly possible [122].

If exenatide is to be combined with sulfonylureas [120,121,124,125], the benefit of better glycemic control has to be weighed against the risk of hypoglycemia and less weight reduction.

A combination of a short-acting incretin mimetic (to control postprandial rises in glycemia) and a long-acting insulin (to titrate fasting glucose into the target range [180,181]) may theoretically appear to make sense, but no studies are available to report experience with this particular combination.

DPP-4 Inhibitors

DPP-4 inhibitors can safely be combined with metformin and thiazolidinediones. A combination with sulfonylureas does not suggest particular advantages, since both agents, through different mechanisms, enhance insulin secretion. This combination would, most likely, not be as safe regarding hypoglycemic episodes [182]. No studies are available regarding a potential combination with α-glucosidase inhibitors or insulin treatment.

Measures to Assure Metabolic Control (Self-Blood-Glucose Monitoring)

Although exenatide was approved by the FDA and introduced for use in the USA in 2005 (and other countries since) and sitagliptin has been approved in the USA and elsewhere in late 2006, no recommendations regarding metabolic control have been issued. The following suggestions, therefore, are based on the known properties of incretin mimetics and DPP-4 inhibitors.

Incretin Mimetics

Since incretin mimetics will be used at fairly standardized doses (vide supra), and not based on individual titration (like in the case of insulin), and since incretin mimetics alone do not provoke hypoglycemic episodes, there will be a rather limited need for blood-glucose self-control in addition to regular determinations of HbA_{1c}. The frequency of glucose control will primarily depend on other antidiabetic agents used in combination and their potential to elicit hypoglycemia. Certainly, in comparison with any insulin regimen, the requirement for blood glucose-self control will be much smaller. This could affect the acceptability of such treatment regimens to patients and on the overall cost–benefit relationship.

DPP-4 Inhibitors

DPP-4 inhibitors, in their most likely use, in combination with metformin, do not require additional measures of blood-glucose self-control, since they are administered at a standard dosage and do not provoke hypoglycemia. Thus, only occasional profiles to assess glycemic control are adequate.

Discontinuation of Treatment

With randomized clinical trials concerning incretin mimetics and DPP-4 inhibitors lasting up to 1 year [125,155], and open-label follow-up reported up to 2 years [183], it is obvious that these studies cannot provide an estimate of how long treatment with incretin mimetics and DPP-4 inhibitors can meaningfully control glycemia. It is, however, obvious that not all patients treated with such agents achieve their glycemic target, even within the time frame of the studies that have been reported. Therefore, preliminary thoughts on when incretin mimetics or DPP-4 inhibitors should be discontinued, and what the treatment alternatives would be, seem adequate, even in the absence of studies that would provide any firm guidance.

Incretin Mimetics

Treatment with exenatide results in fairly stable fasting glucose and HbA_{1c} concentrations after approximately 3 months [119–121,124,125]. If by then HbA_{1c} targets (e.g., <7.0% [166,167]) have not been met, intensification of treatment has to be considered. Since weight loss associated with the use of exenatide progresses at least up to a duration of 2 years [183], a secondary improvement of glycemic control appears possible with further weight reduction, although this is not clearly confirmed by serial HbA_{1c} measurements [163]. Certainly, once weight becomes stable and HbA_{1c} remains outside the target range, antidiabetic therapy needs to be intensified.

Adding more or other oral antidiabetic agents at this stage of type 2 diabetes does not seem to be helpful in achieving adequate glycemic control. Rather, insulin-based treatment regimens will most likely be needed. Since there is no reported experience with a combination of exenatide and insulin, this cannot be recommended. Established treatment regimens ranging from a combination of once-daily basal insulin and oral agents, twice-daily premixed insulin, or intensified regimens with multiple daily insulin injections should be initiated instead.

DPP-4 Inhibitors

When a DPP-4 inhibitor added to metformin no longer adequately controls glycemia, the options for intensifying therapy include the start of basal insulin or an incretin mimetic. It is not known what continued treatment with DPP-4 inhibitors would add to a combination of metformin (continued) and basal insulin (newly initiated). In addition, there has been no published experience with a combination of a DPP-4 inhibitor and an incretin mimetic. Such studies are needed to justify a continuation of DPP-4 inhibitor treatment under these circumstances. Since there have been no head-to-head comparisons of the antihyperglycemic efficacy between DPP-4 inhibitors and incretin mimetics, one can only speculate whether switching from a DPP-4 to an incretin mimetic would improve glycemic control. Based on comparisons of the effects on fasting glucose and HbA_{1c} concentrations (Fig. 5), one might assume that longer-acting incretin mimetics (exenatide LAR, liraglutide) would probably provide a better glycemic control than a DPP-4 inhibitor.

Side Effects of Treatment

Side Effects of Incretin Mimetics

Side Effects of Exenatide

As is typical for the administration of native GLP-1 [184], a considerable proportion of patients receiving exenatide experience gastrointestinal side effects, such as nausea and more rarely vomiting or diarrhea [119–121]. In the phase 3 trials with exenatide, the frequence of these adverse effects was reported to be as high as 48% during treatment with 10 μg of exenatide [119–121]. However, it should be noted that, though frequent, these side effects were mostly mild to moderate in intensity and usually transient. Overall, the percentage of patients who discontinued exenatide treatment as a result of side effects was low. When considering all patients enrolled in the exenatide phase 3 trials, there also seemed to be an increase in the frequency of hypoglycemic events [119–121], but this was limited to the patients receiving additional treatment with sulfonylurea drugs [185]. In contrast, the incidence of hypoglycemia was unchanged in patients treated with metformin [119,121].

Antibody formation has been reported in ~40–50% of patients receiving Exenatide treatment [119–121]. However, these antibodies seemed to exhibit a weak binding affinity and have not been associated with severely impaired antidiabetic effectiveness of exenatide in the majority of treated subjects.

Side Effects of Liraglutide

In the published phase 2 trials with liraglutide, nausea, vomiting, and diarrhea were the most frequent adverse events reported, with the incidence of events being dose-related [131]. Only a small proportion of patients (<5%) discontinued treatment due to these side effects [131,132]. The frequency of hypoglycemia was not increased during liraglutide treatment. Side reactions of urticarial injection were reported in 1 out of 135 patients exposed to liraglutide in one trial and did not occur in the other published studies [131]. No antibody formation has been reported after exposure to liraglutide.

Side Effects of DPP-4 Inhibitors (Sitagliptin and Vildagliptin)

A number of theoretical concerns have been expressed regarding potential adverse effects of DPP-4 inhibitors. In particular, the large number of physiological substrates of DPP-4 [39,140] gave rise to speculations that inhibiting the action of this protease might interfere with numerous other hormonal axes, thereby potentially causing adverse reactions. Furthermore, since DPP-4 is also expressed on T-lymphocytes as CD26, it was speculated that chronic DPP-4 inhibition might alter immune functions [186]. Against these theoretical considerations, the DPP-4 inhibitors have so far proven to be safe and well tolerated in clinical studies, and no characteristic pattern of adverse events has been observed [150,153,159–161]. Thus, in patients with diabetes pretreated with metformin, the incidence of adverse effects during 12 weeks of treatment with sitagliptin was similar to the placebo group [153]. Likewise, the frequency of side effects was not different from the placebo group in diabetic patients previously treated with a dietary regimen [151]. With sitagliptin, the frequency of gastrointestinal side effects was slightly higher compared with placebo in one [148], but not all studies [149,156,187]. Overall, the gastrointestinal side effects typically reported during the treatment with GLP-1 analogues do not represent a problem during DPP-4 inhibitor administration. Nevertheless, further long-term studies will be required to confirm the absence of a potential to cause clinically important adverse reactions before these drugs can unequivocally be accepted as safe, especially with regard to their potential effects on other hormonal axes and immune functions.

Key Issues in the Treatment Strategy

Based on presently available study results, the clinical benefit of using incretin mimetics is determined by their ability to control glycemia (i.e., lower HbA_{1c}), their inability to cause hypoglycemia unless combined with other antidiabetic agents that have the potential to initiate hypoglycemia, their weight effects (promotion of weight loss in the case of incretin mimetics, weight neutrality in the case of DPP-4 inhibitors), and their safety and tolerability, especially the absence of a potential to cause specific severe adverse events.

The novel classes of antidiabetic agents, incretin mimetics and DPP-4 inhibitors, may hold two additional promises: A reduction in cardiovascular complications typically associated with type 2 diabetes [188] and the metabolic syndrome, and a positive influence on the natural history of type 2 diabetes, which with current treatment options is characterized by a steady loss of β-cell function [189,190], which in turn determines a rather short "durability" of successful glycemic control with any choice of antidiabetic agents [191,192].

Possible Effects of Incretin Mimetics and DPP-4 Inhibitors on β-Cell Mass

Both type 1 and type 2 diabetes are caused by a significant deficit in β-cell mass, caused by increased β-cell apoptosis [193–195]. Strategies to inhibit β-cell apoptosis and/or increase the rate of β-cell replication may therefore allow for the prevention or even reversal of diabetes [196]. A number of studies have suggested that GLP-1 might exhibit such properties. Thus, in β-cell lines (INS-1 cells), GLP-1 increased the rate of proliferation through induction of phosphatidylinositol 3-kinase, protein kinase C zeta, and activation of PDX1 gene expression [197,198]. In rodent models of diabetes, GLP-1 led to an increase in β-cell replication, a stimulation of islet neogenesis, and an inhibition of β-cell apoptosis [199–203]. An inhibition of β-cell apoptosis by GLP-1 was also noted in isolated human islets [65]. These actions therefore raised hopes that GLP-1 analogues and DPP-4 inhibitors might halt or even reverse the progression of diabetes.

With exenatide, an increase in β-cell replication and neogenesis resulting in increased β-cell mass has been reported after partial pancreatectomy in rats [199], and a diminished recovery of β-cell mass after partial pancreatectomy was shown in GLP-1 receptor knock-out mice [204]. Likewise, exendin-4 stimulated β-cell neogenesis in streptozotocin-induced diabetic rats [200] as well as in Goto–Kakizaki diabetic rats [201].

The effects of liraglutide on β-cell mass and turnover were studied as well. In db/db mice, liraglutide treatment significantly increased β-cell mass and proliferation resulting in improved diabetes control [205]. In addition, liraglutide inhibited both cytokine- and free fatty acid-induced apoptosis in isolated rat islets [206].

Not only GLP-1 and its analogues, but also the DPP-4 inhibitors have been shown to exert beneficial effects on β-cell mass and turnover. Along these lines, Pospisilik and colleagues reported a significant increase in β-cell mass in strepozotocin-induced diabetic rats following 7 weeks of treatment with the DPP-4 inhibitor P32/98 [207], and recently a significant increase in β-cell mass was reported after treatment with des-fluoro-sitagliptin in high-fat diet (HFD)/streptozotocin (STZ)-induced diabetic mice [208].

Taken together, these studies suggest that both incretin mimetics and DPP-4 inhibitors might indeed have a potential to induce β-cell regeneration in patients with diabetes during long-term treatment. It is, however, difficult to draw firm conclusions from these studies in rodents or in vitro for the situation in humans. In fact, the rates of β-cell turnover seem to be much lower in humans than in rodents [193,209], and the overall capacity for islet regeneration in humans appears to be limited [196]. Furthermore, it is yet impossible to directly measure changes in β-cell mass or turnover, since the human pancreas are inaccessible for repeated biopsy sampling, and since the functional assessment of insulin secretion might only partly relate to the actual β-cell mass [210]. Therefore, while current evidence strongly suggest that the GLP-1 analogues and DPP-4 inhibitors will indeed induce β-cell regeneration in patients with diabetes, this question will ultimately have to be answered in further long-term trials.

The recommendation of an extended and perhaps earlier use of incretin mimetics, for example, starting an injection therapy instead of using oral antidiabetic agents although oral agents would provide adequate glycemic control, would require the demonstration of unique benefits. In principle, the demonstration that exenatide and liraglutide, like GLP-1, can inhibit β-cell apoptosis and increase β-cell mass in isolated pancreatic islets [211–213] and rodents [199,205], would provide a rationale to counteract the progressive loss of β-cell function [189] (and presumably, β-cell mass [193]) typical of type 2 diabetes. However, although some experiments with human islets or islet cell precursors have reported similar findings [65,214], only preliminary hints have been gained from clinical studies examining the long-term effect of incretin mimetics on parameters of "β-cell health." Whether the reported decreases in the proportion of proinsulin (relative to insulin) [119,120] can be used as makers of improvements in "functional β-cell mass," and whether these changes reflect specific actions of the treatment with incretin mimetics or mainly the removal of gluco-lipotoxicity as a consequence of improved metabolic control, remain to be demonstrated in long-term studies. Islet and β-cell turnover appear to be much slower in human subjects than in rodents [215]. Certainly, the demonstration of profound improvements in β-cell mass and function, possibly associated with a longer durability of anti-hyperglycemic effects of incretin mimetics relative to other antidiabetic agents [192], would suggest their use at earlier stages of type 2 diabetes, perhaps even including prediabetes.

A similar reasoning seem to apply to DPP-4 inhibitors: In selected animal models, effects of using sitagliptin [208] or vildagliptin [216] on the rate of β-cell apoptosis and β-cell mass have been demonstrated. In one clinical study an improvement in meal-related β-cell function after a year of treatment has been reported [152]. If substantial benefits in terms of "β-cell health" could be demonstrated, this could broaden the indications for the use of DPP-4 inhibitors.

Cardiac Effects of GLP-1: Consequences of the Treatment with Incretin Mimetics and DPP-4 Inhibitors

The GLP-1 receptor is expressed in the heart [56]. In GLP-1 receptor knock-out mice structural and functional cardiac abnormalities are typical [217]. In animals, exposure to GLP-1 reduces the size of myocardial necroses in the case of induced infarction [218]. In a pilot study with patients treated for acute myocardial infarction, a 48-h infusion of GLP-1 improved left-ventricular function and a wall-motility index [219]. In a dog model of dilated cardiomyopathy, GLP-1 increased glucose uptake and left-ventricular function [220]. These findings, together with the cardiovascular benefit expected from significant weight loss, make it appear possible, that incretin mimetics and/or DPP-4 inhibitors may be agents with the potential to reduce the incidence of cardiovascular events in patients with type 2 diabetes, thus targeting one of the main clinical problems of this metabolic disease. Such potential benefits should be studied in randomized controlled trials of appropriate size and duration.

With incretin mimetics and DPP-4 inhibitors, two novel classes of antidiabetic agents have been developed and are in the course of being approved for the treatment of patients with type 2 diabetes, which will certainly broaden the armamentarium of anti-hyperglycemic therapy. This is valid based on their properties that have already been characterized in clinical trials. Some additional properties need to be explored in future studies, but hold the promise to make a substantial contribution to changing the course of type 2 diabetes, from the prevention of the transition between the prediabetic state to manifest diabetes, to improved and more durable metabolic control with less unwanted side effects and the prevention of diabetic complications.

Summary

GLP-1 is an intestinal incretin hormone that stimulates insulin ("incretin") and suppresses glucagon secretion, inhibits gastric emptying, and reduces appetite and food intake. In contrast to the other incretin hormone, GIP, GLP-1 remains active in patients with type 2 diabetes. GLP-1 itself, however, cannot be used for therapeutic purposes because of its rapid proteolytic degradation and inactivation (DPP-4) and renal elimination, leading to a $t_{1/2}$ of 1–2 min. Therapeutic use of the antidiabetic properties of incretins, especially GLP-1, can be made using degradation-resistant GLP-1 receptor agonists ("incretin mimetics"), or inhibitors of DPP-4 activity ("incretin enhancers"). Clinical studies with exenatide (two injections per day or long-acting release form administered once-weekly) and liraglutide (one injection per day) have proven the antidiabetic efficacy with reductions in fasting and postprandial glucose concentrations and HbA_{1c} (~1–2%), associated with weight loss (2–5 kg). Treatment with incretin mimetics is associated with mild nausea, which occurs early, mostly transiently, after initiation. Orally administered DPP-4 inhibitors (e.g., sitagliptin, vildagliptin) reduce HbA_{1c} by approximately 0.6–1.0%. DPP-4 inhibitors are weight-neutral. There are no specific safety of tolerability concerns emerging from clinical trials. Both incretin mimetics and DPP-4 inhibitors have the potential to increase β-cell mass as shown in animal studies. However, long-term clinical studies are required to ascertain specific benefits of using novel antidiabetic agents derived from the entero-insular axis, in particular incretin hormones like GLP-1, in the treatment of type 2 diabetes.

References

1. UK Prospective Diabetes Study (UKPDS) Group. Intensive blood-glucose control with sulfonylureas or insulin compared with conventional treatment and risk of complications in patients with type 2 diabetes (UKPDS 33). Lancet 1998;352:837–853.
2. Gromada J, Dissing S, Kofod H, Frokjaer-Jensen J. Effects of the hypoglycaemic drugs repaglinide and glibenclamide on ATP-sensitive potassium channels and cytosolic calcium levels in β TC3 cells and rat pancreatic beta cells. Diabetologia 1995;38:1025–1032.
3. Creutzfeldt W. The incretin concept today. Diabetologia 1979;16:75–85.
4. Creutzfeldt W, Nauck M. Gut hormones and diabetes mellitus. Diabetes/Metab Rev 1992;8:149–177.
5. Brown JC, Pederson RA. GI hormones and insulin secretion. Endocrinology. Proceedings of the Vth International Congress Endocrinol 1976;2:568–570.
6. Brown JC, Dahl M, McIntosh CHS, Otte SC, Pedeson RA. Actions of GIP. Peptides 1981;2:241–245.
7. Brown JC. Gastric Inhibitory Polypeptide. Heidelberg: Springer-Verlag; 1982.
8. Pederson RA, Brown JC. The insulinotropic action of gastric inhibitory polypeptide in the perfused rat pancreas. Endocrinology 1976;99:780–785.
9. Dupré J, Ross SA, Watson D, Brown JC. Stimulation of insulin secretion by gastric inhibitory polypeptide in man. J Clin Endocrinol Metab 1973;37:826–828.
10. Krarup T, Saurbrey N, Moody AJ, Kühl C, Madsbad S. Effect of porcine gastric inhibitory polypeptide on β-cell function in Type 1 and Type II diabetes mellitus. Metabolism 1988;36:677–682.
11. Nauck MA, Heimesaat MM, Ørskov C, Holst JJ, Ebert R, Creutzfeldt W. Preserved incretin activity

of glucagon-like peptide 1 [7–36 amide] but not of synthetic human gastric inhibitory polypeptide in patients with type-2 diabetes mellitus. J Clin Invest 1993;91:301–307.
12. Meier JJ, Hücking K, Holst JJ, Deacon CF, Schmiegel WH, Nauck MA. Reduced insulinotropic effect of gastric inhibitory polypeptide in first-degree relatives of patients with type 2 diabetes. Diabetes 2001;50:2497–2504.
13. Vilsbøll T, Krarup T, Madsbad S, Holst JJ. Defective amplification of the late phase insulin response to glucose by GIP in obese Type II diabetic patients. Diabetologia 2002;45:1111–1119.
14. Bell GI, Sanchez-Pescador R, Laybourn PJ, Najarian RC. Exon duplication and divergence in the human preproglucagon gene. Nature 1983;304:368–371.
15. Holst JJ, Ørskov C, Vagn-Nielsen O, Schwartz TW. Truncated glucagon-like peptide 1, an insulin-releasing hormone from the distal gut. FEBS Letters 1987;211:169–174.
16. Mojsov S, Weir GC, Habener JF. Insulinotropin: glucagon-like peptide I (7–37) co-encoded in the glucagon gene is a potent stimulator of insulin release in the perfused rat pancreas. J Clin Invest 1987;79:616–619.
17. Kreymann B, Williams G, Ghatei MA, Bloom SR. Glucagon-like peptide-1 [7–36]: a physiological incretin in man. Lancet 1987;2:1300–1304.
18. Nauck MA, Bartels E, Ørskov C, Ebert R, Creutzfeldt W. Additive insulinotropic effects of exogenous synthetic human gastric inhibitory polypeptide and glucagon-like peptide-1-(7–36) amide infused at near-physiological insulinotropic hormone and glucose concentrations. J Clin Endocrinol Metab 1993;76:912–917.
19. Nathan DM, Schreiber E, Fogel H, Mojsov S, Habener JF. Insulinotropic action of glucagon-like peptide 1 (7–37) in diabetic and non-diabetic subjects. Diabetes Care 1992;15:270–276.
20. Gutniak MK, Holst JJ, Ørskov C, Åhren B, Efendic S. Antidiabetogenic effect of glucagon-like peptide-1 (7–36) amide in normal subjects and patients with diabetes mellitus. N Engl J Med 1992;326:1316–1322.
21. Elrick H, Stimmler L, Hlad CJ, Arai Y. Plasma insulin response to oral and intravenous glucose administration. J Clin Endocrinol Metab 1964;24:1076–1082.
22. McIntyre N, Holdsworth CD, Turner DS. Intestinal factors in the control of insulin secretion. J Clin Endocrinol 1965;25:1317–1324.
23. Perley MJ, Kipnis DM. Plasma insulin responses to oral and intravenous glucose: studies in normal and diabetic subjects. J Clin Invest 1967;46:1954–1962.
24. Brown JC, Dryburgh JR. A gastric inhibitory polypeptide II. The complete amino acid sequence. Can J Biochem 1971;49:867–872.
25. Pederson RA, Schubert HE, Brown JC. Gastric inhibitory polypeptide. Its physiologic release and insulinotropic action in the dog. Diabetes 1975;24:1050–1056.
26. Buchan AMJ, Polak JM, Capella C, Solcia E, Pearse AGE. Electron immunocytochemical evidence of the K cell localisation of gastric inhibitory polypeptide (GIP) in man. Histochemistry 1978;56:37–44.
27. Bell GI. The glucagon super family: Precursor structure and gene organization. Peptides 1986;7(Suppl. 1):27–36.
28. Eissele R, Göke R, Willemer S, Harthus HP, Vermeer H, Arnold R, et al. Glucagon-like peptide-1 cells in the gastrointestinal tract and pancreas of rat, pig and man. Eur J Clin Invest 1992;22:283–291.
29. Ørskov C, Knuhtsen S, Baldissera FG, Poulsen SS, Nielsen OV, Holst JJ. Glucagon-like peptides GLP-1 and GLP-2, predicted products of the glucagon gene, are secreted separately from pig small intestine but not pancreas. Endocrinology 1986;119:1467–1475.
30. Ørskov C, Holst JJ, Seier-Poulsen S, Kirkegaard P. Pancreatic and intestinal processing of proglucagon in man. Diabetologia 1987;30:874–881.
31. Blackmore PF, Mojsov S, Exton JH, Habener JF. Absence of insulinotropic glucagon-like peptide-I (7–37) receptors on isolated rat liver hepatocytes. FEBS Lett 1991;283:7–10.
32. Ørskov C, Rabenhøj L, Wettergren A, Kofod H, Holst JJ. Tissue and plasma concentrations of amidated and glycine-extended glucagon-like peptide 1 in humans. Diabetes 1994;43:535–539.
33. Brubaker PL. Regulation of intestinal proglucagon-derived peptide secretion by intestinal regulatory peptides. Endocrinol 1991;128:3175–3182.
34. Mortensen K, Petersen LL, Orskov C. Colocalization of GLP-1 and GIP in human and porcine intestine. Ann N Y Acad Sci 2000;921:469–472.
35. Nauck MA. Glucagon-like peptide 1 (GLP-1): a potent gut hormone with a possible therapeutic perspective. Acta Diabetol 1998;35:117–129.
36. Vilsbøll T, Krarup T, Deacon CF, Madsbad S, Holst JJ. Reduced postprandial concentrations of intact biologically active glucagon-like peptide 1 in type 2 diabetic patients. Diabetes 2001;50:609–613.
37. Deacon CF, Nauck MA, Toft-Nielsen M, Pridal L, Willms B, Host JJ. Both subcutaneously and intravenously administered glucagon-like peptide 1 are rapidly degraded from the NH_2-terminus in type 2-diabetic patients and in healthy subjects. Diabetes 1995;44:1126–1131.

38. Mentlein R, Gallwitz B, Schmidt WE. Dipeptidyl-peptidase IV hydrolyses gastric inhibitory polypeptide, glucagon-like peptide-1 (7–36) amide, peptide histidine methionine and is responsible for their degradation in human serum. Eur J Biochem 1993;214:829–835.
39. Mentlein R. Dipeptidyl-peptidase IV (CD26) -role in the inactivation of regulatory peptides. Regul Pept 1999;85:9–24.
40. Grandt D, Sieburg B, Sievert J, Schimiczek M, Becker U, Holtmann D. Is GLP-1 (9–36) amide an endogenous antagonist at GLP-1 receptors? (abstract). Digestion 1994;55:302.
41. Knudsen LB, Pridal L. Glucagon-like peptide-1-(9–36) amide is a major metabolite of glucagon-like peptide-1-(7–36) amide after in vivo administration to dogs, and it acts as an antagonist on the pancreatic receptor. Eur J Pharmacol 1996;318:429–435.
42. Deacon CF, Plamboeck A, Moller S, Holst JJ. GLP-1-(9–36) amide reduces blood glucose in anesthetized pigs by a mechanism that does not involve insulin secretion. Am J Physiol (Endocrinol Metab) 2002;282:E873–9.
43. Vahl TP, Paty BW, Fuller BD, Prigeon RL, D'Alessio DA. Effects of GLP-1-(7–36) NH2, GLP-1-(7–37), and GLP-1-(9–36)NH2 on intravenous glucose tolerance and glucose-induced insulin secretion in healthy humans. J Clin Endocrinol Metab 2003;88:1772–1779.
44. Meier JJ, Gethmann A, Nauck MA, Götze O, Schmitz F, Deacon CF, et al. The glucagon-like peptide-1 metabolite GLP-1-(9–36) amide reduces postprandial glycemia independently of gastric emptying and insulin secretion in humans. Am J Physiol (Endocrinol Metab) 2006;290:E 1118–1123.
45. Ørskov C, Wettergren A, Holst JJ. Biological effects and metabolic rates of glucagonlike peptide-1 7–36 amide and glucagonlike peptide-1 7–37 in healthy subjects are indistinguishable. Diabetes 1993;42:658–661.
46. Meier JJ, Nauck MA, Kranz D, Holst JJ, Deacon CF, Gaeckler D, et al. Secretion, degradation, and elimination of glucagon-like peptide 1 and gastric inhibitory polypeptide in patients with chronic renal insufficiency and healthy control subjects. Diabetes 2004;53:654–662.
47. Plamboeck A, Holst JJ, Carr RD, Deacon CF. Neutral endopeptidase 24.11 and dipeptidyl peptidase IV are both mediators of the degradation of glucagon-like peptide 1 in the anaesthetised pig. Diabetologia 2005;48:1882–1890.
48. Plamboeck A, Holst JJ, Carr RD, Deacon CF. Neutral endopeptidase 24.11 and dipeptidyl peptidase IV are both involved in regulating the metabolic stability of glucagon-like peptide-1 in vivo. Adv Exp Med Biol 2003;524:303–312.
49. Marguet D, Baggio L, Kobayashi T, Bernard AM, Pierres M, Nielsen PF, et al. Enhanced insulin secretion and improved glucose tolerance in mice lacking CD26. Proc Natl Acad Sci U S A 2000;97(12):6874–6879.
50. Yamada Y, Hayami T, Nakamura K, Kaisaki PJ, Someya Y, Wang CZ, et al. Human gastric inhibitory polypeptide receptor: cloning of the gene (GIPR) and cDNA. Genomics 1995;29:773–776.
51. Yamada Y, Seino Y. Physiology of GIP -a lesson from GIP receptor knockout mice. Horm Metab Res 2004;36:771–774.
52. Yamada Y, Miyawaki K, Tsukiyama K, Harada N, Yamada C, Seino Y. Pancreatic and extrapancreatic effects of gastric inhibitory polypeptide. Diabetes 2006;55(Suppl. 2):S86–91.
53. Miyawaki K, Yamada Y, Ban N, Ihara Y, Tsukiyama K, Zhou H, et al. Inhibition of gastric inhibitory polypeptide signaling prevents obesity. Nat Med 2002;8:738–742.
54. Thorens B. Expression cloning of the pancreatic beta cell receptor for the gluco-incretin hormone glucagon-like peptide 1. Proc Natl Acad Sci U S A 1992;89:8641–8645.
55. Thorens B, Porret A, Buhler L, Deng SP, Morel P, Widmann C. Cloning and functional expression of the human islet GLP-1 receptor. Demonstration that exendin-4 is an agonist and exendin-(9–39) an antagonist of the receptor. Diabetes 1993;42:1678–1682.
56. Wei Y, Mojsov S. Tissue-specific expression of the human receptor for glucagon-like peptide-I: brain, heart and pancreatic forms have the same deduced amino acid sequences. FEBS Lett 1995;358:219–224.
57. Wei Y, Mojsov S. Distribution of GLP-1 and PACAP receptors in human tissues. Acta Physiol Scand 1996;157:355–357.
58. Drucker DJ, Philippe J, Mojsov S, Chick WL, Habener JF. Glucagon-like peptide I stimulates insulin gene expression and increases cyclic AMP levels in a rat islet cell line. Proc Natl Acad Sci U S A 1987;84:3434–3438.
59. Fehmann H-C, Habener JF. Insulinotropic hormone glucagon-like peptide-I (7–37) stimulation of proinsulin gene expression and proinsulin biosynthesis in insulinoma β TC-1 cells. Endocrinology 1992;130:159–166.
60. Brubaker PL, Drucker DJ. Minireview: Glucagon-like peptides regulate cell proliferation and apoptosis in the pancreas, gut, and central nervous system. Endocrinology 2004;145:2653–2659. Epub 2004 Mar 24.

61. Drucker DJ. The biology of incretin hormones. Cell Metabolism 2006;3:153–165.
62. Perfetti R, Zhou J, Doyle ME, Egan JM. Glucagon-like peptide-1 induces cell proliferation and pancreatic-duodenum homeobox-1 expression and increases endocrine cell mass in the pancreas of old, glucose-intolerant rats. Endocrinology 2000; 141:4600–4605.
63. Li Y, Hansotia T, Yusta B, Ris F, Halban PA, Drucker DJ. Glucagon-like peptide-1 receptor signaling modulates beta cell apoptosis. J Biol Chem 2003;278:471–478.
64. Buteau J, El-Assaad W, Rhodes CJ, Rosenberg L, Joly E, Prentki M. Glucagon-like peptide-1 prevents beta cell glucolipotoxicity. Diabetologia 2004;47:806–815.
65. Farilla L, Bulotta A, Hirshberg B, Li Calzi S, Khoury N, Noushmehr H, et al. Glucagon-like peptide 1 inhibits cell apoptosis and improves glucose responsiveness of freshly isolated human islets. Endocrinology 2003;144:5149–5158.
66. Miyawaki K, Yamada Y, Yano H, Niwa H, Ban N, Ihara Y, et al. Glucose intolerance caused by a defect in the entero-insular axis: A study in gastric inhibitory polypeptide receptor knockout mice. Proc Natl Acad Sci USA 1999;96:14843–14847.
67. Preitner F, Ibberson M, Franklin I, Binnert C, Pende M, Gjinovci A, et al. Gluco-incretins control insulin secretion at multiple levels as revealed in mice lacking GLP-1 and GIP receptors. J Clin Invest 2004;113:635–645.
68. Nauck MA, Heimesaat MM, Behle K, Holst JJ, Nauck MS, Ritzel R, et al. Effects of glucagon-like peptide 1 on counterregulatory hormone responses, cognitive functions, and insulin secretion during hyperinsulinemic, stepped hypoglycemic clamp experiments in healthy volunteers. J Clin Endocrinol Metab 2002;87:1239–1246.
69. Ørskov C, Holst JJ, Nielsen OV. Effect of truncated glucagon-like peptide-1 [proglucagon-(78–107) amide] on endocrine secretion from pig pancreas, antrum, and nonantral stomach. Endocrinology 1988;123:2009–2013.
70. Wettergren A, Schjoldager B, Mortensen PE, Myhre J, Christiansen J, Holst JJ. Truncated GLP-1 (proglucagon 78–107-amide) inhibits gastric and pancreatic functions in man. Dig Dis Sci 1993;38:665–673.
71. Nauck MA, Niedereichholz U, Ettler R, Holst JJ, Ørskov C, Ritzel R, et al. Glucagon-like peptide 1 inhibition of gastric emptying outweighs its insulinotropic effects in healthy humans. Am J Physiol (Endocrinol Metab) 1997;273: E 981–988.
72. Meier JJ, Kemmeries G, Holst JJ, Nauck MA. Erythromycin antagonizes the deceleration of gastric emptying by glucagon-like peptide 1 and unmasks its insulinotropic effect in healthy subjects. Diabetes 2005;54:2212–2218.
73. Little TJ, Pilichiewicz AN, Russo A, Phillips L, Jones KL, Nauck MA, et al. Effects of intravenous glucagon-like peptide-1 on gastric emptying and intragastric distribution in healthy subjects: relationships with postprandial glycemic and insulinemic responses. J Clin Endocrinol Metab 2006;91:1916–1923.
74. Flint A, Raben A, Astrup A, Holst JJ. Glucagon-like peptide-1 promotes satiety and suppresses energy intake in humans. J Clin Invest 1998;101:515–520.
75. Flint A, Raben A, Ersboll AK, Holst JJ, Astrup A. The effect of physiological levels of glucagon-like peptide-1 on appetite, gastric emptying, energy and substrate metabolism in obesity. Int J Obes Relat Metab Disord 2001;25:781–792.
76. Gutzwiller JP, Drewe J, Göke B, Schmidt H, Rohrer B, Lareida J, et al. Glucagon-like peptide-1 promotes satiety and reduces food intake in patients with diabetes mellitus type 2. Am J Physiol (Integr Regul Physiol) 1999;276:R 1541–1544.
77. Gutzwiller JP, Göke B, Drewe J, Hildebrand P, Ketterer S, Handschin D, et al. Glucagon-like peptide-1: a potent regulator of food intake in humans. Gut 1999;44:81–86.
78. Verdich C, Flint A, Gutzwiller JP, Naslund E, Beglinger C, Hellstrom PM, et al. A meta-analysis of the effect of glucagon-like peptide-1 (7–36) amide on ad libitum energy intake in humans. J Clin Endocrinol Metab 2001;86:4382–4389.
79. Burcelin R, Da Costa A, Drucker D, Thorens B. Glucose competence of the hepatoportal vein sensor requires the presence of an activated glucagon-like peptide-1 receptor. Diabetes 2001;50:1720–1728.
80. Wang Z, Wang RM, Owji AA, Smith DM, Ghatei MA, Bloom SR. Glucagon-like peptide-1 is a physiological incretin in rat. J Clin Invest 1995;95:417–421.
81. Kolligs F, Fehmann HC, Göke R, Göke B. Reduction of the incretin effect in rats by the glucagon-like peptide 1 receptor antagonist exendin (9–39) amide. Diabetes 1995;44:16–19.
82. Scrocchi LA, Brown TJ, MaClusky N, Brubaker PL, Auerbach AB, Joyner AL, et al. Glucose intolerance but normal satiety in mice with a null mutation in the glucagon-like peptide 1 receptor gene. Nat Med 1996;2:1254–1258.
83. Schirra J, Sturm K, Leicht P, Arnold R, Göke B, Katschinski M. Exendin (9–39) amide is an antagonist

of glucagon-like peptide-1 (7–36) amide in humans. J Clin Invest 1998;101:1421–1430.
84. Schirra J, Nicolaus M, Roggel R, Katschinski M, Storr M, Woerle HJ, et al. Endogenous glucagon-like peptide 1 controls endocrine pancreatic secretion and antro-pyloro-duodenal motility in humans. Gut 2006;55:243–251.
85. Edwards CMB, Todd JF, Mahmoudi M, Wang Z, Wang RM, Ghatei MA, et al. GLP-1 has a physiological role in the control of postprandial glucose in man. Studies with the antagonist exendin 9–39. Diabetes 1999;48:86–93.
86. Nauck M, Stöckmann F, Ebert R, Creutzfeldt W. Reduced incretin effect in Type 2 (non-insulin-dependent) diabetes. Diabetologia 1986;29:46–54.
87. Krarup T, Vilsbøll T, Madsbad S, Larsen S, Holst JJ, Højberg PV, et al. The incretin effect is preserved in glucose tolerant patients with chronic pancreatitis -but reduced in patients with chronic pancreatitis and secondary diabetes (abstract 0657). Diabetologia 2006;49(Suppl. 1):399.
88. Toft-Nielsen MB, Damholt MB, Madsbad S, Hilsted LM, Hughes TE, Michelsen BK, et al. Determinants of the impaired secretion of glucagon-like peptide-1 in type 2 diabetic patients. J Clin Endocrinol Metab 2001;86:3717–3723.
89. Mitrakou A, Kelley D, Veneman T, Jenssen T, Pangburn T, Reilly J, et al. Contribution of abnormal muscle and liver glucose metabolism to postprandial hyperglycemia in NIDDM. Diabetes 1990;39:1381–1390.
90. Jones IR, Owens DR, Luzio S, Williams S, Hayes TM. The glucose dependent insulinotropic polypeptide response to oral glucose and mixed meals is increased in patients with type 2 (non-insulin-dependent) diabetes mellitus. Diabetologia 1989;32:668–677.
91. Creutzfeldt W, Ebert R, Nauck M, Stöckmann F. Disturbances of the entero-insular axis. Scand J Gastroenterol 1983;82(Suppl.):111–119.
92. Ding WG, Renström E, Rorsman P, Buschard K, Gromada J. Glucagon-like peptide I and glucose-dependent insulinotropic polypeptide stimulate Ca2+-induced secretion in rat alpha-cells by a protein kinase A-mediated mechanism. Diabetes 1997;46:792–800.
93. Jones IR, Owens DR, Moody AJ, Luzio SD, Morris T, Hayes TM. The effects of glucose-dependent insulinotropic polypeptide infused at physiological concentrations in normal subjects and Type 2 (non-insulin-dependent) diabetic patients on glucose tolerance and B-cell secretion. Diabetologia 1987;30:707–712.
94. Nauck MA, Baller B, Meier JJ. Gastric inhibitory polypeptide and glucagon-like peptide-1 in the pathogenesis of type 2 diabetes. Diabetes 2004;53(Suppl. 3):S190–6.
95. Meier JJ, Nauck MA. Incretins and the development of type 2 diabetes. Curr Diab Rep 2006;6:194–201.
96. Kjems LL, Holst JJ, Vølund A, Madsbad S. The influence of GLP-1 on glucose-stimulated insulin secretion: effects on beta-cell sensitivity in type 2 and nondiabetic subjects. Diabetes 2003;52:380–386.
97. Meier JJ, Gallwitz B, Salmen S, Goetze O, Holst JJ, Schmidt WE, et al. Normalization of glucose concentrations and deceleration of gastric emptying after solid meals during intravenous glucagon-like peptide 1 in patients with type 2 diabetes. J Clin Endocrinol Metab 2003;88:2719–2725.
98. Nauck MA. Therapeutic potential of glucagon-like peptide 1 in type 2 diabetes. Diabetic Medicine 1996;13(Suppl.):S39–S43.
99. Amland PF, Jorde R, Aanderup S, Burhol PG, Giercksky K-E. Effects of intravenously infused porcine GIP on serum insulin, plasma C-peptide, and pancreatic polypeptide in non-insulin-dependent diabetes in the fasting state. Scand J Gastroenterol 1985;20:315–320.
100. Nauck MA, Schmidt WE, Ebert R, Striezel J, Cantor P, Hoffmann G, et al. Insulinotropic properties of synthetic gastric inhibitory peptide in man: interactions with glucose, phenylalanine, and cholezystokinin-8. J. Clin. Endocrinol. Metab. 1989;69:654–662.
101. Nauck MA, Homberger E, Siegel EG, Allen RC, Eaton RP, Ebert R, et al. Incretin effects of increasing glucose loads in man calculated from venous insulin and C-peptide responses. J Clin Endocrinol Metab 1986;63:492–498.
102. Holst JJ, Gromada J, Nauck MA. The pathogenesis of NIDDM involves a defective expression of the GIP receptor. Diabetologia 1997;40:984–986.
103. Meier JJ, Nauck MA. Incretins and the development of type 2 diabetes. Curr Diab Rep 2006;6:194–201.
104. Vilsbøll T, Knop FK, Krarup T, Johansen A, Madsbad S, Larsen S, et al. The pathophysiology of diabetes involves a defective amplification of the late-phase insulin response to glucose by glucose-dependent insulinotropic polypeptide-regardless of etiology and phenotype. J Clin Endocrinol Metab. 2003;88:4897–4903.
105. Hinke SA, Lynn F, Ehses J, Pamir N, Manhart S, Kuhn-Wache K, et al. Glucose-dependent insulinotropic polypeptide (GIP): development of

DP IV-resistant analogues with therapeutic potential. Adv Exp Med Biol 2003;524:293–301.
106. Gault VA, O'Harte FP, Harriott P, Mooney MH, Green BD, Flatt PR. Effects of the novel (Pro3) GIP antagonist and exendin (9–39) amide on GIP- and GLP-1-induced cyclic AMP generation, insulin secretion and postprandial insulin release in obese diabetic (ob/ob) mice: evidence that GIP is the major physiological incretin. Diabetologia 2003;46:222–230.
107. Irwin N, Gault VA, Green BD, Greer B, Harriott P, Bailey CJ, et al. Antidiabetic potential of two novel fatty acid derivatised, N-terminally modified analogues of glucose-dependent insulinotropic polypeptide (GIP): N-AcGIP(LysPAL16) and N-AcGIP(LysPAL37). Biol Chem 2005;386:679–687.
108. Pederson RA, Brown JC. Interaction of gastric inhibitory polypeptide, glucose, and arginine on insulin and glucagon secretion from the perfused rat pancreas. Endocrinol 1978;103:610–615.
109. Meier JJ, Gallwitz B, Siepmann N, Holst JJ, Deacon CF, Schmidt WE, et al. Gastric inhibitory polypeptide (GIP) dose-dependently stimulates glucagon secretion in healthy human subjects at euglycaemia. Diabetologia 2003;46:798–801.
110. Nauck MA, Kleine N, Ørskov C, Holst JJ, Willms B, Creutzfeldt W. Normalization of fasting hyperglycaemia by exogenous glucagon-like peptide 1 (7–36 amide) in type 2 (non-insulin-dependent) diabetic patients. Diabetologia 1993;36:741–744.
111. Toft-Nielsen MB, Madsbad S, Holst JJ. Determinants of the effectiveness of glucagon-like peptide-1 in type 2 diabetes. J Clin Endocrinol Metab 2001;86:3853–3860.
112. Nauck MA, Meier JJ. Glucagon-like peptide 1 (GLP-1) and its derivatives in the treatment of diabetes. Regul Pept 2005;128:135–148.
113. Willms B, Werner J, Holst JJ, Ørskov C, Creutzfeldt W, Nauck MA. Gastric emptying, glucose responses, and insulin secretion after a liquid test meal: effects of exogenous glucagon-like peptide-1 (GLP-1)-(7–36) amide in type 2 (noninsulin-dependent) diabetic patients. J Clin Endocrinol Metab 1996;81:327–332.
114. Zander M, Madsbad S, Madsen JL, Holst JJ. Effect of 6-week course of glucagon-like peptide 1 on glycaemic control, insulin sensitivity, and beta-cell function in type 2 diabetes: a parallel-group study. Lancet 2002;359:824–830.
115. Meier JJ, Weyhe D, Michaely M, Senkal M, Zumtobel V, Nauck MA, et al. Intravenous glucagon-like peptide 1 normalizes blood glucose after major surgery in patients with type 2 diabetes. Crit Care Med 2004;32:848–851.
116. Nauck MA, Walberg J, Vethacke A, El Ouaghlidi A, Senkal M, Holst JJ, et al. Blood glucose control in healthy subject and patients receiving intravenous glucose infusion or total parenteral nutrition using glucagon-like peptide 1. Regul Pept 2004;118:89–97.
117. Eng J, Kleinman WA, Singh L, Singh G, Raufman JP. Isolation and characterization of exendin-4, an exendin-3 analogue, from Heloderma suspectum venom. Further evidence for an exendin receptor on dispersed acini from guinea pig pancreas. J Biol Chem 1992;267:7402–7405.
118. Fehmann HC, Jiang J, Schweinfurth J, Wheeler MB, Boyd AE, 3rd, Goke B. Stable expression of the rat GLP-I receptor in CHO cells: activation and binding characteristics utilizing GLP-I(7–36)-amide, oxyntomodulin, exendin-4, and exendin(9–39). Peptides. 1994;15(3):453–456.
119. DeFronzo RA, Ratner RE, Han J, Kim DD, Fineman MS, Baron AD. Effects of exenatide (exendin-4) on glycemic control and weight over 30 weeks in metformin-treated patients with type 2 diabetes. Diabetes Care 2005;28:1092–1100.
120. Buse JB, Henry RR, Han J, Kim DD, Fineman M, Baron AD, et al. Effects of exenatide (exendin-4) on glycemic control over 30 weeks in sulfonylurea-treated patients with type 2 diabetes. Diabetes Care 2004;27:2628–2635.
121. Kendall DM, Riddle MC, Rosenstock J, Zhuang D, Kim DD, Fineman MS, et al. Effects of exenatide (exendin-4) on glycemic control over 30 weeks in patients with type 2 diabetes treated with metformin and a sulfonylurea. Diabetes Care 2005;28: 1083–1091.
122. Zinman B, Hoogwerf B, Garcia SG, Milton D, Giaconia J, Kim D, et al. Safety and efficacy of exenatide in patients with type 2 diabetes mellitus using thiazolidindiones with or without metformin (abstract 117-OR). Diabetes 2006; 55(Suppl. 1):A 28.
123. Ratner RE, Stonehouse A, Gao H-Y, Poon T, Kim D. Exenatide maintains glycaemic control for 2 years in patients with type 2 diabetes: data from an ongoing, open-label study (abstract). Diabetologia 2005;48(Suppl. 1):A 288–289.
124. Heine RJ, Van Gaal LF, Johns D, Mihm MJ, Widel MH, Brodows RG. Exenatide versus insulin glargine in patients with suboptimally controlled type 2 diabetes: a randomized trial. Ann Intern Med 2005;143:559–569.
125. Nauck MA, Duran S, Kim D, Johns D, Northrup J, Festa A, et al. A comparison of twice-daily exenatide and biphasic insulin aspart in patients with type 2

diabetes who were suboptimally controlled with sulfonylurea and metformin: a non-inferiority study. Diabetologia 2006;50:259–267. Epub Dec. 8, 2006.
126. Knudsen LB, Nielsen PF, Huusfeldt PO, Johansen NL, Madsen K, Pedersen FZ, et al. Potent derivatives of glucagon-like peptide-1 with pharmacokinetic properties suitable for once daily administration. J Med Chem 2000;43:1664–1669.
127. Agersø H, Jensen LB, Elbrond B, Rolan P, Zdravkovic M. The pharmacokinetics, pharmacodynamics, safety and tolerability of NN2211, a new long-acting GLP-1 derivative, in healthy men. Diabetologia 2002;45:195–202.
128. Elbrønd B, Jakobsen G, Larsen S, Agersø H, Jensen LB, Rolan P, et al. Pharmacokinetics, pharmacodynamics, safety, and tolerability of a single-dose of NN2211, a long-acting glucagon-like peptide 1 derivative, in healthy male subjects. Diabetes Care 2002;25:1398–1404.
129. Bjerre Knudsen L, Møller Knudsen S, Wilken M, Colding-Jørgensen M, Plum A, Agersø H, et al. Plasma protein binding of NN2211, a long-acting derivative of GLP-1, is important for its efficacy. Diabetes 2005;52(Suppl. 1):A 321–322.
130. Vilsbøll T, Zdravkovic M, Le-Thi T, Krarup T, Schmitz O, Courreges J, et al. Liraglutide significantly improves glycemic control, and lowers body weight without risk of either major or minor hypoglycemic episodes in subjects with type 2 diabetes (abstract 115-OR). Diabetes 2006;55(Suppl. 1):A 27–28.
131. Madsbad S, Schmitz O, Ranstam J, Jakobsen G, Matthews DR. Improved glycemic control with no weight increase in patients with type 2 diabetes after once-daily treatment with the long-acting glucagon-like peptide 1 analog liraglutide (NN2211): A 12-week, double-blind, randomized, controlled trial. Diabetes Care 2004;27:1335–1342.
132. Nauck MA, Hompesch M, Filipczak R, Le TD, Zdravkovic M, Gumprecht J. Five weeks of treatment with the GLP-1 analogue liraglutide improves glycaemic control and lowers body weight in subjects with type 2 diabetes. Exp Clin Endocrinol Diabetes. 2006;114:417–423.
133. Feinglos MN, Saad MF, Pi-Sunyer FX, An B, Santiago O. Effects of liraglutide (NN2211), a long-acting GLP-1 analogue, on glycaemic control and bodyweight in subjects with Type 2 diabetes. Diabetic Med 2005;22:1016–1023.
134. Gedulin BR, Smith P, Prickett KS, Tryon M, Barnhill S, Reynolds J, et al. Dose-response for glycaemic and metabolic changes 28 days after single injection of long-acting release exenatide in diabetic fatty Zucker rats. Diabetologia 2005;48:1380–1385.
135. Kim D, MacConnell L, Zhuang D, Scnabel C, Taylor K, Li W-I, et al. Safety and efficacy of a once-weekly, long-acting release formulation of exenatide over 15 weeks in patients with type 2 diabetes (abstract 487-P). Diabetes 2006;55(Suppl 1):A 116.
136. Kim JG, Baggio LL, Bridon DP, Castaigne JP, Robitaille MF, Jette L, et al. Development and characterization of a glucagon-like peptide 1-albumin conjugate: the ability to activate the glucagon-like peptide 1 receptor in vivo. Diabetes 2003;52:751–759.
137. Baggio LL, Huang Q, Brown TJ, Drucker DJ. A recombinant human glucagon-like peptide (GLP)-1-albumin protein (albugon) mimics peptidergic activation of GLP-1 receptor-dependent pathways coupled with satiety, gastrointestinal motility, and glucose homeostasis. Diabetes 2004;53:2492–2500.
138. Kieffer TJ, McIntosh CH, Pederson RA. Degradation of glucose-dependent insulinotropic polypeptide and truncated glucagon-like peptide 1 in vitro and in vivo by dipeptidyl peptidase IV. Endocrinology 1995;136:3585–3596.
139. De Meester I, Durinx C, Bal G, Proost P, Struyf S, Goossens F, et al. Natural substrates of dipeptidyl peptidase IV. Adv Exp Med Biol 2000;477:67–87.
140. De Meester I, Lambeir AM, Proost P, Scharpe S. Dipeptidyl peptidase IV substrates. An update on in vitro peptide hydrolysis by human DPPIV. Adv Exp Med Biol 2003;524:3–17.
141. Deacon CF, Nauck MA, Meier J, Hücking K, Holst JJ. Degradation of endogenous and exogenous gastric inhibitory polypeptide in healthy and in type 2 diabetic subjects as revealed using a new assay for the intact peptide. J Clin Endocrinol Metab 2000;85:3575–3581.
142. Deacon CF, Johnsen AH, Holst JJ. Degradation of glucagon-like peptide-1 by human plasma in vitro yields an N-terminally truncated peptide that is a major endogenous metabolite in vivo. J Clin Endocrinol Metab 1995;80:952–957.
143. Ørskov C, Wettergren A, Holst JJ. Secretion of the incretin hormones glucagon-like peptide-1 and gastric inhibitory polypeptide correlates with insulin secretion in normal man throughout the day. Scand J Gastroenterol 1996;31:665–670.
144. Nauck MA, El-Ouaghlidi A, Gabrys B, Hücking K, Holst JJ, Deacon CF, et al. Secretion of incretin hormones (GIP and GLP-1) and incretin effect after oral glucose in first-degree relatives of patients with type 2 diabetes. Regul Pept 2004;122:209–217.
145. Drucker DJ, Nauck MA. The incretin system: glucagon-like peptide-1 receptor agonists and dipeptidyl peptidase-4 inhibitors in type 2 diabetes. Lancet 2006;368:1696–1705.

146. Åhren B, Simonsson E, Larsson H, Landin-Olsson M, Torgeirsson H, Jansson P-A, et al. Inhibition of dipeptidyl peptidase IV improves metabolic control over a 4-week study period in type 2 diabetes. Diabetes Care 2002;25:869–875.
147. Herman GA, Stevens C, Van Dyck K, Bergman A, Yi B, De Smet M, et al. Pharmacokinetics and pharmacodynamics of sitagliptin, an inhibitor of dipeptidyl peptidase IV, in healthy subjects: results from two randomized, double-blind, placebo-controlled studies with single oral doses. Clin Pharmacol Ther 2005;78:675–688.
148. Aschner P, Kipnes M, Lunceford J, Mickel C, Davies M, Williams-Herman D. Sitagliptin monotherapy improved glycemic control in the fasting and postprandial states and beta-cell function after 24 weeks in patients with type 2 diabetes (T2DM) (abstract 1995-PO). Diabetes 2006;55 (Suppl. 1):A 462.
149. Charbonnel B, Karasik A, Liu J, Wu M, Meininger G. Efficacy and safety of the dipeptidyl peptidase-4 inhibitor sitagliptin added to ongoing metformin therapy in patients with type 2 diabetes inadequately controlled with metformin alone. Diabetes Care. 2006;29:2638–2643.
150. Åhren B, Landin-Olsson M, Jansson PA, Svensson M, Holmes D, Schweizer A. Inhibition of dipeptidyl peptidase-4 reduces glycemia, sustains insulin levels, and reduces glucagon levels in type 2 diabetes. J Clin Endocrinol Metab 2004;89:2078–2084.
151. Pratley RE, Jauffret-Kamel S, Galbreath E, Holmes D. Twelve-week monotherapy with the DPP-4 inhibitor vildagliptin improves glycemic control in subjects with type 2 diabetes. Horm Metab Res. 2006;38:423–428.
152. Åhren B, Pacini G, Foley JE, Schweizer A. Improved meal-related beta-cell function and insulin sensitivity by the dipeptidyl peptidase-IV inhibitor vildagliptin in metformin-treated patients with type 2 diabetes over 1 year. Diabetes Care 2005;28:1936–1940.
153. Åhren B, Gomis R, Standl E, Mills D, Schweizer A. Twelve- and 52-week efficacy of the dipeptidyl peptidase IV inhibitor LAF237 in metformin-treated patients with type 2 diabetes. Diabetes Care 2004;27:2874–2880.
154. Matikainen N, Manttari S, Schweizer A, Ulvestad A, Mills D, Dunning BE, et al. Vildagliptin therapy reduces postprandial intestinal triglyceride-rich lipoprotein particles in patients with type 2 diabetes. Diabetologia. 2006;49:2049–2057. Epub 2006 Jul 1.
155. Dejager S, Lebeaut A, Couturier A, Schweizer A. Sustained reduction in HbA_{1c} during one-year treatment with vildagliptin in patients with type 2 diabetes (T2DM) (abstract 120-OR). Diabetes 2006;55(Suppl. 1):A 29.
156. Rosenstock J, Baron MA, Schweizer A, Mills D, Dejager S. Vildagliptin is as effective as rosiglitazone in lowering HbA_{1c} but without weight gain in drug-naive patients with type 2 diabetes (T2DM) (abstract 557-P). Diabetes 2006;55(Suppl. 1):A 133.
157. Hansen BC, Bjenning C, Bjerrre Knudsen L. Sustained appetite suppression and weight loss in obese rhesus monkeys treated with a long-acting GLP-1 derivative, NN2211 (abstract). Diabetologia 2001;44(Suppl. 1):A 196.
158. Nauck MA, Hompesch M, Filipicazak R, Le TDT, Nielsen LL, Zdravkovic M, et al. Liraglutide significantly improves glycemic control and reduces body weight compared with glimepiride as add-on to metformin in type 2 diabetes (abstract). Diabetes 2004;53(Suppl. 2):A 83.
159. Scott R, Herman G, Zhao P, Chen X, Wu M, Stein P. Twelve-week efficacy and tolerability of MK-0431, a dipeptidyl peptidase IV (DPP-IV) inhibitor, in the treatment of type 2 diabetes (T2D) (abstract 41-OR). Diabetes 2005;54(Suppl. 1):A 10–11.
160. Hanefeld M, Herman G, Mickel C, McGowan A, Wu M, Zhao P, et al. Effect of MK-0431, a dipeptidyl peptidase IV (DPP-IV) inhibitor, on glycemic control after 12 weeks in patients with type 2 diabetes (abstract 791). Diabetologia 2005;48(Suppl. 1):A 287–288.
161. Brazg R, Thomas K, Zhao P, Xu L, Chen X, Stein P. Effect of adding MK-0431 to ongoing metformin therapy in type 2 diabetic patients who have inadequate glycemic control on metformin (abstract). Diabetes 2005;54(Suppl. 1):A 3.
162. Demuth HU, McIntosh CH, Pederson RA. Type 2 diabetes -therapy with dipeptidyl peptidase IV inhibitors. Biochim Biophys Acta 2005;1751:33–44.
163. Blonde L, Klein EJ, Han J, Zhang B, Mac SM, Poon TH, et al. Interim analysis of the effects of exenatide treatment on A1C, weight and cardiovascular risk factors over 82 weeks in 314 overweight patients with type 2 diabetes. Diabetes Obes Metab 2006;8:436–447.
164. Kolterman O, Gottlieb A, Prickett K, Gaines E, Young A. Dose–response for inhibition of glucagon secretion and gastric emptying by synthetic exendin-4 (AC2993) in subjects with Type 2 diabetes (abstract). Diabetes 2000;49 (Suppl. 1):A 114.
165. Dardik B, Valentin M, Schwartzkopf C, Gutierrez C, Stevens D, Russell ME, et al. NVP-LAF237, a dipeptidyl peptidase IV inhibitor,

improves glucose tolerance and delays gastric emptying in obese insulin resistant Cynomolgus monkeys (abstract 1292-P). Diabetes 2003;52(Suppl. 1):A 322.
166. Nathan DM, Buse JB, Davidson MB, Heine RJ, Holman RR, Sherwin R, et al. Management of hyperglycemia in type 2 diabetes: A consensus algorithm for the initiation and adjustment of therapy: a consensus statement from the American Diabetes Association and the European Association for the Study of Diabetes. Diabetes Care 2006;29:1963–1972.
167. Nathan DM, Buse JB, Davidson MB, Heine RJ, Holman RR, Sherwin R, et al. Management of hyperglycaemia in type 2 diabetes: a consensus algorithm for the initiation and adjustment of therapy. A consensus statement from the American Diabetes Association and the European Association for the Study of Diabetes. Diabetologia 2006;49:1711–1721.
168. Yki-Järvinen H. Combination therapies with insulin in type 2 diabetes. Diabetes Care 2001;24:758–767.
169. UK prospective diabetes study (UKPDS) group. Effect of intensive blood-glucose control with metformin on complications in overweight patients with type 2 diabetes (UKPDS 34). Lancet 1998;352:854–865.
170. Williams-Herman D, Goldstein BJ, Feinglos MN, Lunceford J, Johnson J. Initial combination therapy with sitagliptin, a dipeptidyl peptidase-4 inhibitor, and metformin provides substantial glycemic improvement and HBA1c goal attainment in patients with type 2 diabetes mellitus (T2DM) (abstract P880). Diabetic Med 2006;23(Suppl. 4):319.
171. Yki-Järvinen H. Thiazolidinediones. N Engl J Med 2004;351:1106–1118.
172. Yki-Järvinen H. The PROactive study: some answers, many questions. Lancet 2005;366:1241–1242.
173. Fineman MS, Shen LZ, Taylor K, Kim DD, Baron AD. Effectiveness of progressive dose-escalation of exenatide (exendin-4) in reducing dose-limiting side effects in subjects with type 2 diabetes. Diabetes Metab Res Rev 2004;20:411–417.
174. Nauck MA, Hompesch M, Filipczak R, Le TD, Zdravkovic M, Gumprecht J. Five weeks of treatment with the GLP-1 analogue liraglutide improves glycaemic control and lowers body weight in subjects with Type 2 diabetes. Exp Clin Endocrinol Diabetes 2006;114:417–423.
175. Kolterman OG, Kim DD, Shen L, Ruggles JA, Nielsen LL, Fineman MS, et al. Pharmacokinetics, pharmacodynamics, and safety of exenatide in patients with type 2 diabetes mellitus. Am Health Syst Pharm 2005;62:173–181.
176. Linnebjerg H, Kothare PA, Skrivanek Z, de la Pena A, Atkins M, Ernest CS, et al. Exenatide: effect of injection time on postprandial glucose in patients with Type 2 diabetes. Diabet Med 2006;23:240–245.
177. Linnebjerg H, Park S, Kothare P, Trautmann M, Mace K, Fineman M, et al. Effects of exenatide on gastric emptying and postprandial glucose in type 2 diabetes (abstract 116-OR). Diabetes 2006;55 (Suppl. 1):A 28.
178. Fineman MS, Bicsak TA, Shen LZ, Taylor K, Gaines E, Varns A, et al. Effect on glycemic control of exenatide (synthetic exendin-4) additive to existing metformin and/or sulfonylurea treatment in patients with type 2 diabetes. Diabetes Care 2003;26:2370–2377.
179. Herman GA, Bergman A, Stevens C, Kotey P, Yi B, Zhao P, et al. Effect of single oral doses of sitagliptin, a dipeptidyl peptidase-4 inhibitor, on incretin and plasma glucose levels after an oral glucose tolerance test in patients with type 2 diabetes. J Clin Endocrinol Metab 2006;91:4612–4619.
180. Riddle MC, Rosenstock J, Gerich J. The treat-to-target trial: randomized addition of glargine or human NPH insulin to oral therapy of type 2 diabetic patients. Diabetes Care 2003;26:3080–3086.
181. Yki-Järvinen H, Kauppinen-Makelin R, Tiikkainen M, Vahatalo M, Virtamo H, Nikkila K, et al. Insulin glargine or NPH combined with metformin in type 2 diabetes: the LANMET study. Diabetologia 2006;49:442–451.
182. El-Ouaghlidi A, Rehring E, Schweizer A, Holmes D, Nauck MA. The dipeptidyl peptidase IV inhibitor LAF237 does not accentuate reactive hypoglycaemia caused by the sulfonylurea glibenclamide administered before an oral glucose load in healthy subjects (abstract 507-P). Diabetes 2003;52(Suppl. 1):A 118.
183. Henry RR, Ratner RE, Stonehouse AH, Guan X, Poon T, Malone JK, et al. Exenatide maintained glycemic control with associated weight reduction over 2 years in patients with type 2 diabetes (abstract 485-P). Diabetes 2006;55(Suppl. 1):A 116.
184. Ritzel R, Ørskov C, Holst JJ, Nauck MA. Pharmacokinetic, insulinotropic, and glucagonostatic properties of GLP-1 [7–36 amide] after subcutaneous injection in healthy volunteers. Dose–response-relationships. Diabetologia 1995;38:720–725.
185. Buse JB, Henry R, Han J, Kim DD, Fineman MS, Baron AD. Effect of exenatide (exendin-4) on glycemic control and safety over 30 weeks in sulfonylurea-treated patients with type 2 diabetes (abstract 352-OR). Diabetes 2004;53(Suppl. 2):A 82.
186. Dang NH, Morimoto C. CD26: an expanding role in immune regulation and cancer. Histol. Histopathol. 2002;17(4):1213–1226.

187. Raz I, Hanefeld M, Xu L, Caria C, Williams-Herman D, Khatami H. Efficacy and safety of the dipeptidyl peptidase-4 inhibitor sitagliptin as monotherapy in patients with type 2 diabetes mellitus. Diabetologia 2006;49:2564–2571. [Epub 2006 Sep 26.]
188. Haffner SM, Lehto S, Ronnemaa T, Pyorälä K, Laakso M. Mortality from coronary heart disease in subjects with type 2 diabetes and in nondiabetic subjects with and without prior myocardial infarction. N Engl J Med 1998;339:229–234.
189. U.K. prospective diabetes study group. U.K. prospective diabetes study 16: Overview of 6 years therapy of type II diabetes: A progressive disease (Perspectives in diabetes). Diabetes 1995;44:1249–1258.
190. Levy J, Atkinson AB, Bell PM, McCance DR, Hadden DR. Beta-cell deterioration determines the onset and rate of progression of secondary dietary failure in type 2 diabetes mellitus: the 10-year follow-up of the Belfast Diet Study. Diabet Med 1998;15:290–296.
191. Turner RC, Cull CA, Frighi V, Holman RR. Glycemic control with diet, sulfonylurea, metformin, or insulin in patients with type 2 diabetes mellitus: progressive requirement for multiple therapies (UKPDS 49). UK Prospective Diabetes Study (UKPDS) Group. J Am Med Ass 1999;281:2005–2012.
192. Kahn SE, Haffner SM, Heise MA, Herman WH, Holman RR, Jones NP, et al. Glycemic durability of rosiglitazone, metformin, or glyburide monotherapy. N Engl J Med 2006;355:2427–2443.
193. Butler AE, Janson J, Bonner-Weir S, Ritzel R, Rizza RA, Butler PC. Beta-cell deficit and increased beta-cell apoptosis in humans with type 2 diabetes. Diabetes 2003;52:102–110.
194. Gepts W. Pathologic anatomy of the pancreas in juvenile diabetes mellitus. Diabetes. 1965;14(10):619–633.
195. Meier JJ, Bhushan A, Butler AE, Rizza RA, Butler PC. Sustained beta cell apoptosis in patients with long-standing type 1 diabetes: indirect evidence for islet regeneration? Diabetologia. 2005;48:2221–2228. [Epub 2005 Oct 5.]
196. Meier JJ, Bhushan A, Butler PC. The potential for stem cell therapy in diabetes. Pediatr Res. 2006;59:65R–73R.
197. Buteau J, Roduit R, Susini S, Prentki M. Glucagon-like peptide-1 promotes DNA synthesis, activates phosphatidylinositol 3-kinase and increases transcription factor pancreatic and duodenal homeobox gene 1 (PDX-1) DNA binding activity in beta (INS-1)-cells. Diabetologia 1999;42:856–864.
198. Buteau J, Foisy S, Joly E, Prentki M. Glucagon-like peptide 1 induces pancreatic beta-cell proliferation via transactivation of the epidermal growth factor receptor. Diabetes 2003;52:124–132.
199. Xu G, Stoffers DA, Habener JF, Bonner-Weir S. Exendin-4 stimulates both beta-cell replication and neogenesis, resulting in increased beta-cell mass and improved glucose tolerance in diabetic rats. Diabetes 1999;48:2270–2276.
200. Tourrel C, Bailbe D, Meile MJ, Kergoat M, Portha B. Glucagon-like peptide-1 and exendin-4 stimulate beta-cell neogenesis in streptozotocin-treated newborn rats resulting in persistently improved glucose homeostasis at adult age. Diabetes 2001;50:1562–1570.
201. Tourrel C, Bailbe D, Lacorne M, Meile MJ, Kergoat M, Portha B. Persistent improvement of type 2 diabetes in the Goto-Kakizaki rat model by expansion of the beta-cell mass during the prediabetic period with glucagon-like peptide-1 or exendin-4. Diabetes 2002;51:1443–1452.
202. Stoffers DA, Desai BM, DeLeon DD, Simmons RA. Neonatal exendin-4 prevents the development of diabetes in the intrauterine growth retarded rat. Diabetes 2003;52:734–740.
203. Farilla L, Hui H, Bertolotto C, Kang E, Bulotta A, Di Mario U, et al. Glucagon-like peptide-1 promotes islet cell growth and inhibits apoptosis in Zucker diabetic rats. Endocrinology 2002;143:4397–4408.
204. De Leon DD, Deng S, Madani R, Ahima RS, Drucker DJ, Stoffers DA. Role of endogenous glucagon-like peptide-1 in islet regeneration after partial pancreatectomy. Diabetes 2003;52:365–371.
205. Rolin B, Larsen MO, Gotfredsen CF, Deacon CF, Carr RD, Wilken M, et al. The long-acting GLP-1 derivative NN2211 ameliorates glycemia and increases beta-cell mass in diabetic mice. Am J Physiol (Endocrinol Metab) 2002;283:E 745–752.
206. Bregenholt S, Moldrup A, Blume N, Karlsen AE, Nissen Friedrichsen B, Tornhave D, et al. The long-acting glucagon-like peptide-1 analogue, liraglutide, inhibits beta-cell apoptosis in vitro. Biochem Biophys Res Commun. 2005;330:577–584.
207. Pospisilik JA, Martin J, Doty T, Ehses JA, Pamir N, Lynn FC, et al. Dipeptidyl peptidase IV inhibitor treatment stimulates beta-cell survival and islet neogenesis in streptozotocin-induced diabetic rats. Diabetes 2003;52:741–750.
208. Mu J, Woods J, Zhou YP, Roy RS, Li Z, Zycband E, et al. Chronic inhibition of dipeptidyl peptidase-4 with a sitagliptin analog preserves pancreatic β-cell mass and function in a rodent model of type 2 diabetes. Diabetes 2006;55:1695–1704.
209. Butler AE, Janson J, Soeller WC, Butler PC. Increased beta-cell apoptosis prevents adaptive increase in beta-cell mass in mouse model of type 2 diabetes: evidence for role of islet amyloid formation rather than direct action of amyloid. Diabetes. 2003;52(9):2304–2314.

210. Larsen MO, Rolin B, Sturis J, Wilken M, Carr RD, Porksen N, et al. Measurements of insulin responses as predictive markers of pancreatic beta-cell mass in normal and beta-cell-reduced lean and obese Gottingen minipigs in vivo. Am J Physiol Endocrinol Metab. 2006;290:E670–7. [Epub 2005 Nov 8.]
211. Stoffers DA, Kieffer TJ, Hussain MA, Drucker DJ, Bonner-Weir S, Habener JF, et al. Insulinotropic glucagon-like peptide 1 agonists stimulate expression of homeodomain protein IDX-1 and increase islet size in mouse pancreas. Diabetes 2000;49:741–748.
212. Hui H, Wright C, Perfetti R. Glucagon-like peptide 1 induces differentiation of islet duodenal homeobox-1-positive pancreatic ductal cells into insulin-secreting cells. Diabetes 2001;50:785–796.
213. Hui H, Nourparvar A, Zhao X, Perfetti R. Glucagon-like peptide-1 inhibits apoptosis of insulin-secreting cells via a cyclic 5′-adenosine monophosphate-dependent protein kinase A- and a phosphatidylinositol 3-kinase-dependent pathway. Endocrinology 2003;144:1444–1455.
214. Abraham EJ, Leech CA, Lin JC, Zulewski H, Habener JF. Insulinotropic hormone glucagon-like peptide-1 differentiation of human pancreatic islet-derived progenitor cells into insulin-producing cells. Endocrinology 2002;143:3152–3161.
215. Ritzel RA, Butler AE, Rizza RA, Veldhuis JD, Butler PC. Relationship between beta-cell mass and fasting blood glucose concentration in humans. Diabetes Care 2006;29:717–718.
216. Duttaroy A, Voelker F, Zhang X, Ren X, Merriam K, Qiu L, et al. The DPP-4 inhibitor vildagliptin increases pancreatic beta cell mass in rodents (abstract 481). Diabetologia 2005;48(Suppl. 1):A 178.
217. Gros R, You X, Baggio LL, Kabir MG, Sadi AM, Mungrue IN, et al. Cardiac function in mice lacking the glucagon-like peptide-1 receptor. Endocrinology 2003;144:2242–2252.
218. Bose AK, Mocanu MM, Carr RD, Brand CL, Yellon DM. Glucagon-like peptide 1 can directly protect the heart against ischemia/reperfusion injury. Diabetes 2005;54:146–151.
219. Nikolaidis LA, Mankad S, Sokos GG, Miske G, Shah A, Elahi D, et al. Effects of glucagon-like peptide-1 in patients with acute myocardial infarction and left ventricular dysfunction after successful reperfusion. Circulation 2004;109:962–965. [Epub 2004 Feb 23.]
220. Nikolaidis LA, Elahi D, Hentosz T, Doverspike A, Huerbin R, Zourelias L, et al. Recombinant glucagon-like peptide-1 increases myocardial glucose uptake and improves left ventricular performance in conscious dogs with pacing-induced dilated cardiomyopathy. Circulation 2004;110:955–961.
221. Kolterman OG, Buse JB, Fineman MS, Gaines E, Heintz S, Bicsak TA, et al. Synthetic exendin-4 (exenatide) significantly reduces postprandial and fasting plasma glucose in subjects with type 2 diabetes. J Clin Endocrinol Metab 2003;88:3082–3089.
222. Juhl CB, Hollingdal M, Sturis J, Jakobsen G, Agerso H, Veldhuis J, et al. Bedtime administration of NN2211, a long-acting GLP-1 derivative, substantially reduces fasting and postprandial glycemia in type 2 diabetes. Diabetes 2002;51:424–429.
223. Quddusi S, Vahl TP, Hanson K, Prigeon RL, D'Alessio DA. Differential effects of acute and extended infusions of glucagon-like peptide-1 on first- and second-phase insulin secretion in diabetic and nondiabetic humans. Diabetes Care 2003;26:791–798.
224. Fehse FC, Trautmann M, Holst JJ, Halseth AE, Fineman MS, Kim D, et al. Effects of exenatide on first and second phase insulin secretion in response to intravenous glucose in subjects with type 2 diabetes (Abstract). Diabetes 2004;53(Suppl. 2):A 83.
225. Polonsky KS, Given BD, Hirsch LJ, Tillil H, Shapiro ET, Frank BH, et al. Abnormal patterns of insulin secretion in non-insulin-dependent diabetes mellitus. N Engl J Med 1988;318:1231–1239.
226. Rachman J, Gribble FM, Levy JC, Turner RC. Near-normalization of diurnal glucose concentrations by continuous administration of glucagon-like peptide 1 (GLP-1) in subjects with NIDDM. Diabetologia 1997;40:205–211.
227. Gerich JE. Abnormal glucagon secretion in type 2 (noninsulin-dependent) diabetes mellitus: Causes and consequences. In: Creutzfeldt W, Lefèbvre P, editors. Diabetes mellitus: Pathophysiology and therapy. Berlin, Heidelberg: Springer Verlag; 1989, 127–133.
228. Degn KB, Brock B, Juhl CB, Djurhuus CB, Grubert J, Kim D, et al. Effect of intravenous infusion of exenatide (synthetic exendin-4) on glucose-dependent insulin secretion and counterregulation during hypoglycemia. Diabetes 2004;53:2397–2403.
229. Nauck M, El-Ouaghlidi A, Hompesch M, Jacobsen J, Elbrønd B. No impairment of hypoglycemia counterregulation via glucagon with NN2211, a GLP-1 derivative, in subjects with type 2 diabetes (abstract 550-P). Diabetes 2003;52(Suppl. 1)(A 128).
230. Fehmann HC, Göke R, Göke B. Cell and molecular biology of the incretin hormones glucagon-like peptide-I and glucose-dependent insulin releasing polypeptide. Endocr Rev 1995;16:390–410.
231. Rahier J, Goebbels RM, Henquin JC. Cellular composition of the human diabetic pancreas. Diabetologia 1983;24:366–371.

232. Buteau J, Foisy S, Rhodes CJ, Carpenter L, Biden TJ, Prentki M. Protein kinase C_{zeta} activation mediates glucagon-like peptide-1-induced pancreatic beta-cell proliferation. Diabetes 2001;50:2237–2243.
233. Li Y, Cao X, Li LX, Brubaker PL, Edlund H, Drucker DJ. β-cell PDX1 expression is essential for the glucoregulatory, proliferative, and cytoprotective actions of glucagon-like peptide-1. Diabetes 2005;54:482–491.
234. Bregenholdt S, Moldrup A, B. Knudsen L, Petersen JS. The GLP-1 derivative NN2211 inhibits cytokine-induced apoptosis in primary rat β-cells (abstracts). Diabetes 2001;50(Suppl. 1):A 31.
235. Phillips WT, Salman UA, McMahan CA, Schwartz JG. Accelerated gastric emptying in hypertensive subjects. J Nucl Med 1997;38:207–211.
236. Colditz GA, Willett WC, Rotnitzky A, Manson JE. Weight gain as a risk factor for clinical diabetes mellitus in women. Ann Intern Med 1995;122:481–486.
237. Poon T, Nelson P, Shen L, Mihm M, Taylor K, Fineman M, et al. Exenatide improves glycemic control and reduces body weight in subjects with type 2 diabetes: a dose-ranging study. Diabetes Technol Ther 2005;7:467–477.
238. Harder H, Nielsen L, Tu DT, Astrup A. The effect of liraglutide, a long-acting glucagon-like peptide 1 derivative, on glycemic control, body composition, and 24-h energy expenditure in patients with type 2 diabetes. Diabetes Care 2004;27:1915–1921.
239. Raz I, Hanefeld M, Xu L, Caria C, Davies M, Williams-Herman D, et al. Sitagliptin monotherapy improved glycemic control and beta-cell function after 18 weeks in patients with type 2 diabetes (T2DM) (abstract 1996-PO). Diabetes 2006;55(Suppl. 1):A 462.
240. Nonoka K, Kakikawa T, Sato A, Okuyama K, Fujimoto G, Hayashi N, et al. Twelve-week efficacy and tolerability of sitagliptin, a dipeptidyl peptidase-4 (DPP-4) inhibitor, in Japanese patients with type 2 diabetes (Abstract 0038). Diabetologia 2006;49(Suppl. 1):25.
241. Karasik A, Charbonnell B, Liu J, Wu M, Meehan A, Meininger G. Sitagliptin added to ongoing metformin therapy enhanced glycemic control and beta-cell function in patients with type 2 diabetes (abstract 501-P). Diabetes 2006;55(Suppl. 1):A 119–120.
242. Nauck MA, Meininger G, Sheng D, Terranella L, Stein P. Efficacy and safety of the dipeptidyl peptidase-4 inhibitor, sitagliptin, compared to the sulfonylurea, glipizide, in patients with type 2 diabetes inadequately controlled on metformin alone: A randomized, double-blind, non-inferiority trial. Diabetes Obesity Metab 2007;9:194–205.
243. Rosenstock J, Brazg R, Andryuk PJ, McCrary Sisk C, Lu K, Stein P. Addition of sitagliptin to pioglitazone improved glycemic control with neutral weight effect over 24 weeks in inadequately controlled type 2 diabetes (T2DM) (abstract 556-P). Diabetes 2006;55(Suppl. 1):A 132–133.
244. Pratley R, Galbreath E. Twelve-week monotherapy with the DPP-4 inhibitor, LAF 237 improves glycemic control in patients with type 2 diabetes (T2DM) (abstract 355-OR). Diabetes 2004;53(Suppl. 2):A 83.
245. Kikuchi M, Abe N, Kato M, Terao S, Holmes D, Mimori N. Vildagliptin decreases HbA1c after 12 weeks treatment in Japanese patients with type 2 diabetes (abstract 0789). Diabetologia 2006;49(Suppl. 1):478.
246. Dejager S, Baron MA, Razac S, Foley JE, Dickinson S, Schweizer A. Efficacy of vildagliptin in drug-naïve patients with type 2 diabetes (abstract 0791). Diabetologia 2006;49(Suppl. 1):479.
247. Garber A, Camisasca RP, Ehrsam E, Collober-Maugeais C, Rochotte E, Lebeaut A. Vildagliptin added to metformin improves glycemic control and may mitigate metformin-induced GI side effects in patients with type 2 diabetes (T2DM) (abstract 121-OR). Diabetes 2006;55(Suppl. 1):A 29.

13
The Role of Alpha-Glucosidase Inhibitors (Acarbose)

Markolf Hanefeld and Frank Schaper

Keywords: acarbose, pharmacology, diabetes, metabolic syndrome, primary prevention, cardiovascular disease.

Introduction

There is now a bulk of evidence that excessive postprandial or postchallenge hyperglycemia is an independent risk factor for cardiovascular disease [1–3], stroke [4], and all-cause mortality [5]. Rapid increase in postprandial glucose concentrations has harmful effects on endothelial function as indicated by reduced flow-mediated vasodilatation of the forearm [6] and myocardial blood-flow measurements by contrast echocardiography [7]. Excessive postprandial glucose excursion initiates a cascade of proatherogenic and prothrombotic events (Fig. 1). Recently it has been shown that rapid rise in glucose level increases the activity of low-grade inflammation [8]. Furthermore, a direct correlation between oxidative stress measured by urinary 8-iso $PGF_2\alpha$ excretion and mean amplitude of glucose excursion in circadian blood-glucose profile measurement was demonstrated by Monnier et al. [9]. On the other hand excessive postprandial hyperglycemia may also have harmful effects on the beta-cell (glucotoxicity) and has been shown to deteriorate insulin sensitivity of the musculature [10]. As shown for fasting hyperglycemia, postprandial hyperglycemia is a continuous risk factor with a linear relationship to cardiovascular event rate up to the normal range [11]. Therefore, near to normal control of postprandial glucose with 2 h postprandial levels below 6–8 mmol/L is nowadays recommended by many national and international boards. In modern diabetes treatment strict normalization of the gluco-triad (Fig. 2) should be the target.

This however may lead to a higher risk of hypoglycemia as long as long-acting oral insulin secretagogues such as glibenclamide/glimepride or regular insulin are used to control postprandial hyperglycemia. Another problem of strict control of hyperglycemia is weight gain in the case of advanced type 2 diabetes [12,13].

Postprandial hyperglycemia strongly depends on the amount of absorbed monosaccharides and the velocity of absorption in the small intestine. Carbohydrates are recommended to account for ~50% of the daily supply of calories in type 2 diabetes. Monosaccharides play only a minor role as dietary carbohydrates. They consist mainly of complex carbohydrates, such as starch (~60%), and disaccharides, such as sucrose (~30%). Complex carbohydrates and disaccharides must be hydrolyzed by intestinal and pancreatic enzymes before they can be transported through the mucosa of the bowel. Thus, any medication that delays breakdown of complex carbohydrates should decrease postprandial hyperglycemia and improve insulin sensitivity, as well as protecting the beta cells of the pancreas.

Alpha-glucosidase inhibitors (AGIs) were the first drugs developed to meet the needs of better postprandial glucose control when sulfonylureas and biguanides were the only available oral antidiabetics that did not show any vasoprotective effect in the UGDP study [14].

The digestion of complex carbohydrates in the lower parts of the small intestine and upper part of colon, as is the case with natural eating habits, has a stronger stimulating effect on gastrointestinal

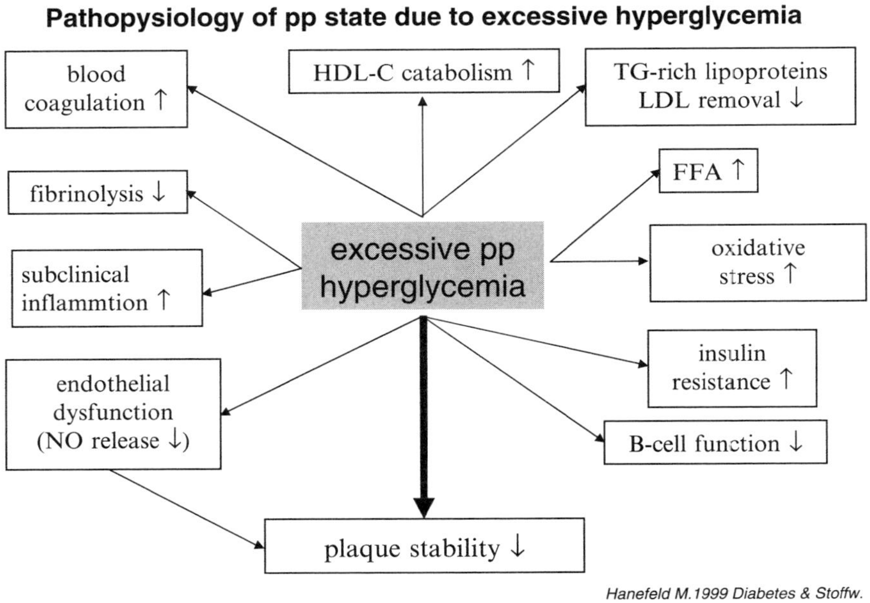

FIG. 1. Pathology of postprandial state due to excessive hyperglycemia.

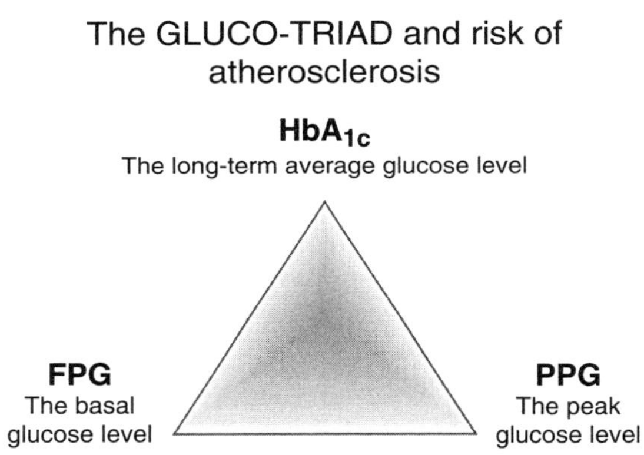

FIG. 2. The gluco-triad and the risk of atherosclerosis.

hormones, such as glucagon-like peptide 1 (GLP_1), than the consumption of refined carbohydrates as typical for modern fast food [15]. AGIs – acarbose, miglitol, voglibose – are oral antidiabetics that specifically inhibit alpha-glucosidases in the brush border of the small intestine. These enzymes are essential for the release of glucose from more complex carbohydrates [16].

Transit of food from the stomach along the bowel has stimulatory effects on incretins, which regulate insulin secretion and beta-cell regeneration as well as glucagon release.

Pharmacology of Alpha-Glucosidase Inhibitors

AGIs were developed by Puls et al. [17] to control diabetes by inhibition of glucose release from starch and disaccharides, the major carbohydrate components in the food.

An appropriate agent (acarbose) of microbial origin (culture filtrates of actinoplanes) was first described by Schmidt in 1977 [18], and this inhibitor was introduced onto the market in 1990. Three AGIs are now in therapeutic use worldwide (Table 1) and are frequently prescribed in Asia and Central and South Europe.

Acarbose is a pseudotetrasaccharide with nitrogen bound between the first and second glucose unit. This modification of a natural tetrasaccharide is important for its high affinity for active centers of alpha-glucosidases of the brush border of the small intestine and for its stability. 1-Desoxynojirimycin is the parent compound of other AGIs such as miglitol, which, in contrast to acarbose, is a small molecule, similar to glucose. Voglibose is produced by reductive alkylation of valiolamine [19].

TABLE 1. Summary of pharmacological characteristics of AGBs in clinical use.

Drug	Acarbose	Miglitol	Voglibose
Extent of absorption	Low	High, dose-dependent	Low, dose-dependent
Unchanged drug	<2%	>96%	<6%
Metabolites	<35%		
Bioavailability	<2%	>96%	<6%
Clearance	Mainly renal by glomerular filtration	Mainly renal by glomerular filtration	Mainly renal
Protein binding	Low to high, species-dependent, saturable	Low	Low to high, species-dependent, saturable
Distribution	Extracellular, low tissue affinity	Extracellular, low tissue affinity	Low tissue affinity
Metabolism	Extrasystemic in the intestine	None	None
Excretion			
Fecal	>65%	Low	Almost complete
Renal	<35%	>96%	<5%
Biliary	<5%	<0.2%	–

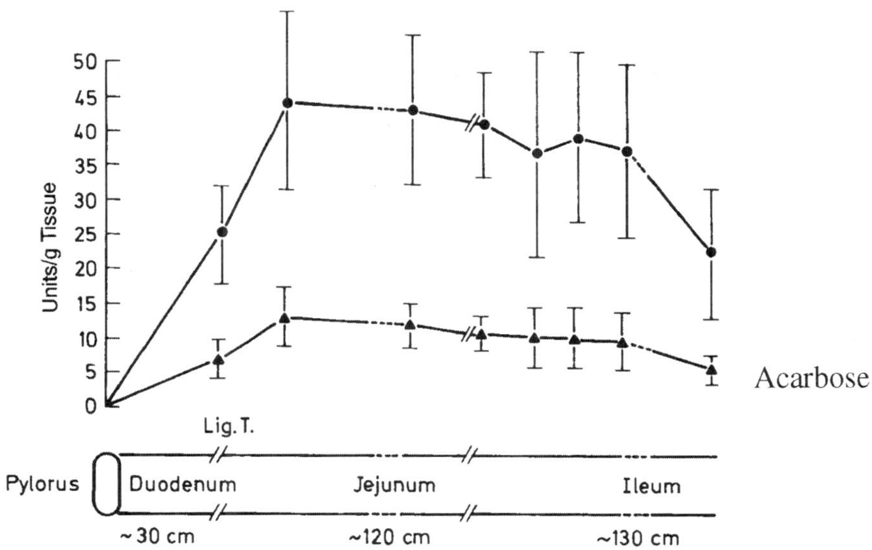

FIG. 3. Effect on postload glucose and insulin excursions after a mixed meal.

AGIs act as competitive inhibitors because of their high affinity for alpha-glucosidases; they block the enzymatic reaction particularly because of their nitrogen component. Thus, AGIs must be present at the site of enzymatic action at the same time as the carbohydrates. The effect on postload glucose excursion and insulin after a starch-containing mixed meal is shown in Fig. 3. In principle, all three AGIs act in the same way, by inhibiting alpha-glucosidase enzymes in the brush border of the upper part of the small intestine. There are, however, some differences with respect to the inhibitory efficiency on various alpha-glucosidases, which may be responsible for differences in the frequency of side effects. Acarbose is most effective on glucoamylase, followed by sucrase, maltase, and dextranase [16]. It also inhibits the alpha-amylase, but has no effect on beta-glucosidases, such as lactase. Miglitol is a more potent inhibitor of disaccharide-digesting enzymes, such as sucrase and maltase, than acarbose, and is also active on isomaltase but has no effect on alpha-amylase [20]. It also weakly interacts as a pseudo monosaccharide with the intestinal sodium-dependent glucose transporter, without having a clinically relevant effect on glucose absorption [21]. Voglibose is isolated from

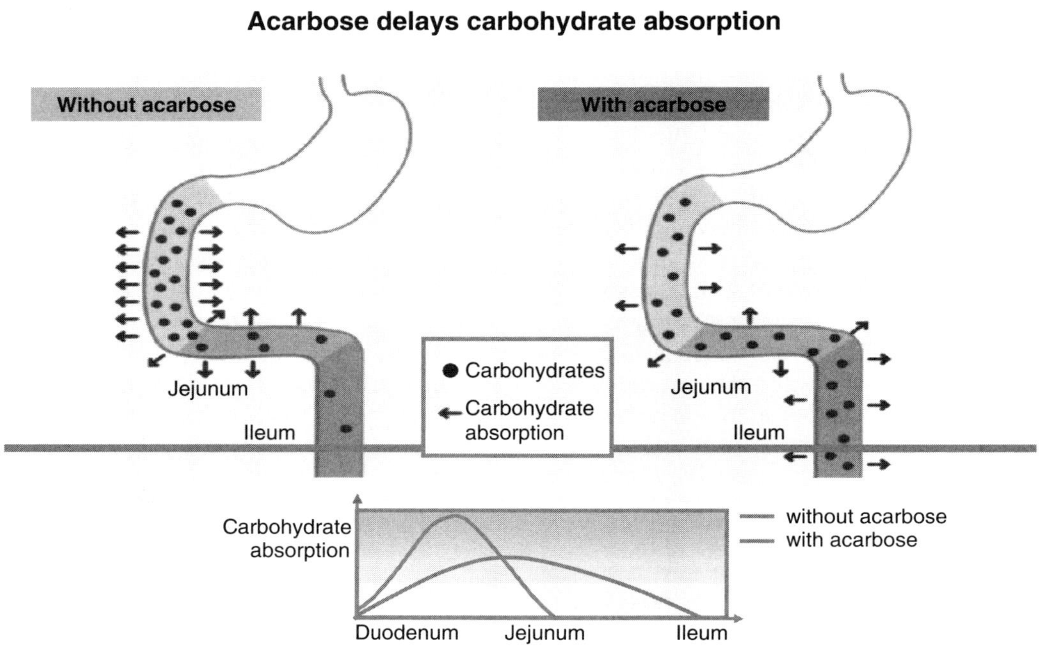

FIG. 4. Acarbose delays carbohydrate absorption.

Streptomyces culture broths. It is a strong AGI with minor effect on alpha-amylase.

Acarbose is absorbed unchanged only by 0.5–1.7%. About 98% is degraded to glucose, maltose, and acarviosine by bacterial enzymes (Table 1); about 35% of degradation products appear in the urine. Miglitol remains unchanged and is excreted dose-dependently by the kidneys. Only 3–5% of voglibose is absorbed, and it is almost completely excreted via feces. After oral administration, about 90% unchanged drug remains. By extrapolation, the most striking differences between AGIs in clinical use are with respect to absorption. Neither acarbose nor voglibose are absorbed in their active form; whereas miglitol is almost completely absorbed in the upper part of the small intestine, it has a long-lasting presence in the mucosa. Intake of acarbose has profound effects on a complex pattern of intestinal enzymes and gene expression regulating immune response to food (unpublished data). AGIs primarily act on the alpha-glucosidases of the jejunum. Thus, larger proportions of undigested carbohydrates reach the ileum and colon ascends (Fig. 4). There they are hydrolyzed by bacterial enzymes with no malabsorption. The consequence is formation of gases and short-chain fatty acids leading to meteorism and flatulence. The intensity of gas formation together with increased motility strongly depends on the amount and type of carbohydrates in the food.

There exist striking differences in the regional use of AGIs as oral antidiabetics. It has been found that acarbose is more effective in a diet rich in starch as it is the case in Asian type of nutrition since it preferentially inhibits glucoamylase [22]. By contrast AGIs are seldom prescribed in the USA and Northern Europe with a diet rich in fat and proteins. However, in many Asian countries with nutrition rich in complex carbohydrates AGIs are frequently used as first-line drugs and/or in combination with metformin with less gastrointestinal complaints.

Effects on Hormonal Regulation

AGIs neither have a direct effect on insulin secretion nor on insulin sensitivity of target tissues. However, as reported by Meneilly et al. [23] acarbose significantly improves insulin sensitivity in elderly patients with type 2 diabetes as measured by euglycemic CLAMP. This may mainly be due to reduction of postprandial hyperglycemia. Consistent data on postprandial insulin excursion [24,25] prove a diminished postprandial insulin excursion. After AGI intake, reduction in postprandial glucose load may lead to improved beta-cell function. Accordingly, it could be shown in people with IGT [26,27] and patients with type 2 diabetes that proinsulin output is lower after acarbose treatment [28]. This fits well to the results of the STOP-NIDDM trial where treatment with acarbose reduced the incidence of newly diagnosed diabetes by 36% [29]. A new insight on possible actions of AGIs on hormonal regulation is provided by the incretin concept. The slowing down of gastric emptying observed in men after intake of AGIs causes a decrease in gastric inhibitory polypeptide (GIP) release. Even more important, the fact that larger amounts of undigested carbohydrates reach the lower part of the small intestine rich in C-cells producing GLP_1 stimulates a long-lasting increase in this incretin [15,30].

A slower emptying of the stomach and subsequent GLP_1 increase after mixed meals have been demonstrated for acarbose [31] as well as for voglibose [30]. GLP_1 (60–240 min) and – to less extent – GIP are natural insulin secretagogues and play a key role in the entero-insulinar axis. This may support the therapeutic effect of AGIs behind their direct effects on postprandial hyperglycemia.

Synergistic Effects on Metabolic Syndrome

In long-term studies in patients with IGT and type 2 diabetes, respectively, a significant reduction of body weight in the range of 0.7–0.9 kg was observed with acarbose [32,33]. In the STOP-NIDDM trial in patients with prediabetes, individuals receiving acarbose had lost about 1.2 kg, compared with individuals receiving placebo [29]. This weight loss cannot be explained by changes in dietary habits [33] and malabsorption [16], than may be rather a consequence of changes in release of incretins as seen in recent results of treatment with GLP_1 analoges. The strongest effect on traits of the metabolic syndrome has been shown for elevated blood pressure. A double-blind, randomized, placebo-controlled study in 44 patients with type 2 diabetes found that achievement of good glycemic control with acarbose was accompanied by significant reductions in diurnal systolic, diastolic, and mean blood-pressure values ($p < 0.05$) [34]. Similarly, a randomized 6-month study in obese patients with diabetes found that acarbose treatment reduced the mean 24-h systolic blood pressure by a mean of 5.2 mmHg, compared with only 1.6 mmHg with glibenclamide ($p = 0.0001$) [35].

In the STOP-NIDDM trial the incidence of newly diagnosed hypertension was reduced by 34%. In a meta-analysis of controlled long-term studies with acarbose (MeRIA), systolic blood pressure was reduced by 2.7 mmHg ($p = 0.024$) [36]. The synergistic effect of AGIs on blood pressure may be the result of improved endothelial function due to protection from vasotoxic postprandial glucose spikes [37].

AGIs have no significant effect on total and LDL-cholesterol [38]. However, recently published investigations in patients with IGT analyzing LDL-subfractions reveal a decrease in small dense LDL [39]. No significant effects have been shown on HDL-cholesterol in the STOP-NIDDM study [29] and the MeRIA meta-analysis [36]. The major effect is on fasting and postprandial triglycerides with a reduction of about 15% [40]. As discussed in a review, effect on postprandial hypertriglyceridemia may add to vasoprotective power of acarbose [41].

Low-grade inflammation is closely associated with the metabolic syndrome and is an accepted new cardiovascular risk factor. Reductions in postprandial glucose excursion by treatment with acarbose in patients with type 2 diabetes have shown to reduce the activity ($p = 0.045$) and nuclear localization ($p = 0.02$) of the proinflammatory transcription factor NFκB, suggesting a mechanism by which the anti-inflammatory effects of acarbose may be mediated [8]. This mechanism would be consistent with reductions in the level of coagulation factors seen with acarbose treatment. For example, acarbose has been shown to reduce the level of fibrinogen in patients with type 2 diabetes ($p = 0.013$ vs. placebo) [42] and serum C-reactive protein levels in individuals with IGT ($p < 0.01$ vs. placebo) [43]. We found a significant reduction in postprandial leukocyte excursion another indicator of low grade inflammation by acarbose treatment compared with placebo (Hanefeld et al., unpublished results). These data suggest that acarbose, for reasons that are not yet fully understood, has a beneficial effect on low-grade inflammation activity and immune response to food.

AGIs have beneficial pleiotropic effects on major components of the metabolic syndrome, which should add to their therapeutic benefit in the treatment of IGT and type 2 diabetes.

Indications for AGIs and Clinical Practice

AGIs can be used as first-line drugs in newly diagnosed type 2 diabetes insufficiently treated with diet and exercise alone, as well as in combination with all oral antidiabetics and insulin if monotherapy with these drugs fails to achieve the targets for HbAlc and postprandial blood glucose [25,44]. As first-line drugs, AGIs are particularly useful in newly diagnosed type 2 diabetes with an excessive postprandial hyperglycemia, because of their unique mode of action in controlling the release of glucose from complex carbohydrates and disaccharides. In these cases, they lower postprandial blood-glucose level peaks by >50 mg dL^{-1}, resulting in an average reduction of HbAlc by 0.7–1.2%. Table 2 summarizes subgroups of type 2 diabetes that may preferentially benefit from the use of AGIs as first-line treatment. Especially elderly obese women exhibit postchallenge hyperglycemia as the dominant abnormality of glucose homeostasis. Since AGIs are very safe and have very few contraindications and drug interactions, they also may be considered in polymorbid patients with beginning renal and hepatic dysfunction. Their weak weight-reducing effect could be an advantage over oral insulin secretagogues for some patients. AGIs have no risk of causing hypoglycemia; they are therefore a rational alternative for patients who experience hypoglycemic episodes with insulin secretagogues. In early type 2 diabetes with both high fasting plasma glucose and high postprandial glucose, a combination of acarbose either with metformin or long-acting insulin secretagogues, such as glibenclamide and glimepiride, should be considered. This approach has the advantage of increasing efficacy and reducing side-effects, if low doses of either drug are used for the combination.

TABLE 2. Indications for AGIs as first-line drug in type 2 diabetes.

Newly diagnosed patients insufficiently treated with diet and dominating postprandial hyperglycemia
Elderly multimorbid patients
Elderly patients with weight gain or hypoglycemia under treatment with insulin secretagogues
Patients with hepatic or renal disorders

Many patients on monotherapy with either metformin or sulfonylureas do not reach HbAlc levels <6.5–7%. A further reduction of HbAlc of 0.5–1% can be achieved by add-on therapy with AGIs [45,46]. There is increasing evidence that postprandial hyperglycemic excursions add to the risk of progression of type 2 diabetes and its cardiovascular complications [47,48]. In this context, AGIs are also useful adjuncts if postprandial glucose levels cannot be controlled sufficiently with metformin, sulfonylureas, or insulin. A meta-analysis revealed an additional effect of 0.7% of acarbose given after metformin pretreatment, and 0.85% when added to sulfonylurea treatment [46]. Extrapolation of controlled clinical trials with AGIs as add-on therapy showed an additional reduction in postprandial glucose of >40 mg dL^{-1}. The additional reduction in fasting blood glucose is >20 mg dL^{-1}. Little is known so far about combination therapy with thiazolidindiones and "prandial oral insulin secretagogues," such as nateglinide and repaglinide. Scarce information also exists on the clinical use of AGIs in combination with bed-time administered long-acting insulin injections in type 2 diabetes. This combination may be useful in avoiding weight gain and to achieve better control of postprandial hyperglycemia. As shown by Monnier et al. [49] postprandial hyperglycemia accounts for 60% of variance HbA1c in patients with a HbA1c level below 7.5%.

Practicalities

Efficacy, side-effects, and compliance with AGIs strongly depend on rational indication, education of patients on how to use the drug, and good dietary advice. Even with good clinical practice, a considerable variation in response and side-effects is seen. Side-effects depend, among other things, on the

TABLE 3. Advice to patients to overcome difficulties with AGSs.

Start low, go slow
Prefer nutrients with complex carbohydrates (rice, pasta, full bread, vegetables, fruits)
Avoid refined carbohydrates (sugar, sweets). Take only three meals
Avoid laxatives, such as sugar alcohols (sorbitol)
Control your postprandial blood glucose to experience the efficacy of treatment
In most cases gastrointestinal side-effects are transient

dose and time intervals for titration of optimal therapeutic dosage. It is essential to start with low doses of 25 mg of acarbose or miglitol twice a day, with a stepwise increase in 2–3 week intervals. A study in type 2 diabetes patients treated with sulfonylurea compared the tolerability of stepwise increase with an initial dose of 100 mg three times per day of acarbose [50]. The stepwise increase in dosage reduced specific side-effects from 70% to 31%. The maximum dosage for acarbose and miglitol is usually 100 mg three times per day. There are, however, controlled studies that show that 200 mg three times per day is more effective, but has a higher rate of gastrointestinal side-effects [51].

After 3–4 weeks gastrointestinal side-effects diminish to <20% in almost all studies. In long-term studies, the great majority of discontinuations because of side-effects happens during the first 3 months. It is important to reinforce dietary advice before treatment and if side-effects occur. A high content of refined carbohydrates and a diet rich in fat and protein are causes of gastrointestinal discomfort. Patients should be made aware that side-effects are due to the mode of action, are mostly transient, and can be prevented by prudent diet. Table 3 summarizes some guidelines for patients to help overcome difficulties.

Patients should also take blood-glucose levels twice a week at 2 h postprandial to see the benefit of the treatment, because the fasting blood-glucose levels are not indicative of therapy success in the first month of treatment.

AGIs in the Primary Prevention of Type 2 Diabetes

IGT is prediabetic category and an established risk factor for cardiovascular disease. Prevalence of IGT in all nations with a westernized lifestyle is >15% in subjects aged >40 years. Primary prevention efforts with life-style modification are therefore of high priority [52]. In terms of medical intervention in subjects with IGT, AGIs have been shown to improve insulin sensitivity and reduce proinsulin secretion [26,27]. In the STOP-NIDDM trial, a large placebo-controlled multinational study of 1,429 subjects with IGT, acarbose reduced the annual incidence of diabetes by 36% in the intention to treat analysis [29]. No serious adverse event associated with acarbose was observed during the 3.4-year follow-up.

AGIs in the Prevention of Cardiovascular Disease

Acarbose has favorable effects on a broad spectrum of established cardiovascular risk factors: it lowers blood pressure, improves atherogenic lipoprotein profile, has antithrombotic actions, reduces parameters of low-grade inflammation, and downregulates insulin resistance as already described. In this respect less data are available for miglitol and voglibose. In a study by Wascher et al. [37] reduction of postprandial glucose excursion by acarbose was associated with improved flow-mediated vasodilation. The cardiovascular benefits of acarbose were shown by the STOP-NIDDM study. The study found that treatment of people with IGT with acarbose was associated with a 49% reduction in the incidence of newly diagnosed cardiovascular events over a mean follow-up of 3.3 years, including a 12:1 myocardial infarction in favor of acarbose ($p = 0.02$) [53]. Compared with placebo, acarbose treatment reduced the annual progress of intima media thickness (IMT) by approximately 50% ($p < 0.027$) [54]. The treatment with acarbose reduced the risk of any cardiovascular event by 35% ($p = 0.006$) as shown in a meta-analysis of seven long-term placebo-controlled trials in patients with type 2 diabetes (MeRIA) [36]. Again the strongest effect was on incidence of myocardial infarction, which was reduced by 64% ($p = 0.012$, Fig. 5). In both studies a trend for reduction of cardiac failure was observed.

Thus in conclusion, acarbose improves endothelial function, reduces progression of IMT, lowers incidence of newly diagnosed hypertension, and prevents any cardiovascular events in particular myocardial infarction in patients with IGT and type 2 diabetes, respectively.

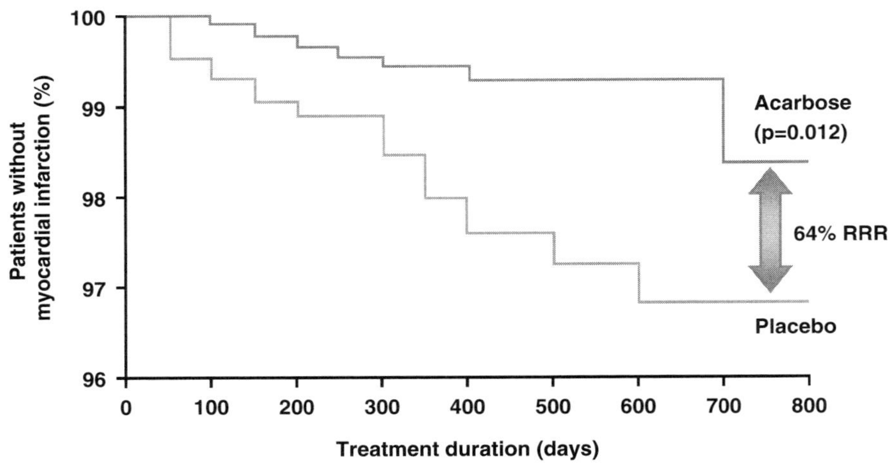

FIG. 5. Acarbose reduces the risk of myocardial infarction in patients with type 2 diabetes.

Conclusions

AGIs have been in clinical use for 15 years and are now registered worldwide. They are among the best-studied oral antidiabetics, with data from controlled studies and long-term clinical investigations for all three clinically used compounds. AGIs are used as first-line drugs in early type 2 diabetes, as well as in combination with nearly all established oral antidiabetics and insulin. In some cases of type 1 diabetes, with rapid postprandial glucose rise, and in cases of premeal hypoglycemia, AGIs may be introduced as adjunct therapy. Numerous trials have demonstrated that acarbose is a safe and effective oral antidiabetic agent in patients with diabetes and IGT. Furthermore, acarbose reduces the risk of cardiovascular events, improves different cardiovascular risk factors, and may have long-term benefits for patients with metabolic syndrome. So far acarbose is the only antidiabetic drug in the treatment of prediabetes with evidence for reduction of cardiovascular disease. These properties can be attributed to the mode of action of acarbose, which directly targets postprandial hyperglycamia and avoids several common side-effects associated with other blood-sugar-lowering medications. AGIs are very safe drugs. The most common side-effects are mild-to-moderate GI events, and these can be minimized if appropriate stepwise-dosing regimens are used at the start of the treatment. AGIs are therefore a valuable option for the management of type 2 diabetes, and particularly acarbose, the only oral antidiabetic agent approved for the treatment of prediabetes, can help to improve clinical management across the dysglycamic disease continuum.

References

1. Wallander M, Bartnik M, Efendic S et al. Beta cell dysfunction in patients with acute myocardial infarction but without previously known type 2 diabetes: a report from the GAMI study. Diabetologia 2005;48(11):2229–2235.
2. Hanefeld M, Fischer S, Julius U et al. Risk factors for myocardial infarction and death in newly detected NIDDM: The Diabetes Intervention Study, 11 years follow-up. Diabetologia 1996;39(12):1577–1583.
3. Ceriello A, Hanefeld M, Leiter L et al. Postprandial glucose regulation and diabetic complications. Arch Intern Med 2004;164(19):2090–2095.
4. Burchfiel CM, Curb JD, Rodriguez BL et al. Glucose intolerance and 22-year stroke incidence. The Honolulu Heart Program. Stroke 1994;25(5):951–957.
5. DECODE Study Group, European Diabetes Epidemiology Group. Is the current definition for diabetes relevant to mortality risk from all causes and cardiovascular and noncardiovascular diseases? Diabetes Care 2003;26(3):688–696.
6. Kawano H, Motoyama T, Hirashima O et al. Hyperglycemia rapidly suppresses flow-mediated

endothelium-dependent vasodilation of brachial artery. J Am Coll Cardiol 1999;34(1):146–154.
7. Scognamiglio R, Negut C, De Kreutzenberg SV et al. Postprandial myocardial perfusion in healthy subjects and in type 2 diabetic patients. Circulation 2005; 112(2):179–184.
8. Rudofsky G, Reismann P, Schiekofer S et al. Reduction of postprandial hyperglycemia in patients with type 2 diabetes reduces NF-κB activation in PBMCs. Horm Met Res 2004;36:630–638.
9. Monnier L, Mas E, Ginet C et al. Activation of oxidative stress by acute glucose fluctuations compared with sustained chronic hyperglycemia in patients with type 2 diabetes. JAMA 2006;295(14):1681–1687.
10. Woerle HJ, Szoke E, Meyer C et al. Mechanisms for abnormal postprandial glucose metabolism in type 2 diabetes. Am J Physiol Endocrinol Metab 2006; 290(1):E67–E77.
11. Coutinho M, Gerstein HC, Wang Y et al. The relationship between glucose and incident cardiovascular events. A meta-regression analysis of published data from 20 studies of 95,783 individuals followed for 12.4 years. Diabetes Care 1999;22(2):233–240.
12. UK Prospective Diabetes Study (UKPDS) Group. Intensive blood-glucose control with sulfonylureas or insulin compared with conventional treatment and risk of complications in patients with type 2 diabetes (UKPDS 33). Lancet 1998; 352:837–853.
13. Kahn SE, Haffner SM, Heise MA et al. Glycemic durability of rosiglitazone, metformin, or glyburide monotherapy. N Engl J Med 2006;355(23):2427–2443.
14. Salsburg DS. The UGDP study. JAMA 1971;218(11):1704–1705.
15. Goke B, Herrmann C, Goke R et al. Intestinal effects of alpha-glucosidase inhibitors: absorption of nutrients and enterohormonal changes. Eur J Clin Invest 1994;24(Suppl 3):25–30.
16. Puls W. Pharmacology of glucosidase inhibitors. Oral Antidiabetics. Berlin: Springer, 1996;119:497–525.
17. Puls W, Keup U, Krause HP et al. Glucosidase inhibition. A new approach to the treatment of diabetes, obesity and hyperlipoproteinemia. Naturwissenschaften 1977;64:536–537.
18. Schmidt DD, Frommer W, Junge B et al. Alpha-glucosidase inhibitors. New complex oligosaccharides of microbial origin. Naturwissenschaften 1977;64: 535–536.
19. Krause HP, Ahr HJ. Pharmacokinetics and metabolism of glucosidase inhibitors. In: Kuhlmann J, Puls W, editors. Handbook of Experimental Pharma–cology: Oral Antidiabetics. Vol. 119. Berlin: Springer, 1996;541–545.
20. Junge B, Matzke M, Stoltefuss J. Chemistry and structure–activity relationships of glucosidase inhibitors. In: Kuhlmann J, Puls W, editors. Handbook of Experimental Pharmacology: Oral Antidiabetics. Vol. 119. Berlin: Springer, 1996;541–545.
21. Joubert PH, Venter HL, Foukaridis GN. The effect of miglitol and acarbose after an oral glucose load: a novel hypoglycaemic mechanism. Br J Clin Pharmacol 1990;30:391–396.
22. Toeller M. Modulation of intestinal glucose absorption: postponement of glucose absorption by alpha-glucosidase inhibitors. In: Mogensen CE, Standl E, editors. Pharmacology of Diabetes. Berlin: De Gruyter, 1991;93–112.
23. Meneilly G, Ryan EA, Radziuk J et al. Effect of acarbose on insulin sensitivity in elderly patients with diabetes. Diabetes Care 2000;23:1162–1167.
24. Hillebrand I, Boehme K, Frank G et al. Effects of the glycoside hydrolase inhibitor (BAY g 5421) on postprandial blood glucose, serum insulin and triglycerides levels in man. In: Creutzfeldt W, editor. Frontiers of Hormone Research, the Entero-insular Axis. Basel: Karger, 1979;7:290–291.
25. Hanefeld M, Fischer S, Schulze J et al. Therapeutic potentials of acarbose as first-line drug in NIDDM insufficiently treated with diet alone. Diabetes Care 1991;14:732–737.
26. Chiasson JL, Josse RG, Leiter LA et al. The effect of acarbose on insulin sensitivity in subjects with impaired glucose tolerance. Diabetes Care 1996;19:1190–1193.
27. Laube H, Linn T, Heyen P. The effects of acarbose on insulin sensitivity and proinsulin in overweight subjects with impaired glucose tolerance. Exp Clin Endocrinol Diabetes 1998;106:231–233.
28. Hanefeld M, Haffner SM, Menschikowski M et al. Different effects of acarbose and glibenclamide on proinsulin and insulin profiles in people with type 2 diabetes. Diabetes Res Clin Pract 2002;55:221–227.
29. Chiasson JL, Josse RG, Gomis R et al. Acarbose for prevention of type 2 diabetes mellitus: the STOP-NIDDM randomised trial. Lancet 2002;359(9323): 2072–2077.
30. Goke B, Fuder H, Wieckhorst G et al. Voglibose is an efficient alpha-glucosidase inhibitor and mobilize the endogenous GLP-1 reserve. Digestion 1995;56: 493–501.
31. Qualmann C, Nauck MA, Hoist JJ et al. Glucagon-like peptide 1 (GLP-1) [17–36 amide] secretion in response to luminal sucrose from the upper and lower gut: a study using α-glucosidase inhibition (acarbose). Scand J Gastroenterol 1995;30:892–896.
32. Holman RR, Turner RC, Cull CA et al. A randomised double-blind trial of acarbose in type 2 diabetes shows improved glycemic control over 3 years (UK Prospective Diabetes Study 44). Diabetes Care 1999;22:960–964.

33. Wolever TMS, Chiasson JL, Josse RG et al. Small weight loss on long-term acarbose therapy with no change in dietary pattern or nutrient intake of individuals with non-insulin-dependent diabetes. Int J Obes Relat Metab Disord 1997;21:756–763.
34. Lindström J, Tuomilehto J, Spengler M. Acarbose treatment does not change the habitual diet of patients with type 2 diabetes mellitus. The Finnish Acarbose Study Group. Diabet Med 2000;17(1):20–25.
35. Rosenthal JH, Mauersberger H. Effects on blood pressure of the alpha-glucosidase inhibitor acarbose compared with the insulin enhancer glibenclamide in patients with hypertension and type 2 diabetes mellitus. Clin Drug Invest 2002;22(10):695–701.
36. Hanefeld M, Cagatay M, Petrowitsch T et al. Acarbose reduces the risk for myocardial infarction in type 2 diabetic patients: meta-analysis of seven long-term studies. Eur Heart J 2004;25(1):10–16.
37. Wascher TC, Schmoelzer I, Wiegratz A et al. Reduction of postchallenge hyperglycaemia prevents acute endothelial dysfunction in subjects with impaired glucose tolerance. Eur J Clin Invest 2005;35(9):551–557.
38. Leonhardt W, Hanefeld M, Fischer S et al. Efficacy of alpha-glucosidase inhibitors on lipids in NIDDM subjects with moderate hyperlipidaemia. Eur J Clin Invest 1994;24(Suppl 3):45–49.
39. Inoue I, Shinoda Y, Nakano T et al. Acarbose ameliorates atherogenecity of low-density lipoprotein in patients with impaired glucose tolerance. Metabolism 2006;55(7):946–952.
40. Hanefeld M, Fischer S, Schulze J et al. Therapeutic potentials of acarbose as first-line drug in NIDDM insufficiently treated with diet alone. Diabetes Care 1991;14:732–737.
41. Heine RJ, Dekker JM. Beyond postprandial hyperglycaemia: metabolic factors associated with cardiovascular disease. Diabetologia 2002;45(4):461–475.
42. Tschoepe D. Decreased fibrinogen by treatment with the alpha-glucosidase inhibitor acarbose. Diabetes 2004;53(Suppl 2):A189.
43. Wang X, Lu J, Pan C. Comparison of serum C-reactive protein level in different glucose tolerance subjects and the change in serum CRP level in IGT subjects with acarbose. EASD 2003. Published in Chinese: Lu JM et al. Chin J Endocrinol Metab 2003;19:254–256.
44. Drent ML. Miglitol as single oral hypoglycemic agent in type 2 diabetes [Abstract]. Diabetologia 1994;37(Suppl 1):211.
45. Mertes G. Safety and efficacy of acarbose in the treatment of Type 2 diabetes: data from 5-year surveillance study. Diabetes Res Clin Pract 2001;2:193–204.
46. Leboritz HE. α-Glucosidase inhibitors as agents in the treatment of diabetes. Diabetes Rev 1998;6:132–145.
47. Hanefeld M, Fischer S, Julius U et al. and the DIS Group. Risk factors for myocardial infarction and death in newly detected NIDDM: the Diabetes Intervention Study, 11-year follow-up. Diabetologia 1996;39:1577–1583.
48. Temelkova-Kurktschiev T, Kohler C, Henkel E et al. Post-challenge plasma glucose and glycemic spikes are more strongly associated with atherosclerosis than fasting glucose or HbAlc level. Diabetes Care 2000;23:1830–1834.
49. Monnier L, Lapinski H, Colette C. Contributions of fasting and postprandial plasma glucose increments to the overall diurnal hyperglycemia of type 2 diabetic patients: variations with increasing levels of HbA(1c). Diabetes Care 2003;26(3):881–885.
50. May C. Efficacy and tolerability of step wise increasing dosage of acarbose in patients with non-insulin-dependent diabetes (NIDDM) treated with sulfonylureas. Diabetes Stoffwechsel 1995;4:3–7.
51. Fischer S, Hanefeld M, Spengler M et al. European study on dose–response relationship of acarbose as a first-line drug in non-insulin-dependent diabetes mellitus: efficacy and safety of low and high doses. 1998;35:34.
52. Knowler WC, Barrett-Connor E, Fowler SE et al. Reduction in the incidence of type 2 diabetes with lifestyle intervention or metformin. N Engl J Med 2002;346(6):393–403.
53. Chiasson JL, Josse RG, Gomis R et al. Acarbose treatment and the risk of cardiovascular disease and hypertension in patients with impaired glucose tolerance: the STOP-NIDDM trial. JAMA 2003;290(4):486–494.
54. Hanefeld M, Chiasson JL, Koehler C et al. Acarbose slows progression of intima-media thickness of the carotid arteries in subjects with impaired glucose tolerance. Stroke 2004;35(5):1073–1078.

14 Multifactorial Intervention in Type 2 Diabetes

Oluf Pedersen

Keywords: Diabetes, cardiovascular disorder, microangiopathy, macroangiopathy, risk factors, health behaviour, polypharmacy, drug concordance, patient, motivation, patient education.

Treatment of Type 2 Diabetes: from a Glucocentric Approach Towards Global Vascular Protection

For long, type 2 diabetes mellitus was considered to be a relatively benign disorder, at least in the elderly [1]. Insights have, however, become deeper. From epidemiological surveys it is well documented that the age-adjusted prevalence of coronary heart disease in white adults who have diabetes is about 45% compared to about 25% in individuals without diabetes [2]. Cardiovascular disorders (CVD i.e. coronary heart disease, stroke, and peripheral vascular disease) may account for about 70% of all deaths in people with diabetes mellitus and all manifestations of CVD are also substantially more common in patients with type 2 diabetes than in non-diabetic individuals [3]. Therefore, type 2 diabetes is not 'just another risk factor' for a poor cardiovascular prognosis; at the population level it per se defines maximal risk for target organ damage, primarily the cardiovascular system [4].

During recent years numerous prospective studies have identified several modifiable risk factors for CVD in patients with type 2 diabetes. On top of hyperglycaemia these factors include hypertension, dyslipidaemia, microalbuminuria, a pro-thrombotic state, visceral fat accumulation, and associated chronic low-grade inflammation, smoking, diets rich in saturated or *trans*-fatty acids, and lack of physical activity [5–9].

Even though at present there are no data from controlled long-term clinical trials to provide definite answers to the impact on CVD outcome of each of the individual behavioural factors, there is overwhelming epidemiological evidence that an integrated healthy life performance including no smoking, daily physical activity, a low-fat, vegetable-/fruit- and seafood-enriched diet and mental stress coping reduces insulin resistance and helps preventing CVD in the general population. It is reasonable to expect that the same will be the case in patients with type 2 diabetes. When it comes to the practicality and impact of sustained weight loss a randomized controlled trial sponsored by the National Institute of Diabetes and Digestive and Kidney Diseases termed Look AHEAD: Action for Health in Diabetes has been initiated [10]. Five thousand one hundred and forty-five obese type 2 diabetic patients are enrolled for an estimated period of 10 years to evaluate if an average weight loss of 7% of body weight induced by altered diet and exercise habits reduces risk of CVD.

Importantly, crucial information has been gained from individual risk factor intervention trials in both diabetic and non-diabetic subjects. Based upon the results of these interventions in diabetic patients (for review see [11–14]), the degree of CVD relative risk reduction with each individual risk factor target ranges from small (e.g. non-significant for hyperglycaemia lowering using insulin or sulphonylurea in the UKPDS), to moderate (e.g. about 10% with aspirin therapy) to substantial (e.g. 25–40% with blood pressure reduction or statin-induced lipid lowering). in addition, treatment with ACE inhibitors as secondary prevention of CVD is convincingly demonstrated. Based upon the indisputable results from clinical endpoint trials, the pharmacotherapy of type 2 diabetes as reflected in national guidelines including those from the American Diabetes Association [15] has changed from the glucocentric tradition towards an approach of more global vascular protection.

The outcome of this intensive and integrated vascular treatment approach aiming at multiple sources of risk has, however, only been evaluated in a few studies of patients with type 2 diabetes (for review see 12–14). By targeting several risk factors simultaneously using treatment goals in many respects comparable to current guidelines from the American Diabetes Association [15], the Steno-2 study, which was initiated 15 years ago, demonstrated an overall 50% relative risk reduction of CVD in a high-risk population of type 2 diabetic patients with microalbuminuria (a marker of a generalized vasculopathy), thus underscoring the benefits of an intensified intervention integrating both a target-driven polypharmacological therapy and a focused behaviour modification [16,17].

Steno-2 Demonstrates that an Intensive and Multi-Targeted Intervention Makes a Major Difference

The Steno-2 study [16,17] was the first long-term type 2 diabetes trial that compared the impact of an intensified, multi-targeted intervention with that of a usual multifactorial treatment on risk factors for angiopathy. In a randomized, open, parallel trial, 80 patients with type 2 diabetes and microalbuminuria were randomized to receive usual care in accordance with national guidelines, while another 80 patients with type 2 diabetes were assigned to receive an intensified, comprehensive approach targeting a series of modifiable risk factors. The primary composite endpoint was death from CVD, non-fatal MI, non-fatal stroke, percutaneous coronary intervention (PCI), coronary artery bypass grafting, revascularization, and amputation. At a mean follow-up of 7.8 years, patients receiving the intensive therapy had a 53% (95% CI: 27–76%) lower relative risk of CVD. Shown graphically, the difference began to be observed within the first year with a continuous widening gap over time (Fig. 1). More detailed information on the impact of intensified interventions on the various components of the primary CVD endpoint is given in Fig. 2.

Also the secondary endpoints of microvascular complications were markedly altered: 61% (CI: 13–83%) lower relative risk of nephropathy, 58% (CI: 14–79%) lower risk of retinopathy, and 63% (CI: 21–82%) lower risk of autonomic neuropathy. For the primary CVD endpoint risk reductions were seen for all the different components except for mortality. It may be added that this trial was not statistically powered to evaluate the interventional impact on mortality.

Compared to the majority of individual risk factor intervention trials, the absolute risk reduction in the Steno-2 trial was considerable. The absolute risk reduction for the primary endpoint was 20% meaning that one CVD event was prevented for every five patients treated intensively for 7.8 years. In comparison, the absolute risk reductions for most of the other intervention studies are typically about 5% giving a number needed to treat of 20. The outcome of the Steno-2 study may have implications for type 2 diabetes care generally, adding to the accumulating knowledge and practical experiences that integrating several pieces of now evidence-based interventions cut the risk of macro- and microangiopathy by half – at least in high-risk patients.

How were the Angiopathy-Risk Reductions Achieved in the Steno-2 Trial?

Patients randomized to intensive therapy were followed by a diabetes care team consisting of a nurse, a clinical dietician, and a physician. In this group each patient paid a visit to the clinic at least every third month. Individual risk assessments and prioritizations of risk factor targeting were made at the start of the trial and whenever appropriate but as a minimum annually throughout the trial period. At each consultation measurements of clinical (blood pressure, body mass index, waist and hip circumference, smoking status) and biochemical variables (HbA_{1c}, fasting serum levels of total cholesterol, High-density lipoprotein-cholesterol

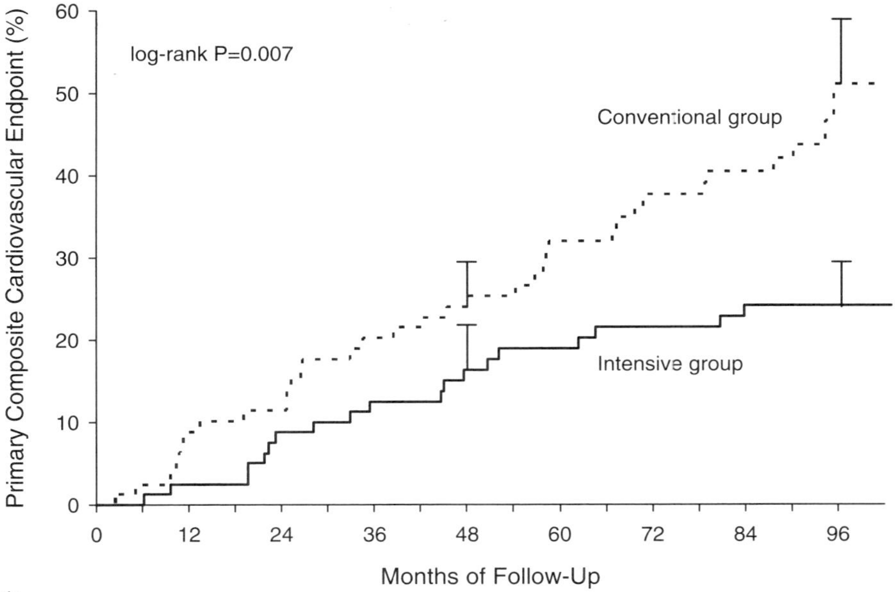

No. at risk									
Conventional	80	72	70	63	59	50	44	41	13
Intensive	80	78	74	71	66	63	61	59	19

FIG. 1. Kaplan–Meier estimates of time to first CVD event in the intensive therapy and conventional therapy group (reproduced from ref. 16).

(HDL-cholesterol), and triglycerides as well as urinary albumin excretion rate) were performed and the treatment was adjusted accordingly.

The intensive intervention involved a stepwise introduction of lifestyle and pharmacological interventions aimed at keeping glycated haemoglobin (<6.5%), blood pressure (<130/80 mmHg), total fasting serum cholesterol (<175 mg/dL) and fasting serum triglycerides (<150 mg/dL) at strict targets close to what was considered normal physiology. It should be emphasized that the treatment goals in the intensive arm were made more ambitious throughout the study concomitantly with the gain of novel insights from published single risk factor intervention studies. A *stepwise* introduction of the pharmacotherapeutic package was chosen to facilitate concordance. The details of the treatment algorithms have previously been reported [12–17]. To keep up the long-term motivation for this integrated and aggressive approach, at each consultation the patients were educated about the rationale for the prescribed polypharmacy and the behaviour modification.

A diet interview was performed annually or whenever patients or the diabetes educators found it necessary. In this way continuity in diet education was maintained. The dietary intervention was concentrated on qualitative changes of the diet including a reduction in the intake of animal fat, an increase in omega-3 fatty acid-rich food items (seafood, walnuts and almonds), and an increase in daily intake of vegetables and fruits. At each consultation patients were encouraged to stop smoking. Structured stop-smoking courses for smoking patients in the intensive therapy group and their spouses were organized throughout the follow-up period. Nicotine substitution was offered for free. The patients were continuously inspired to increase the level of leisure-time physical activity of any type. Otherwise, treatment goals for smoking and exercise were similar in the two treatment arms.

Treat to Target in Type 2 Diabetes– is it that Easy?

In evidence-based medicine what seems to be common sense still has to be documented. The Steno-2 study proved what many diabetes educators for years had thought to be obvious: that type 2 diabetes is a treatable disorder and that the angiopathy

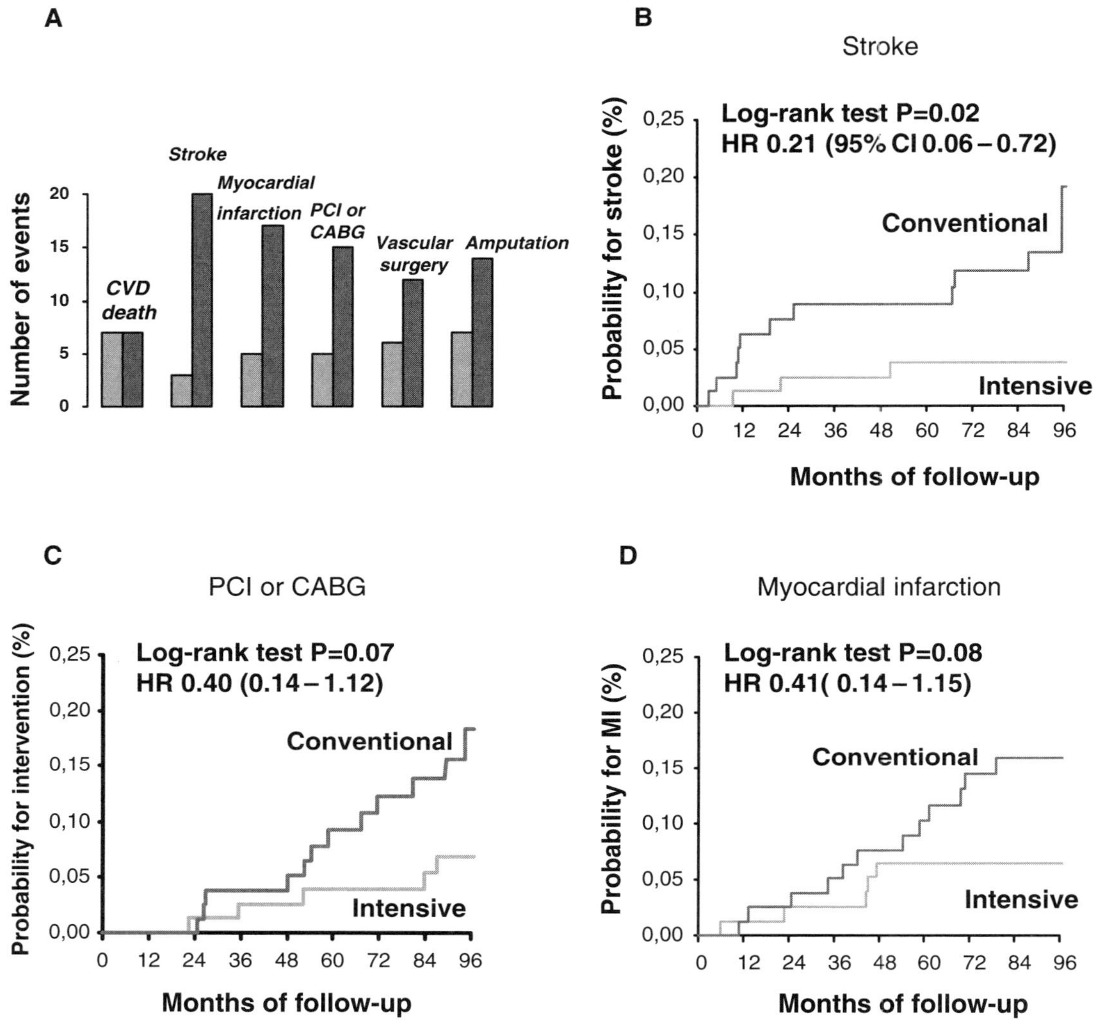

FIG. 2. (A) Distribution of the total number of cardiovascular events in the intensive therapy group in the Steno-2 Study [16] (light gray) and the conventional therapy group (dark gray). (B) Kaplan–Meier estimates of time to first stroke in the intensive therapy and conventional therapy group. HR denotes hazard ratio. 95%CI denotes confidence interval. (C) Kaplan–Meier estimates of time to first percutaneous coronary intervention (PCI) or coronary bypass graft (CABG) in the intensive therapy and conventional therapy group. (D) Kaplan–Meier estimates of time to first myocardial infarction in the intensive therapy and conventional therapy group (reproduced from ref. 13).

prognosis of these patients can be dramatically improved if the intervention is aggressively directed against a series of modifiable risk factors and if the patients are offered a continuous education and motivation.

A major strength of the Steno-2 study is the pragmatic treatment approach to the everyday clinical challenges that patients with type 2 diabetes present. Although the protocol was limited to patients who had microalbuminuria, this subgroup of patients may constitute up to one third of all patients with type 2 diabetes. It may be reasonable, however, to expect lower absolute risk reductions for type 2 diabetic patients at lower risk than with patients included in the Steno-2 trial.

Even in a clinical trial setting such as the Steno-2 study it is, however, quite thought-provoking that treatment goals were not obtained to greater extents in the intensive therapy group. Only 15% of patients in this group achieved an HbA_{1c} value

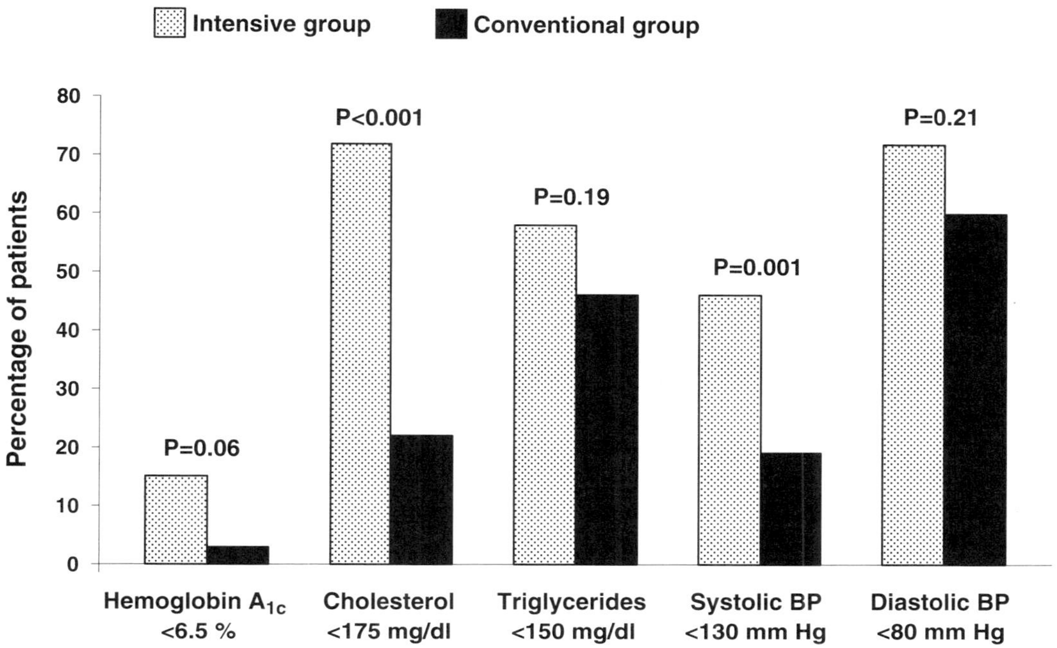

FIG. 3. The percentage of patients in each treatment group who reached the intensive treatment goals at the end of the Steno-2 Study (reproduced from ref. 16).

below 6.5%, which was the upper normal value for the applied assay and only about half achieved the target for systolic blood pressure [16] (Fig. 3). In addition, it turned out to be extremely difficult in a long-term perspective to change health behaviour in middle-aged and elderly overweight people despite the investment of relatively many educational resources [16].

Should Every Type 2 Diabetic Patient be Offered a Steno-2 Like Treatment Algorithm?

An ongoing trial with a treatment concept and clinical endpoints similar to the Steno-2 protocol is examining the effect in a low-risk population of screen-detected type 2 diabetic patients [18]. If significant vascular risk reductions are demonstrated in these low-risk patients, the intensified approach might be offered to all patients with type 2 diabetes. However, until then it seems reasonable to confine the intensified approach primarily to type 2 diabetic patients with elevated levels of albumin excretion rate or known CVD. Such patient categories may well comprise more than half of the type 2 diabetes population.

The Gap between Clinical Reality and Guidelines Recommending the Multi-targeted Therapeutic Package

A recent Swedish survey [19] involving more than 40,000 patients with type 2 diabetes from both primary care units and diabetes clinics reported that the new European treatment targets of HbA_{1c} < or = 6.1%, blood pressure <130/80 mmHg, and total serum cholesterol <4.5 mmol/L were attained by 16%, 13%, and 28% of the patients in 2003, respectively. Aspirin was prescribed in 36% of cases. These findings are compatible with reports from the USA [20] calling for much more focus on the implementation of current guidelines at the community level and changes in today's strategies. Moreover, since a review from the Cochrane Library [21] concluded that unstructured care in the community is associated with poor follow-up, worse glycaemic regulation, and a greater mortality than specialist care of type 2 diabetes, it is obvious that diabetes care professionals have to reconsider their CVD risk reduction approaches. That structured care can be implemented in a community setting has been demonstrated in a 6-year randomized intervention study enrolling more than 1,200 patients with newly diagnosed type 2 diabetes who were treated by general practitioners [22].

Also nurse-led type 2 diabetes care might well be a major innovation in the field of successful CVD risk intervention. The results from a British protocol-driven, nurse-led cardiovascular risk reduction clinic using an open clinical algorithm were recently reported [23]. The primary aim of the study was in 110 patients with type 2 diabetes and hypertension to optimize blood pressure control; secondary aims were to reduce modifiable CVD risk factors. Patients taking one or more antihypertensive drugs were selected for referral to the nurse-led clinic if blood pressure was >140/85 mmHg. An open clinical algorithm was designed to direct the nurse on the use of antihypertensive, statin, and aspirin therapy plus lifestyle advice. Blood pressure was reduced to 130/68 mmHg ($p < 0.001$), this reduction being sustained at review 9 months later (mean BP 133/67 mmHg), with 87 (79%) achieving BP < or = 140/85 mmHg. Treatment modalities were adjusted to reduce CVD risk, including antihypertensive medication, lipid-lowering therapy, and antiplatelet therapy. HDL-cholesterol improved from 1.2 ± 0.5 mmol/L to 1.4 ± 0.5 mmol/L ($p = 0.004$). The number of patients with microalbuminuria decreased from 41 (47%) to 25 (28%) ($p = 0.02$), with a fall in urinary albumin:creatinine ratio from 3.0 (1.3–7.9) to 1.8 (1.0–5.0) mg/mmol ($p = 0.01$). The number of smokers decreased from 22 (20%) to 14 (13%) ($p = 0.01$). Although not included as an intervention in the protocol, HbA_{1c} improved to 8.1 ± 1.6% from 8.7 ± 1.6% ($p < 0.001$).

The Patient-centred Approach – the Essentials of Continued Education and Motivation

It is the experience of the Steno-2 investigators that repetitive teaching about the rationale for the individual interventions and their expected health benefits is of utmost significance for the long-term motivation and therapy adherence of the patients. A similar experience was recently reported by Dr Ravid and co-workers who examined whether motivating patients to gain expertise and closely follow their risk factors would attenuate the course of vascular sequelae of diabetes [24]. A randomized, prospective study was conducted involving 165 patients who had type 2 diabetes, hypertension, and hyperlipidemia and were referred for consultation to a diabetes clinic in an academic hospital. Patients were randomly allocated to standard consultation (SC) or to a patient participation (PP) programme. Both groups were followed by their primary care physicians. The mean follow-up was 7.7 years, a period similar to the one of the Steno-2 study. The SC group attended eight annual consultations. The PP patients initiated on average one additional consultation per year. There were 80 cardiovascular events (eight deaths) in the SC group versus 47 events (five deaths) in the PP group ($p = 0.001$). The relative risk (RR) over 8 years for a cardiovascular event in the intervention (PP) versus the control (SC) group was 0.65 (95%CI, 0.89 to 0.41). There were 17 and 8 cases of stroke in the SC and PP groups, respectively ($p = 0.05$). RR for stroke was 0.47 (95%CI, 0.85 to 0.32). In the SC group, 14 patients developed overt nephropathy (four ESRD) versus seven (one ESRD) in the PP group ($p = 0.05$) (Fig. 3). Throughout the study period blood pressure, serum level of LDL-cholesterol, and HbA_{1c} were significantly lower in the PP than in the SC patients. The investigators therefore concluded that well-informed and motivated patients are more successful in obtaining and adequately coping with their risk factors, resulting in reduced CVD risk as well as slower progression of microvascular disease.

Also a recent randomized controlled trial in Canada sought to determine whether a 1-year intensive multi-therapy programme resulted in greater goal attainment than usual care among patients with poorly regulated type 2 diabetes [25]. It was demonstrated that an intensive multifactorial intervention was successful in helping patients meet most of the ambitious treatment goals. However, 6 months after intensive therapy and education, treatment was stopped and patients returned to usual care, the benefits had vanished, again underlining the critical importance of continued motivation and support.

Treatment Barriers

The success of a treatment strategy depends both on the patient's ability or will to adhere to the treatment prescribed as well as possible barriers of the health professional against the treatment. A recent investigation of the adherence to prescribed oral medications in type 2 diabetic patients following a multifactorial approach in a primary care setting demonstrated that only one in three patients had adequate adherence [26]. Factors associated with non-adherence included diabetes duration, complexity of drug regimen and inadequate control of risk factors for vaculopathy.

Many of the therapies given in an intensified multifactorial intervention approach are given as preventive treatments irrespective of the presence of symptoms, and therefore patients without symptoms may find, that the treatment interferes more with their quality of life than the disease itself. In this respect, it is worth noticing, that patients may find that a change in lifestyle and diet can lead to a large reduction in the quality of life and thus be a more severe barrier for the adherence to treatment than taking drugs [27]. Even in case of symptoms, the start of a treatment may not relieve these, thereby in itself being a risk factor for non-adherence to treatment [28].

Many patients with type 2 diabetes and therefore with multiple health issues may be able to handle changes only one step at a time. The long-term therapeutic action plan will, however, require multiple steps but the plan needs to be gradually developed by the physician and the patient together based upon individualized risk assessment, digestible evidence-based information, empathetic motivation and realistic tradeoffs related to benefits and potential undesired effects of the intervention.

Two different pills plus insulin for control of blood glucose, one or two for dyslipidaemia, then three or four for hypertension and on top of this a low-dose aspirin a day. Upwards of eight or more drugs a day for each intensively treated type 2 diabetic patient and that is even before we consider the drug treatment of concomitant diseases. No wonder that patients exposed to life-long intensive treatment of type 2 diabetes to be motivated, need continued and personalized education about indications, mechanisms of actions, and potential side effects of the prescribed medications. Whether the pill burden of polypharmacy in patients with type 2 diabetes may be alleviated through the use of drugs that intrinsically are effective against more aspects of the metabolic abnormalities or by prescription of a single poly-pill per day containing many of the known ingredients needed in the prevention of vasculopathy is an intriguing question that deserves to be pursued [29]. Of course, side effects including drug interactions will also influence drug adherence, and finally cost of treatment may be of major significance [30,31].

On the professional side it has been shown that barriers of the professionals in following guidelines are related to their knowledge of the disease and its rational treatment [32]. One of the obstacles may thus be that some physicians and diabetes educators still think of type 2 diabetes as a relatively benign disease [32] or they may doubt that the impressive results from the clinical trials can be achieved in daily practice or they share the concern of some of the patients that treatment side effects outbalance benefits. Therefore, to facilitate the implementation processes of an aggressive micro- and macroangiopathy risk intervention in patients with diabetes, it appears relevant to offer not only postgraduate training of diabetes care professionals but in order to reveal treatment resistance also to establish a continuous monitoring of the response to treatment including efficacy, concordance, and adverse effects. A proposal for a focused and multifactorial management of type 2 diabetes is given in Table 1.

Residual Risk of Angiopathy and Future Complementary Treatment Approaches

The cardiovascular complications are by far the most threatening for the long-term prognosis in patients with overt type 2 diabetes and the high-risk microalbuminuric patients participating in the standard multi-targeted intervention in the Steno-2 study showed an event rate of the combined CVD endpoint of 7% per year [16]. Although the intensified multifactorial intervention cut this event rate by half, it is still more than three times as high as in the matched background population leaving much room for improvements.

The radical fight back is obviously to intensify the primary prevention of type 2 diabetes [33–36].

TABLE 1. A multifactorial approach to a personalized treatment of type 2 diabetes.

Risk assessment

Several computer-based risk scoring programs are available. One of them is the UKPDS Risk Engine (www.dtu.ox.ac.uk), which has been developed at Oxford University. It can be used to estimate the future risk of the type 2 diabetic patient to develop ischaemic heart disease or stroke. A CVD risk profile at annual intervals may be a useful tool for the repetitive motivating dialogues and prioritization of risk marker interventions.

Therapeutic action plan based upon repetitive patient education, listening-, and motivation sessions.

The long-term therapeutic action plan will require multiple steps but the plan needs to be gradually developed by the diabetes educators and the patient together based upon the individualized risk assessment, digestible evidence-based information, empathetic listening and motivation, and realistic tradeoffs related to benefits and potential undesired effects of the intervention. Obviously, regular and readily understood feedback on progress towards the goals is crucial for sustained patient motivation and treatment success.

An integrated healthy life performance including no smoking, daily physical activity (at least for 1 hour), a low-fat, vegetable-/fruit- and seafood-enriched diet, and mental stress coping is notoriously difficult to implement. Nevertheless, enthusiastic motivation for this first-line therapy should be an essential part of the recurring patient education [15].

Hyperglycaemia

Target: HbA_{1c} <6.0% (referenced to a non-diabetic range of 4.0–6.0% using a DCCT-based assay). The target should, however, be higher in patient with known coronary heart disease or unawareness of hypoglycaemia.

Oral antidiabetic drugs (OAD) are introduced if HbA_{1c} is >6.0% after 3 months of dietary and exercise intervention. Overweight and obese patients are started on metformin to maximum of 2×1 g. If contraindicated or in lean patients, a sulphonylurea or a meglitinide is prescribed.

Combination of the two types of drugs or addition of a glitazone drug is considered when HbA_{1c} target is not met after 6–9 months.

NPH insulin or long-acting insulin analogues at bedtime or mixed short- and long-acting insulin analogues at the main meals 2–3 times a day should be added when HbA_{1c} is >7.0% despite maximal dose of OADs. At the start of insulin treatment, obese patients stop the sulphonylurea/meglitinide and the lean patients stop metformin.

Alternatively, the patient may be prescribed a combination of conventional OADs and a DPP IV inhibitor or a GLP-1 analogue

Hypertension

Target: <130/80 mmHg. In diabetic patients with albuminuria the target should be even lower.

Angiotensin II receptor antagonists or ACE inhibitors as initial treatment. Like the HbA_{1c} target the blood pressure target will often require multiple agents including thiazides, loop diuretics, calcium antagonists and β-blockers.

Dyslipidaemia

Targets: serum LDL-cholesterol <2.6 mmol/L (<100 mg/dL) and fasting serum triglycerides <1.7 mmol/(<150 mg/dL).

Treatment: a statin or a combination of a statin and ezetimibe for raised isolated hypercholesterolaemia or combined dyslipidaemia; fibrates and/or high doses of omega-3 fatty acids (2 g $\times$ 2 daily) in isolated fasting hypertriglyceridemia (>3.4 mmol/L or >350 mg/dL).

Albuminuria

Angiotensin II receptor antagonists or ACE inhibitors are prescribed irrespective of blood pressure values.

Prevention of platelet aggregation

Aspirin 75 mg/daily to all type 2 diabetic patients. For patients with very high CVD risk or in whom aspirin is contraindicated, clopidrogel is an option.

Secondary CVD prevention

Treatment with an ACE inhibitor should be considered.

Depression

About 5% or more of diabetic patients suffer from depression, which should be recognized and therapeutically addressed to ensure that the patient remains an active and motivated partner of the management plan.

Barriers and treatment resistance

A continuous monitoring of the response to treatment including efficacy, concordance, and adverse effects is a key to dissolve treatment resistance.

Perhaps a breakthrough in our understanding of the molecular pathogenesis of abdominal obesity and thereby of targets for antiobesity drug development will be an answer to many of the current shortcomings in the prevention and successful treatment of the majority of type 2 diabetes patients since abdominal obesity is known to cause insulin resistance and an atherogenic low-grade inflammatory state partially due to an excessive secretion of proinflammatory adipokines including tumour necrosis factor alpha.

Another target for major improvement is treatment of resistant hyperglycaemia of type 2 diabetic patients. The UKPDS showed a steady decline in pancreatic beta-cell function with diabetes duration, most likely caused by an accelerated apoptosis induced by numerous factors including chronic exposure to elevated levels of free fatty acids, glucose and proinflammatory cytokines [37]. Any future intervention that might prevent reduction of beta-cell mass or function (e.g. GLP-1 analogues, exanetide and DPPIV inhibitors) is expected to improve glycaemic regulation as are treatments which diminish insulin resistance (glitazones) [38]. Due to the progressive nature of type 2 diabetes more aggressive insulin regimens in combination with oral hypoglycaemic drugs should be applied as well.

Treatment targets for circulating levels of LDL-cholesterol and triglycerides can in most cases rather easily be achieved with statins, ezemtibine, fibrates and omega-3 fatty acids. In contrast, it is much more difficult to improve the low serum level of HDL-cholesterol as a prominent CVD risk factor in type 2 diabetes. Some hope is given to several novel drug candidates [39].

Continued smoking has disastrous effects on the progress of retinopathy and cardiovascular complications. Although much more needs to be explored about how to successfully apply smoking cessation approaches, smoking remains a treatable addiction and in this context one of the most crucial initiatives a care provider can take is to refer the patient (and his spouse) who smokes to repetitive structured programmes including both psychological and drug therapy interventions.

Finally, it is anticipated that progress within the field of pharmacogenomics identifying by genotype those patients who are responders and less responders, respectively, to a given drug treatment of hyperglycaemia, dyslipidaemia, or hypertension greatly will contribute to efficacious 'personalized' interventions improving the risk marker profile and thereby enhancing the health of patients suffering from type 2 diabetes.

Conclusion

Type 2 diabetes is a major risk factor for premature angiopathy equivalent to existing ischaemic coronary disease. The reason appears to be that besides hyperglycaemia a clustering of other interactive but modifiable risk factors for vasculopathy coexists in these patients more often than would be expected by chance. During the last 5–10 years several successful randomized individual risk factor intervention trials have, however, been performed punching the nihilistic attitude to improve the vascular prognosis of type 2 diabetes previously taken on by many physicians and diabetes educators. Thus, to prevent or postpone premature vasculopathy in type 2 diabetes evidence has been provided that at all age groups a structured and intensified long-term approach is required that is far more than just glucocentric – an approach addressing more vascular risk factors including hypertension, dyslipidaemia, platelet aggregation, sedentary behaviour, smoking and dietary habits. The application of such an integrated and focused therapy for almost 8 years to high-risk type 2 diabetic patients cuts the relative risk of micro- and macroangiopathy by half. It is time to take these health benefits of global vascular interventions aimed at all validated targets gained in the controlled clinical trials to the community level, where it has been documented that a gap exists between evidence-based diabetology and daily clinical practice. To facilitate the implementation process it appears relevant to offer not only postgraduate training of diabetes care professionals but in order to identify treatment barriers also to establish a continuous monitoring of the intervention including efficacy, levels of patient motivation and concordance, as well as adverse effects.

References

1. Fabre J, Balant LP, Dayer PG, Fox HM, Vernet AT. The kidney in maturity onset diabetes mellitus: a clinical study of 510 patients. Kidney Int 1982;21:730–738.

2. Wingard DL, Barrett-Connor EL. Heart disease and diabetes. In: Harris MI, Cowie CC, Stern MS, Boyko EJ, Rieber GE, Bennet PH (eds.), Diabetes in America, 2nd ed. Washington: National Institutes of Health: 1995;429–448.
3. Laakso M, Lehto S. Epidemiology of macrovascular disease in diabetes. Diabet Rev 1997;5:294–315.
4. Haffner SM, Lehto S, Ronnemaa T, Pyorala K, Laakso M. Mortality from coronary heart disease in subjects with type 2 diabetes and in nondiabetic subjects with and without prior myocardial infarction. N Engl J Med 1998;339:229–234.
5. Stamler J, Vaccaro O, Neaton JD, Wentworth D. Diabetes, other risk factors, and 12-yr cardiovascular mortality for men screened in the Multiple Risk Factor Intervention Trial. Diabetes Care 1993;16: 434–444.
6. Turner RC, Millns H, Neil HA, Stratton IM, Manley SE, Matthews DR, Holman RR. Risk factors for coronary artery disease in non-insulin dependent diabetes mellitus: United Kingdom Prospective Diabetes Study (UKPDS: 23). BMJ 1998;316:823–828.
7. Standl E, Balletshofer B, Dahl B, Weichenhain B, Stiegler H, Hormann A, Holle R. Predictors of 10-year macrovascular and overall mortality in patients with NIDDM: the Munich General Practitioner Project. Diabetologia 1996;39:1540–1545.
8. Sowers J, Stump C. Insights into the biology of diabetic vascular disease: what's new? Am J Hypertens 2004;17:2–6.
9. Forman D, Bulwer BE. Cardiovascular disease: optimal approaches to risk factor modification of diet and lifestyle. Curr Treat Opt Cardiovasc Med 2006; 8:47–57.
10. Look AHEAD trial at www.niddkh.nih.gov/patient/show/lookahead//htm2005.
11. Hovens MM, Tamsma JT, Beishuizen ED, Huisman MV. Pharmacological strategies to reduce cardiovascular risk in type 2 diabetes mellitus: an update. Drugs 2005;65:433–445.
12. Gæde P, Pedersen O. Target intervention against multiple risk markers to reduce cardiovascular disease in patients with type 2 diabetes. Ann Med 2004;36: 355–366.
13. Gæde P, Pedersen O. Intensive integrated therapy of type 2 diabetes: implications for long-term prognosis. Diabetes 2004;53:S39–S47.
14. Gæde P, Pedersen O: Multi-targeted and aggressive treatment of patients with type 2 diabetes at high risk: what are we waiting for? Horm Metab Res 2005;37 (Suppl 1):76–82.
15. American Diabetes Association. Standards of Medical Care in Diabetes – 2006. Diabetes Care 2006;29:S4–S42.
16. Gæde P, Vedel P, Larsen N, Jensen GV, Parving HH, Pedersen O. Multifactorial intervention and cardiovascular disease in patients with type 2 diabetes. N Engl J Med 2003;348:383–393.
17. Gæde P, Vedel P, Parving HH, Pedersen O. Intensified multifactorial intervention in patients with type 2 diabetes mellitus and microalbuminuria: the Steno type 2 randomised study. Lancet 1999;353:617–622.
18. Lauritzen T, Griffin S, Borch-Johnsen K, Wareham NJ, Wolffenbuttel BH, Rutten G, Anglo-Danish-Dutch Study of Intensive Treatment in People with Screen Detected Diabetes in Primary Care. The ADDITION study: proposed trial of the cost-effectiveness of an intensive multifactorial intervention on morbidity and mortality among people with type 2 diabetes detected by screening. Int J Obes 2000;24 (Suppl 3):S6–S11.
19. Eliasson B, Cederholm J, Nilsson P, Gudbjornsdottir S, Steering Committee of the Swedish National Diabetes Register. The gap between guidelines and reality: type 2 diabetes in a National Diabetes Register 1996–2003. Diabet Med 2005;10:1420–1426.
20. Saydah SH, Fradkin J, Cowie CC. Poor control of risk factors for vascular disease among adults with previously diagnosed diabetes. JAMA 2004;291: 335–342.
21. Griffin S, Kinmonth AL. Systems for routine surveillance for people with diabetes mellitus (Cochrane Review). In The Cochrane Library. Oxford: Update Software: 2002.
22. Olivarius NF, Beck-Nielsen H, Andreasen AH, Horder M, Pedersen PA. Randomised controlled trial of structured personal care of type 2 diabetes mellitus. BMJ 2001;323:970–975.
23. Woodward A, Wallymahmed M, Wilding J, Gill G. Successful cardiovascular risk reduction in type 2 diabetes by nurse-led care using an open clinical algorithm. Diabet Med 2006;23:780–787.
24. Rachmani R, Slavachevski I, Berla M, Frommer-Shapira R, Ravid M. Teaching and motivating patients to control their risk factors retards progression of cardiovascular as well as microvascular sequelae of type 2 diabetes mellitus – a randomized prospective 8 years follow-up study. Diabet Med 2005;22:410–414.
25. Menard J, Payette H, Baillargeon JP, Maheux P, Lepage S, Tessier D, Ardilouze JL. Efficacy of intensive multitherapy for patients with type 2 diabetes mellitus: a randomized controlled trial. CMAJ 2005; 173:1457–1466.
26. Mateo JF, Gil-Guillen VF, Mateo E, Orozco D, Carbayo JA, Merino J. Multifactorial approach and adherence to prescribed oral medications in patients with type 2 diabetes. Int J Clin Pract 2006;60: 422–428.

27. Glasgow RE, McCaul KD, Schafer LC. Barriers to regimen adherence among persons with insulin-dependent diabetes. J Behav Med 1986;9:65–77.
28. Johansen J, Claudi T, Holtedahl K. Insulin treatment for poorly regulated diabetic patients in general practice. Better regulation and symptom relief? Scand J Prim Health Care 1999;17:244–249.
29. Wald NJ, Law MR. A strategy to reduce cardiovascular disease by more than 80%. BMJ 2003;326:1419.
30. Snoek FJ. Barriers to good glycaemic control: the patient's perspective. Int J Obes 2000;24:S12–S20.
31. Hiss RG. Barriers to care in non-insulin-dependent diabetes mellitus. The Michigan experience. Ann Intern Med 1996;124:146–148.
32. Kenny SJ, Smith PJ, Goldschmid MG, Newman JM, Herman WH. Survey of physician practice behaviors related to diabetes mellitus in the U.S. Physician adherence to consensus recommendations. Diabet Care 1993;16:1507–1510.
33. Pan XR, Li GW, Hu YH, Wang JX, Yang WY, An ZX, Hu ZX, Lin J, Xiao JZ, Cao HB, Liu PA, Jiang XG, Jiang YY, Wang JP, Zeng H, Zhang H, Bennet PH, Howard BV. Effects of diet and exercise in preventing NIDDM in people with impaired glucose tolerance. The Da Qing IGT and Diabetes Study. Diabetes Care 1997;20:537–544.
34. Tuomilehto J, Lindstrom J, Eriksson JG, Valle TT, Hamalainen H, Ilanne-Parikka P, Keinanen-Kiukaanniemi S, Laakso M, Louheranta A, Rastas M, Salminen V, Uusitupa M. Prevention of type 2 diabetes mellitus by changes in lifestyle among subjects with impaired glucose tolerance. N Engl J Med 2001;344:1343–1350.
35. Knowler WC, Barrett-Conor E, Fowler SE, Hamman RF, Lachin JM, Walker EA, Nathan DM: Diabetes Prevention Program Research Group. Reduction in the incidence of type 2 diabetes with lifestyle intervention or metformin. N Engl J Med 2002;346:393–403.
36. DREAM (Diabetes Reduction Assessment with ramipril and rosiglitazone Medication) Trial Investigators, Gerstein HC, Yusuf S, Bosch J, Pogue J, Sheridan P, Dinccag N, Hanefeld M, Hoogwerf B, Laakso M, Mohan V, Shaw J, Zinman B, Holman RR. Effect of rosiglitazone on the frequency of diabetes in patients with impaired glucose tolerance or impaired fasting glucose: a randomised controlled trial. Lancet 2006;368:1096–1105.
37. UKPDS 16. Overview of 6 years' therapy of type II diabetes: a progressive disease. Diabetes 1995;44: 1249–1258.
38. Poulsen MK, Henriksen JE, Hother-Nielsen O, Beck-Nielsen H. The combined effect of triple therapy with rosiglitazone, metformin, and insulin aspart in type 2 diabetic patients. Diabet Care 2003;26:3273–3279.
39. Forrester JS, Shah PK. Emerging strategies for increasing high-density lipoprotein. Am. J. Cardiol 2006;98:1542–1549.

Section: Treating the Comorbid Patient

15
Obesity and Pharmacological Treatment

Bjørn Richelsen

Keywords: Diabetes, Pharmacotherapy, Orlistat, Siblitramine, Rimonabant, Weightloss

In the past 25 years, the rates of obesity have tripled in countries that have adopted a Western lifestyle with decreased physical activity and overconsumption of cheap, easily available, energy-dense food. The prevalence of overweight (BMI > 25 kg/m^2) is 40–60% and the prevalence of obesity (BMI > 30 kg/m^2) is 10–25% in adults in most Western countries. Of special concern, this obesity epidemic also affects children where overweight among them ranges from 10% to 25%, and the prevalence of obesity ranges from 3% to 10%.

Obesity, particularly with abdominally located fatness, is associated with development of type 2 diabetes, cardiovascular diseases, and some cancers. The increase in the prevalence of type 2 diabetes worldwide is closely linked to the increase in obesity. Moreover, obesity is associated with considerable impairment of the quality of personal and social life. About 80–90% of type 2 diabetes is attributable to excess weight. Thus, the best way to prevent or treat type 2 diabetes is to be able to prevent or to treat excess body weight. There are, however, obvious problems both in preventing and in treating excess body weight since most obese patients losing weight regain it and even though most people do not like to be obese the prevalence of obesity is increasing steadily.

Management of obesity should be integrated, aiming to alter the micro-environment of the patient and his family to favour a better lifestyle with more physical activity and a better diet with focus on more fruit, vegetables, and whole-grain products. The general success of lifestyle interventions in obtaining long-lasting weight loss in obese patients is relatively poor. However, minor weight loss in the range of 2.5–10% maintained for more than a year has been shown to improve some of the health complications of obesity. Minor weight loss maintained for a few years together with increased physical activity have been shown particularly to improve glucose-insulin homeostasis by preventing the development of overt diabetes or to improve the diabetic state [1,2].

More pronounced weight losses induced by surgical methods have been shown to reduce most of the obesity-related complications including reducing the development of type 2 diabetes with more than 80% compared with a control group [3]. Furthermore, it has now been demonstrated that pronounced weight loss (induced by surgery), which can be maintained long-term (more than 15 years), is able to reduce the obesity-related mortality by 25–30% (Sjostrom L personal communication).

Pharmacotherapy

Pharmacological intervention is often recommended as an adjunct to dietary modification and physical activity when other approaches have failed for patients with overweight and obesity. Currently only three medications are suitable for long-term therapy – orlistat, sibutramine, and rimonabant. These medications should only be prescribed in combination with lifestyle modifications and a structured long-term follow-up. Clinical practice guidelines suggest a stepped approach to the management of overweight and obesity with only those of significant risk requiring more intensive therapies such as pharmacotherapy. Thus, pharmacotherapy could be considered in patients with obesity (BMI > 30 kg/m^2) or in those with BMI between 27 and 29.9 kg/m^2 with increased risk such as type 2 diabetes, risk of or manifest cardiovascular disease, or obstructive sleep apnoea [4].

Weight regain is common after the medications are discontinued, and long-term drug administration may be required for weight loss maintenance. Weight regain may, however, occur despite continued drug treatment. Weight loss usually reaches a plateau after 6–9 months of treatment. It is unclear whether this is due to biological or more psychological factors. Moreover, some obese patients are refactory to drug treatment and do not respond at all. Thus, if the patient does not obtain any weight loss after treatment for 2–3 months, drug treatment should be stopped. Patients are more likely to be compliant if they receive ongoing counselling and follow-up by a dietician and/or general practitioner. It is also important to discuss realistic expectations for weight loss and the long-term consequences of maintaining a healthy lifestyle with the patients.

Sibutramine

Sibutramine acts centrally as a noradrenalin-serotonin uptake inhibitor and has appetite-suppressing effects. Sibutramine also stimulates thermogenesis but this effect seems to play a minor role in weight reduction. Together with lifestyle modification sibutramine provides a mean weight loss of approximately 4 kg after treatment for 1 year when compared with placebo [5]. The dose of sibutramine used was either 10 or 15 mg once daily. The number of patients reaching 5% and 10% weight loss was 34% and 15% larger with sibutramine than with placebo. Wadden et al [6] have shown that a programme of sibutramine together with lifestyle modification is considerably more successful than either therapy alone. After a significant weight loss sibutramine is better to maintain the weight loss for up to 2 years when compared with placebo [7].

Besides common usually mild side effects such as dry mouth, constipation, insomnia, and headaches, sibutramine produces a dose-dependent minor increase in heart rate and may increase the blood pressure as well, leading to concerns about potential cardiovascular negative effects. Thus, it should be used with caution in patients with hypertension and the blood pressure should be monitored in all patients particularly in the initiation of treatment. Sibutramine is contraindicated in patients with untreated or poorly controlled hypertension, arrhythmias, coronary heart disease, cardiac failure, and severe impairment of the liver and kidney function.

Sibutramine and Diabetes

Several smaller interventions with sibutramine in obese patients with type 2 diabetes have been performed. In 6- to −12-month interventions glycemic control improved in parallel with weight loss and those with a weight loss of ≥10% also achieved significant decreases in HbA1c. Diabetic patients have higher rates of hypertension than non-diabetic patients. At least 10% of the patients will experience a 10 mmHg or more rise in blood pressure using sibutramine [8]. Thus, the drug should be used with caution in diabetic patients. In a Cochrane review concerning pharmacotherapy for weight loss in adults with type 2 diabetes, it is concluded that the magnitude of weight loss is modest and the long-term health benefits of pharamocotherapy remain unclear. Moreover, the safety of sibutramine in these patients is still uncertain [9].

Long-term data on the effect of sibutramine on obesity-related morbidity and mortality are still lacking. However, the current Sibutramine Cardiovascular Outcomes (SCOUT) trial is evaluating the efficacy of sibutramine on major cardiovascular events (myocardial infarction, stroke, and mortality). It is planned that this study should be finished in 2008.

Orlistat

Orlistat binds to intestinal and pancreatic lipases, inhibiting their action and reduces dietary fat absorption by about 30%. The typical dose of orlistat is 120 mg three times per day with meals. Less than 1% of the drug is taken up. Thus, most of the drug is excreted unchanged in faeces.

The mean weight loss after treatment for 1 year with orlistat is around 3 kg when compared with placebo. The number of patients reaching 5% and 10% weight loss was 21% and 12% larger with orlistat than with placebo [10]. In a 3-year trial the placebo-corrected extra weight loss with orlistat was 2.5 kg [11]. In a 4-year intervention the weight loss after treatment with orlistat was 2.7 kg when compared with placebo [12]. In some but not all studies it is found that orlistat treatment leads to more favourable changes in total cholesterol and LDL-cholesterol. Orlistat has been found to reduce blood pressure by 1.8 mmHg systolic and by 1.6 mmHg diastolic. Side effects of orlistat are related to its mode of action and include particularly gastrointestinal problems such as fatty oily stools, faecal urgency, diarrhoea, flatulence, and abdominal pain. These side effects are reduced by following a low fat diet. Fat malabsorption does, however, increase the risk of vitamin D, E, and beta-caroten deficiency, and, therefore, daily supplementation with vitamins is recommended during orlistat treatment. These supplements should be taken between meals.

Orlistat and Diabetes

Beneficial results in the glycemic profile (mean reduction of fasting glucose by about 0.8 mmol/L) have been reported with orlistat-induced weight loss in 6- to 12-month studies in obese type 2 diabetic patients. This has been found also when orlistat was given as an adjunct to antidiabetic treatment such as with metformin and sulphonylurea drugs. Smaller but significant reductions of HbA1c have also been found by orlistat treatment (placebo controlled).

In a 4-year Swedish intervention with orlistat in 3,305 obese patients, it was found that orlistat reduced weight by extra 2.7 kg and decreased the incidence of type 2 diabetes from 9.0% to 6.2% (hazard ratio 0.63). The preventive effect associated with orlistat treatment was almost only in patients with impaired glucose tolerance at baseline (20% of the population) [12].

Apart from diabetes incidence, the effect of orlistat on obesity-related morbidity and mortality is still lacking.

Rimonabant

Rimonabant is the first endocannabinoid–CB [1] blocking drug in the treatment of obesity. The CB1 receptor is widely distributed in CNS and these receptors interact with several pathways involved in appetite regulation (e.g. ghrelin and leptin pathways). Rimonabant may, however, also have peripheral effects on metabolic factors. Endogenous ligands for these receptors, the endocannabinoids, are synthesised from phospholipid derivatives of arachidonic acid and may stimulate the appetite. There are some indications that obesity is associated with an overactivity of the endocannabinoid system, which may be reduced by rimonabant.

Four clinical trials in overweight or obese adults with or without type 2 diabetes have currently been published. Oral rimonabant 20 mg once daily reduces mean weight by around 4–5 kg more than placebo after treatment for 1 year [13–16]. The proportion of patients achieving ≥5% and ≥10% weight loss was 30% and 20% higher in the rimonabant group compared with placebo. The reduction in waist circumference after treatment with rimonabant was closely related to the extra weight loss. After 1 year of rimonabant treatment rerandomisation of the patients to placebo resulted in weight regain. Rimonabant-induced weight loss has only been associated with slightly reduced blood pressure [13]. More pronounced improvements in HDL-cholesterol and in triglyceride have, however, been observed after treatment with rimonabant. From analysing the data from the four trials it is suggested that rimonabant may have weight loss independent effects in improving HDL-cholesterol and triglyceride. However, these possible weight independent effects of rimonabant await further verifications from studies specifically designed to investigate this issue.

The adverse effects of rimonabant are upper respiratory tract infections, nausea, dizziness, and insomnia. The focus has, however, particularly been on mood alterations, depressive disorders, and anxiety, and these symptoms were reported in 3.2% with rimonabant (20 mg) and in 1.6% in placebo-treated patients. Patients with psychiatric illnesses were, however, not included in the published rimonabant trials. Thus, there is limited data available on the safety of rimonabant in patients with mental illness. Therefore, the use of rimonabant is not recommended in patients with depression or in patients on antidepressant medication.

Rimonabant and Diabetes

Only one study investigating the effect of rimonabant in type 2 diabetic patients has been published [16]. The rimonabant-induced weight loss was associated with a reduction of HbA1c by 0.7% after treatment for 1 year in obese diabetic patients who were not well controlled on either metformin or sulphonylurea drugs. The proportion of patients obtaining HbA1c under 6.5% was 43% in the rimonabant treated and 21% with placebo. Rimonabant had similar positive effects on HDL-cholesterol and triglyceride as in the other trials in non-diabetic patients [17].

No data on cardiovascular morbidity or mortality of rimonabant have still been reported but a large study investigating the effect of rimonabant on myocardial infarction, stroke, and cardiovascular death has been started.

Clinical Perspectives

No head-to-head trials of the three major antiobesity drugs on the market exist, which makes the decision of the benefit of one drug over the other for a given patient almost impossible. Therefore, if drug treatment is under consideration the choice among the three drugs may mainly take into account the adverse effects, the patients' preference, the concomitant diseases, and the cost of the drug.

It is shown that orlistat could prevent or retard the development of type 2 diabetes and reduce LDL-cholesterol. Thus, orlistat could be the choice in obese subjects with a high risk of development of type 2 diabetes (e.g. impaired glucose tolerance) and at enhanced risk of cardiovascular disease (e.g. hypertension and high LDL). Orlistat should be avoided in patients who are unable to reduce their fat intake and in patients with chronic diarrhoea.

Sibutramine may be useful in patients where the obese state is characterised by overeating and snacking because of its appetite reducing effects. Sibutramine should not be used in patients with uncontrolled hypertension or with tachy-arrhythmia. Rimonabant may be preferred in obese patients with the metabolic syndrome particularly in those with low HDL and high triglyceride. Because of few data rimonabant should be avoided in patients with psychiatric illness, particularly in patients with major depressions and in patients in antidepressive treatment. These suggestions are not evidence based but the recommendations that can be used until more direct head-to-head investigations have been performed.

If treatment with one of the drugs does not result in weight loss of more than 2–3% after 3 months, it should be stopped and another drug could be initiated. For all three drugs it has been found that when the drugs are stopped weight regain is very common. Treatment with orlistat has been performed up to 4 years without safety problems. For sibutramine and rimonabant data up to 2 years have been published. No data are available that suggest that combination treatment results in better weight losses than just using one drug.

References

1. Tuomilehto J, Lindstrom J, Eriksson JG, Valle TT, Hamalainen H, Ilanne-Parikka P, Keinanen-Kiukaanniemi S, Laakso M, Louheranta A, Rastas M, Salminen V, Uusitupa M: Prevention of type 2 diabetes mellitus by changes in lifestyle among subjects with impaired glucose tolerance. *N. Engl. J. Med.* 344:1343–1350, 2001.
2. Knowler WC, Barrett-Connor E, Fowler SE, Hamman RF, Lachin JM, Walker EA, Nathan DM: Reduction in the incidence of type 2 diabetes with lifestyle intervention or metformin. *N. Engl. J. Med.* 346:393–403, 2002.
3. Sjostrom L, Lindroos AK, Peltonen M, Torgerson J, Bouchard C, Carlsson B, Dahlgren S, Larsson B, Narbro K, Sjostrom CD, Sullivan M, Wedel H: Lifestyle, diabetes, and cardiovascular risk factors 10 years after bariatric surgery. *N. Engl. J. Med.* 351:2683–2693, 2004.
4. Padwal RS, Majumdar SR: Drug treatments for obesity: orlistat, sibutramine, and rimonabant. *Lancet* 369:71–77, 2007.
5. Li Z, Maglione M, Tu W, Mojica W, Arterburn D, Shugarman LR, Hilton L, Suttorp M, Solomon V, Shekelle PG, Morton SC: Meta-analysis: pharmacologic treatment of obesity. *Ann. Intern. Med.* 142:532–546, 2005.
6. Wadden TA, Berkowitz RI, Womble LG, Sarwer DB, Phelan S, Cato RK, Hesson LA, Osei SY, Kaplan R, Stunkard AJ: Randomized trial of lifestyle modification and pharmacotherapy for obesity. *N. Engl. J. Med.* 353:2111–2120, 2005.
7. James WP, Astrup A, Finer N, Hilsted J, Kopelman P, Rossner S, Saris WH, Van Gaal LF: Effect of sibutramine on weight maintenance after weight loss: a randomised trial. STORM Study Group. Sibutramine Trial of Obesity Reduction and Maintenance. *Lancet* 356:2119–2125, 2000.
8. Arterburn DE, Crane PK, Veenstra DL: The efficacy and safety of sibutramine for weight loss: a systematic review. *Arch. Intern. Med.* 164:994–1003, 2004.

9. Norris SL, Zhang X, Avenell A, Gregg E, Brown TJ, Schmid, CH, Lau J: Long-term non-pharmacological weight loss interventions for adults with type 2 diabetes mellitus. Cochrane Database of Systematic Reviews: Reviews 2005 Issue 2 John Wiley and Sons(TRUNCATED), 10.1002/14651858.CD004095.pub2.
10. Padwal R, Li SK, Lau DC: Long-term pharmacotherapy for overweight and obesity: a systematic review and meta-analysis of randomized controlled trials. *Int. J. Obes. Relat. Metab. Disord.* 27:1437–1446, 2003.
11. Richelsen B, Tonstad S, Rossner S, Toubro S, Niskanen L, Madsbad S, Mustajoki P, Rissanen A: Effect of Orlistat on Weight Regain and Cardiovascular Risk Factors Following a Very-Low-Energy Diet in Abdominally Obese Patients: A 3-year randomized, placebo-controlled study. *Diabetes Care* 30:27–32, 2007.
12. Torgerson JS, Hauptman J, Boldrin MN, Sjostrom L: XENical in the prevention of diabetes in obese subjects (XENDOS) study: a randomized study of orlistat as an adjunct to lifestyle changes for the prevention of type 2 diabetes in obese patients. *Diabetes Care* 27:155–161, 2004.
13. Despres JP, Golay A, Sjostrom L: Effects of rimonabant on metabolic risk factors in overweight patients with dyslipidemia. *N. Engl. J. Med.* 353:2121–2134, 2005.
14. Van Gaal LF, Rissanen AM, Scheen AJ, Ziegler O, Rossner S: Effects of the cannabinoid-1 receptor blocker rimonabant on weight reduction and cardiovascular risk factors in overweight patients: 1-year experience from the RIO-Europe study. *Lancet* 365:1389–1397, 2005.
15. Pi-Sunyer FX, Aronne LJ, Heshmati HM, Devin J, Rosenstock J: Effect of rimonabant, a cannabinoid-1 receptor blocker, on weight and cardiometabolic risk factors in overweight or obese patients: RIO-North America: a randomized controlled trial. *JAMA* 295:761–775, 2006.
16. Scheen AJ, Finer N, Hollander P, Jensen MD, Van Gaal LF: Efficacy and tolerability of rimonabant in overweight or obese patients with type 2 diabetes: a randomised controlled study. *Lancet* 368:1660–1672, 2006.
17. Henness S, Robinson DM, Lyseng-Williamson KA: Rimonabant. *Drugs* 66:2109–2119, 2006.

16
Management of Diabetic Dyslipidaemia

D. John Betteridge

Keywords: dyslipidaemia, LDL-cholesterol, small dense LDL, HDL-cholesterol, statins, fibrates, ezetimibe, nicotinic acid.

Introduction

Cardiovascular disease (CVD) remains the most important cause of morbidity and mortality in people with diabetes [1]. This high-risk population is more likely to suffer a fatal event as the first manifestation of myocardial infarction (MI) or stroke, making primary prevention a priority. The pathogenesis of atherosclerosis-related disease is multifactorial but dyslipidaemia is a common and important risk predictor and is open to therapeutic intervention. Pharmacological intervention is supported by major randomised, controlled clinical trials (RCTs) of primary and secondary CVD prevention. RCTs with statin drugs have demonstrated unequivocal benefit in reducing major coronary events and stroke.

Dyslipidaemia is strongly correlated to insulin resistance and hyperinsulinaemia. It is present at the time of diagnosis of diabetes as part of the insulin-resistance syndrome and persists despite treatment of glycaemia. It should be treated in its own right; indeed, given the evidence of benefit from RCTs, effective management of dyslipidaemia needs to move centrestage in the prevention of CVD.

In this chapter, the pathophysiology of diabetic dyslipidaemia and its relation to CVD are described. RCTs, which provide the basis for clinical practice, are discussed together with new information pointing to benefits from more intensive therapy. As a result of this evidence more stringent goals of therapy have been advocated by national and international bodies.

It will become clear that the major goal of therapy is to reduce low-density lipoprotein (LDL) cholesterol with the statin class of drugs. Sadly, audit data point to the fact that many patients are not yet receiving optimal management.

Most trial data relate to patients with type 2 diabetes but the increased lifetime risk in type 1 diabetes should not be overlooked and, although not strictly evidence-based, strategies for lipid-lowering management of this important group have been proposed.

Diabetic Dyslipidaemia

Diabetic dyslipidaemia is a complex phenotype of both quantitative and qualitative lipid and lipoprotein abnormalities [2]. It is present at the time of diagnosis and in the pre-diabetic period. Its expression in an individual patient will be influenced by both genetic and lifestyle factors such as gender, obesity, (particularly central obesity), level of physical activity, cigarette smoking, alcohol intake, diet, and poor glycaemic control; concomitant drug therapies and medical conditions such as primary dyslipidaemias (e.g. familial combined hyperlipidaemia and homozygosity for apoprotein E2, which predisposes to type III hyperlipidaemia) and other secondary causes of dyslipidaemia particularly renal and hepatic dysfunction and hypothyroidism.

It is characterised by moderately raised triglycerides, low high-density lipoprotein (HDL)-cholesterol, and the accumulation of cholesterol-enriched remnant lipoprotein particles. Total and LDL-cholesterol concentrations mainly reflect those of the background population but there are important qualitative changes in LDL particle distribution, which is shifted to smaller, denser particles, so-called small, dense LDL [3].

Depending on the cut points taken, raised triglycerides will be present in up to 60% of patients. In the Prospective Cardiovascular Munster (PROCAM) study in Germany, triglyceride concentrations >2.3 mmol/L were present in 39% of diabetic subjects compared with 21% in the general population and low HDL-cholesterol (<0.9 mmol/L) in 27% compared with 6% [4]. In the Botnia study, involving 4,483 men and women aged 35–70 years, patients with diabetes (n = 1,697) were three-fold more likely to have elevated triglycerides (>1.7 mmol/L) and low HDL-cholesterol (<0.9 mmol/L in men and <1 mmol/L in women). In individuals with impaired glucose tolerance (n = 798), dyslipidaemia was increased two-fold compared with those with normal glucose tolerance [5].

Factors leading to characteristic dyslipidaemia are complex and not fully understood. Insulin resistance is associated with the failure of normal suppression of hormone-sensitive lipase in adipose tissue and increased lipolysis leading to increased flux of non-esterified fatty acids (NEFAs) to the liver; this is partly responsible for increased hepatic output of very low-density lipoprotein (VLDL) [6]. Central obesity is common in insulin resistance and type 2 diabetes and visceral fat is increasingly recognised as an important paracrine and endocrine organ [7]. Adiponectin, an important adipose-specific adipokine, is reduced in insulin resistance and type 2 diabetes [8]. This would favour increased lipolysis as the action of a further important cytokine, TNF-alpha in stimulating lipolysis is unopposed.

Insulin normally suppresses hepatic VLDL assembly and secretion by increasing the degradation of apoprotein B-100, the major apoprotein of VLDL and inhibiting the expression of microsomal transfer protein, important in VLDL assembly [9,10]. In insulin resistance, increased flux of NEFAs together with lack of inhibition of VLDL assembly leads to overproduction of VLDL, mainly large VLDL. VLDL is overproduced in the postprandial state and as chylomicrons are absorbed from the gut, activity of the enzyme, lipoprotein lipase (LPL), is saturated leading to increased and prolonged postprandial lipaemia [11]. Clearance of triglyceride-rich lipoproteins is further affected as the activity of LPL is reduced in the presence of excess NEFAs and apoprotein C-III, a major inhibitor of LPL activity, is increased but this may not be independent of triglyceride levels [11].

Enhanced postprandial lipaemia stimulates lipid exchange between lipoproteins through the action of cholesterol ester transfer protein (CETP) [12]. CETP mediates the mole for mole transfer of cholesterol ester from HDL to lipoproteins of lower density in exchange for triglyceride. This contributes significantly to the qualitative lipoprotein abnormalities. Partially hydrolysed triglyceride-rich lipoproteins or remnant particles become enriched in cholesterol. These particles are thought to be highly atherogenic contributing to foam cell formation, oxidative stress, and endothelial dysfunction [13,14].

HDL becomes triglyceride-enriched through lipid exchange and is a substrate for hepatic lipase, which is increased in insulin resistance. As a result of hydrolysis of HDL triglyceride, smaller, denser HDL particles are formed; these are more rapidly catabolised contributing to the decreased HDL levels [15]. As previously discussed, adiponectin concentrations are reduced and this may contribute not only to decreased production of apo A1 the major protein of HDL, but also to decreased expression of the ATP cassette binding protein, ABC A1, an important peripheral binding site for HDL in the process of reverse cholesterol transport. These effects of adiponectin are probably related to its ability to stimulate peroxysome proliferator-activated receptor gamma (PPAR gamma) activity [8,16]

Hypertriglyceridaemia is a major factor in determining LDL particle size [17,18]. It appears from kinetic studies that it is a large VLDL, which is most strongly related to the generation of small, dense LDL [2]. CETP activity is again involved in lipid exchange producing triglyceride-enriched LDL particles, which are substrates for hepatic lipase, the resultant triglyceride hydrolysis resulting in smaller denser particles. LDL particle size is decreased in IGT with further reductions in frank diabetes, and these effects seem to be more marked in women [19].

Rationale for Lipid-Lowering from Epidemiology Studies

Total and LDL-cholesterol are similar or only slightly elevated in type 2 diabetes compared with the background population but are major determinants of CVD risk. In men, screened for the Multiple Risk Factor Intervention Trial (MRFIT), total cholesterol was an important determinant of CVD mortality in those with diabetes as in those without and, for a given cholesterol concentration, CVD risk was two- to three-fold higher [20].

LDL-cholesterol was the best predictor of MI in the United Kingdom Prospective Diabetes Study (UKPDS) [21]. Based on the observational epidemiology, a 1 mmol/L increase in LDL is associated with a 57% increased risk. LDL-cholesterol was also a strong predictor of CVD in diabetic individuals with insulin resistance and relatively low LDL concentrations in the Strong Heart Study [22].

LDL particle size distribution is shifted to smaller, denser particles in insulin resistance. These particles have less polar lipid leading to increased surface accessibility of apolipoprotein B (apo B), the major apo protein of LDL, including segments with increased binding affinity to glycosaminoglycans. Small dense LDL is a less effective ligand for the LDL receptor, a major determinant of the clearance of LDL from the circulation. More prolonged plasma residence time together with the smaller particle size facilitates penetration to the arterial subintimal space with subsequent increased retention due to binding to glycosaminoglycans. Small dense LDL is also more susceptible to oxidation and it is oxidised LDL that is central to many of the processes of atherogenesis [23,24].

When LDL particles are small and dense, there will be an increased particle number for a given LDL-cholesterol concentration. As there is one molecule of apo B per LDL particle, measurement of plasma apo B helps to identify the presence of small, dense LDL as the level will be higher than expected for the LDL-cholesterol concentration [25].

A further qualitative change in LDL, which may affect its atherogenic potential, is glycation of apo B. Glycated LDL is a less effective ligand for the LDL receptor, which will tend to prolong its plasma residence time and also increase susceptibility to oxidation [26].

HDL-cholesterol concentrations are inversely related to CVD risk in diabetes as in the general population [27]. There are several potential mechanisms by which HDL may protect but the most widely accepted is its roll in reverse cholesterol transport whereby free cholesterol is removed from the periphery, including the arterial wall, to the liver for excretion. This process is becoming increasingly understood at the cellular level with the identification of important receptors on liver and peripheral cells [28,29]. HDL may also protect against atherogenesis in other ways in that it has anti-inflammatory, anti-oxidant, and anti-thrombotic activity. In UKPDS a strong inverse correlation was demonstrated between HDL-cholesterol and risk; a 0.1 mmol increase being associated with a 15% decrease in CVD events [21].

When calculating absolute CVD risk in the individual patient, several guidelines incorporate a measure of total to HDL-cholesterol ratio as a means of assessing atherogenic cholesterol against the protective action of HDL [30]. The INTERHEART study, a multinational, case-control study involving 15,152 patients with MI together with 14,820 controls, assessed the relationship between the major apo proteins involved in cholesterol transport, apo B and apo A1, among other risk factors. In this analysis the strongest predictor of risk was the apo B/apo A1 ratio [31].

The relationship between triglycerides and CVD risk has been debated over many years. A risk factor in many cross-sectional and prospective studies, the relationship between triglycerides and CVD disappeared on multivariate analysis when other important confounders such as HDL-cholesterol were adjusted for [32]. Although one meta-analysis has demonstrated a significant association after adjustment for HDL [33] it is likely that epidemiology will not provide further insights in this area. Given the complexity of the interactions between triglyceride-rich lipoproteins and other lipoproteins, particularly HDL and small, dense LDL, mathematical modelling to determine the independence of a triglyceride CVD relationship is fraught with problems. The inherent variation in triglyceride concentrations will also tend to reduce its strength in multivariate models.

In view of these concerns some investigators have examined CVD risk in relation to triglyceride concentrations taking into account LDL and HDL. In the PROCAM study [34] and the Helsinki Heart Study [35], hypertriglyceridaemia was associated with CVD risk in individuals with an LDL to HDL ratio >5. This clustering of lipid abnormalities is often referred to as the atherogenic lipoprotein profile. Another approach has involved factor and principal component analysis. In a prospective study from Finland, a "hyperinsulinaemia cluster", a factor having high positive loadings for BMI, triglycerides, and insulin together with a high negative loading for HDL-cholesterol, was predictive of CHD death in type 2 diabetes [36].

Rationale for Lipid-Lowering from RCTs

Early lipid-lowering trials were handicapped by lack of well-tolerated and effective therapeutic agents. Clinical trial science was less developed, particularly in relation to the need for sufficient hard clinical end points to ensure statistical power and the need to follow all randomised patients until study completion. These trials suggested benefit for lipid-lowering in reducing non-fatal MI but there was little impact on fatal events and in some a suggestion of increased non-cardiac mortality. These findings led to the so-called cholesterol controversies of the late 1980s and early 1990s [37].

Introduction of the statins in the mid-1980s transformed cholesterol management [38]. Isolated from the culture broths of penicillins in the 1970s, they proved to be specific, competitive inhibitors of HMG CoA reductase (3-hydoxy 3-methylglutaryl coenzyme A reductase). This enzyme converts HMG CoA into mevalonate, the first committed step in cholesterol synthesis and an important site of metabolic control. The reduction in hepatic cholesterol synthesis (approximately 40% in vivo) results in up-regulation of LDL receptor activity with binding and uptake of plasma LDL to restore hepatic cholesterol balance. The activity of the LDL receptor is a major determinant of plasma cholesterol levels. These mechanisms are now well understood at a molecular level.

The statins lived up to expectations and proved to be highly effective in reducing LDL-cholesterol concentrations and to be among the best tolerated of all pharmaceutical agents. These drugs enabled definitive RCTs to be performed with sufficient power to test the cholesterol-lowering hypothesis.

CVD Secondary Prevention Trials with Statins

The first trials were performed in those with symptomatic coronary disease at high risk of subsequent CVD events. No trials have been performed in specific diabetic populations but there is a wealth of information from subgroup analyses, which enable definitive conclusions to be drawn. The excitement was palpable when the results of the first trial were announced to the American Heart Association (AHA) in 1994 and published simultaneously in the *Lancet*.

The Scandinavian Simvastatin Survival Study (4S) recruited patients with established CHD (n = 4,444, 827 females) and total cholesterol concentrations, despite dietary measures, between 5.5 and 8 mmol/L [39]. Patients were randomised to simvastatin, 20 mg/day or matching placebo. The primary end point was overall mortality and the study needed to continue until 440 deaths had occurred to meet power calculations. Secondary end points were fatal and non-fatal MI and sudden death. In the simvastatin group, the treatment goal was total cholesterol concentration of 3.0–5.2 mmol/L and 37% of patients required 40 mg/day.

Simvastatin therapy led to a 35% reduction in LDL-cholesterol, an 8% increase in HDL-cholesterol and a 10% reduction in triglycerides compared with the placebo group. After a mean follow-up of 5.4 years, there were 182 deaths in the simvastatin group compared with 256 deaths in the placebo group, a 30% reduction in overall mortality (HR 0.7; 95% CI 0.59–0.85; $p < 0.0003$). In addition, there were significant reductions in all coronary events.

Two post hoc analyses of 4S have been performed in diabetic patients. There were 202 known diabetic patients (mean age 60years, 78% male) included in the trial, 97 on placebo and 105 on simvastatin [40]. Clearly this is a small number and probably represents an atypical diabetic population in that they were hypercholesterolaemic and baseline triglycerides entry was relatively low at <2.5 mmol/L. Lipid changes in the diabetic subgroup were similar to those observed in non-diabetics. The analysis demonstrated the high risk of diabetic patients with CHD, approximately half suffering a major event during the study period. In the simvastatin group there was a 55% reduction in CVD events ($p = 0.002$). The numbers were too small to assess the effect on overall mortality, although there was a 47%, non-significant reduction.

In a further analysis, additional diabetic patients (n = 483) were identified on the basis of a baseline fasting glucose >7.0 mmol/L [41]. In addition, 678 patients were identified with impaired fasting glucose (IFT) with glucose levels between 6.1 and 6.9 mmol/L. There was a significant reduction in major CHD events of 42% with simvastatin (HR 0.58; 95% CI 0.42–0.81, $p < 0.001$). The 28% reduction in overall mortality did not reach significance. In the group with IFT, the 43% reduction in overall mortality was significant (HR 0.57; 95%CI 0.31–0.91, $p < 0.02$) [42].

The results of 4S have been confirmed in further subgroup analyses from several large RCTs (reviewed in ref. 42). The Heart Protection Study (HPS) included a large diabetes subgroup and its analysis was pre-specified [43]. The conclusion from these studies is that patients with diabetes and CHD respond in a similar way to the non-diabetic population. However, it is clear that a substantial residual vascular risk persists as demonstrated from the HPS study. The residual risk of suffering a major CVD event in diabetic patients with CHD receiving 40 mg/day simvastatin remained higher than in non-diabetic patients with CHD on placebo [43].

The question arose as to whether more intensive statin therapy would result in further risk reduction. This was supported by a relatively small ($n = 1{,}600$) and uncontrolled secondary prevention study performed in Greece [44]. Patients were randomly allocated to atorvastatin in increasing doses (mean dose 24 mg/day) to achieve an LDL-cholesterol below 2.6 mmol/L. This group was compared with a usual care group; at that time statin therapy was not routine in Greece and only 14% of this group received lipid-lowering therapy. As might be expected there was a large difference (46%) in LDL between the two groups, which was associated with a 51% risk reduction in the composite primary end point of death, non-fatal MI, unstable angina, stroke, congestive heart failure and revascularisation. Both groups had similar treatment with other drugs known to be of benefit for secondary prevention; 80% received aspirin and beta-blockers and 50% received ACE inhibitors. In the small diabetic subgroup ($n = 313$) there was a relative risk reduction of 58% ($p < 0.0001$). This trial can be criticised for a variety of reasons but it did suggest that more effective LDL-lowering therapy might be associated with a greater reduction in risk and a lower residual risk [44].

The potential benefit of more intensive therapy has been tested in formal RCTs in both acute coronary syndromes and stable coronary disease. Standard therapy (pravastain 40 mg/day) was compared with more intensive therapy (atorvastatin 80 mg/day) and was compared in patients ($n = 4162$) within 10 days of acute coronary syndrome [45]. The primary end point was a composite of death from any cause, MI, documented unstable angina requiring hospitalisation, revascularisation (performed at least 30 days after randomisation), and stroke. In the pravastatin group mean LDL-cholesterol was 2.46 mmol/L compared with 1.6 mmol/L in the atorvastatin group. After a mean follow-up period of 2 years, more intensive therapy was associated with a 16% risk reduction in CVD events ($p = 0.005$). This benefit occurred as early as 30 days after the start of the study. There were 734 diabetic patients in PROVE-IT and test of heterogeneity of effect was negative, indicating that the most likely outcome in the diabetic group would be the same as that seen in the overall study.

In the Treat to New Targets (TNT) trial, more intensive therapy with atorvastatin, 80 mg/day, was compared with atorvastatin 10 mg/day in 10,001 patients with stable CHD [46] 15,464 patients were originally recruited with LDL-cholesterol 3.4–6.5 mmol/L. All patients received 8-week run-in therapy with atorvastatin 10 mg/day. If an LDL-cholesterol target <3.4 mmol/L was achieved, patients were re-randomised to take 10 or 80 mg/day. About 5461 patients were excluded because of failure to reach this target. Over a mean follow-up of 4.9 years, LDL-cholesterol in the intensively treated group was 2.0 mmol compared with 2.6 mmol/L in the group on standard therapy; this was associated with 22% risk reduction in the primary end point, CHD death, non-fatal MI resuscitated cardiac arrest and stroke.

Two important further analyses of TNT have examined effects of more intensive treatment in the diabetic cohort [47] and also a cohort with metabolic syndrome [48]. In the diabetic subgroup ($n = 1{,}501$) LDL-cholesterol in the intensive group was 2.0 mmol/L compared with 2.55 mmol/L in the standard treatment group; this was associated with a significant risk reduction in the primary end point of 25%, 103 (17.9%) events compared with 135 (13.8%), (HR 0.75; 95% CI 0.58–0.97, $p = 0.026$).

Totally, 5584 patients (56%) were identified with metabolic syndrome [48]. Intensive therapy was associated with a 29% risk reduction in the primary end point, 262 events (9.5%) compared with 367 events (13%), (HR 0.71; 95% CI 0.61–0.84,

$p < 0.0001$). Importantly, irrespective of treatment assignment significantly more patients with metabolic syndrome suffered major CVD events, hazard ratio 1.44, 95% CI 1.26–1.64, $p < 0.0001$.

A meta-analysis has examined data from four recent trials of intensive versus conventional statin therapy in patients with acute coronary syndromes or with stable coronary disease involving 27,584 patients [49]. Intensive statin therapy (higher dose or more potent drug) was associated with a further 16% reduction in coronary death and MI (HR 0.84; 955: CI 0.77–0.91; $p < 0.0001$). This large data base supports the findings from individual trials of the benefits from more intensive therapy and given the high risk in the diabetic population should be translated into routine clinical care for the diabetic patient with established disease.

CVD Primary Prevention Trials with Statins

Higher case fatality in diabetes with the first CVD event argues strongly for effective primary prevention of CVD. Early trials did not include sufficient diabetic patients to assess benefit. The first trial to include a large number of diabetic patients was HPS, which included 2,912 patients (aged 40–80 years) with non-fasting cholesterol >3.5 mmol/L and without CVD [43]. In this pre-specified analysis, the composite primary end point was coronary death, non-fatal MI, revascularisation, and stroke. Simvastatin therapy (40 mg/day), which reduced LDL-cholesterol by 0.9 mmol/L compared to placebo, was associated with a 33% relative risk reduction in CVD events, $p = 0.0003$. This effect was independent of baseline lipids, diabetes duration, glycaemic control, and age. The authors calculated that simvastatin therapy over 5 years should prevent first events in about 45 people per 1,000 treated. They concluded that statin therapy should be considered routinely in all diabetic patients at sufficiently high risk of major vascular events independent of initial cholesterol levels.

Support for the findings of HPS came from the Collaborative Atorvastatin Diabetes Study (CARDS) the first end point trial to be performed in a specific diabetic population [50]. Totally, 2,838 type 2 diabetic patients (aged 40–75 years) without clinical CVD but with one other risk factor, hypertension, current cigarette smoking, retinopathy or albuminuria were randomly allocated to atorvastatin 10 mg/day or matching placebo. Patients were excluded if baseline LDL-cholesterol >4.14 mmol/L, baseline triglyceride levels up to 6.78 mmol/L were permitted. The trial had 90% power to detect a reduction of a third in the primary end point in the atorvastatin group at a significance level of $p < 0.05$; assuming a cumulative annual incidence of 2.35% for the primary end point in the placebo group, a total of 304 primary end points needed to accrue.

The primary end point was a composite of time to first occurrence of acute CVD events, coronary revascularisation or stroke. The trial was terminated 2 years earlier than expected because the pre-specified early stopping rule for efficacy had been met. Atorvastatin reduced LDL-cholesterol by 40% compared with placebo, representing an absolute reduction of 1.2 mmol/L; this reduction was associated with a 37% (95% CI −52 to −17, $p = 0.001$) relative risk reduction in the primary end point, 83 patients with a first event (1.54 per 100 person years at risk) compared with 127 patients (2.46 per 100 person-years at risk). There was a 36% reduction in acute coronary events, a 31% reduction in revascularisations and a 48% reduction in stroke. Although not powered for overall mortality, there was a 27% reduction ($p = 0.059$). No heterogeneity of effect was observed in relation to baseline lipids, age, diabetes duration, glycaemic control, systolic blood pressure, smoking, or albuminuria. The authors concluded that atorvastatin was safe and effective in reducing the risk of first CVD events in patients without high LDL-cholesterol levels (mean baseline 3 mmol/L). On the basis of this trial together with HPS there seems to be no justification for a particular threshold level of LDL to determine which patients should receive statin therapy.

The diabetes subgroup ($n = 2532$) from the Anglo Scandinavian Cardiac Outcomes Trial Lipid-Lowering Arm (ASCOT-LLA) showed a similar trend (test for heterogeneity not significant) to reduction of CVD events as those without diabetes. This trial is of particular interest because the benefits of statin therapy (atorvastatin 10 mg/day) were seen in well-treated hypertensive patients [51].

An important further conclusion from the statin trails for both primary and secondary CVD prevention is the impact on stroke. Meta-analysis of the early statin trials demonstrated a 21.5 risk reduction for every 1 mmol/L decrease in LDL-cholesterol [52]. This reduction in stroke risk was seen in patients without previous stroke. In CARDS the reduction in stroke was 48% [50]. Recently, the results of the first statin trial to recruit a specific population of stroke or TIA survivors (n = 4731) with time to subsequent stroke as the primary end point has been reported [53]. Statin therapy (atorvastatin 80 mg/day) was associated with a reduction in subsequent stroke of 16% (HR 0.84 95% CI 0.71–0.99, $p < 0.03$). As might be predicted, secondary end points of major coronary events showed highly significant reductions. The results of the diabetes subgroup have not yet been published.

Primary and Secondary Prevention Trials with Fibrates

Fibrates are ligands for peroxisome, proliferator-activated receptors alpha, (PPARα) [54]. PPARs are transcription factors that regulate gene expression in response to natural (e.g. fatty acids) and synthetic ligands. On activation, PPARs form heterodimers with retinoid X receptors and activate transcription of target genes. They can also repress gene expression by interfering with other signalling pathways such as NFκβ. These mechanisms increase fatty acid β-oxidation in liver and reduce VLDL synthesis and output. PPARα reduce levels of apo C III an important inhibitor of LPL and increase LPL gene expression. HDL-cholesterol is increased together with apo A1 and apo A2. The main effects of fibrates are to reduce triglycerides and increase HDL-cholesterol with only modest effects on total and LDL-cholesterol [54].

RCTs supporting the benefits of fibrate therapy is not consistent. Gemfibrozil was used in the Helsinki Heart Study, a primary prevention trial in men with raised non-HDL-cholesterol [55], and the Veterans Administration HDL Intervention Trial, VAHIT, a secondary CVD prevention trial in men with low HDL-cholesterol and relatively normal LDL [56]. These studies showed significant positive benefit for the drug overall and in diabetic subgroups. However, the populations studied in these trials also respond well to statin therapy [43]. In the Bezafibrate Infarction Prevention Trial, a CVD secondary prevention trial [57], there was a trend towards reduction in the primary end point but this did not reach statistical significance. In a post hoc analysis it was found that hypertriglyceridamic subjects appeared to benefit. In a more recent analysis, patients fulfilling the criteria for metabolic syndrome showed benefit [58].

The effects of fenofibrate in a specific diabetic population have recently been reported [59]. In this combined primary and secondary CVD outcomes study the primary end point (CHD death and non-fatal MI) did not reach statistical significance. Non-fatal MI was reduced significantly but coronary mortality showed a non-significant increase. Total cardiovascular events, (cardiac death, MI, stroke, coronary and carotid revascularisation) were significantly reduced but total mortality was non-significantly increased.

The conflicting results of FIELD are puzzling. Baseline HDL-cholesterol in FIELD was 1.1 mmol/L, whereas in VAHIT, which showed a positive outcome, it was lower at 0.8 mmol/L. Perhaps this lipid phenotype was better suited for intervention with the fibrate. In FIELD, fenofibrate had a disappointing long-term effect on HDL with barely a 2% increase by the end of the study. Furthermore, the reduction in LDL was only modest. Other confounders may be the adverse effect of fenofibrate in increasing homocysteine levels and higher drop-in statin therapy in the placebo group. However, the major conclusion following the results of FIELD is that statins remain first line therapy [60].

An Approach to Lipid-Lowering Therapy in Diabetes

It is taken for granted that diet and lifestyle have been optimised as far as is practical in the individual patient with special focus on quitting cigarette smoking, weight reduction, diet, and physical activity in addition to the instigation of lipid-lowering drugs.

Statins

Statin therapy should be first line therapy for the overwhelming majority of diabetic patients. Although the characteristic abnormalities are moderate hypertriglyceridaemia and low HDL-cholesterol, total and LDL-cholesterol are the most important predictors of CVD risk. Furthermore, diabetic dyslipidaemia is associated with increased concentrations of apo B-containing particles other than LDL and the plasma concentration of these potentially atherogenic lipoproteins will be reduced along with LDL by statin therapy.

Given the new information pointing to the benefits of more intensive statin therapy, ATP III guidelines in the USA were reviewed [61]. For those at highest risk including diabetic patients with established atherosclerosis-related disease of any type, a new goal of therapy of LDL-cholesterol <1.8 mmol/L is proposed. The new Joint British Societies (JBS 2) guidelines have also adopted a lower LDL goal of 2 mmol/L [30]. In these patients statin therapy should be started regardless of baseline LDL.

In CVD primary prevention a new concept has emerged from the RCTs. The same proportional risk reduction with statin therapy is observed regardless of baseline LDL. In CARDS [50], the mean baseline LDL of 3 mmol/L was until relatively recently the goal of therapy for several guidelines. Therefore, in CVD risk management, the absolute risk of the individual patient rather than the level of LDL is the major determinant of whether to start statin therapy. This concept is reflected in new primary prevention guidelines, which acknowledge that the great majority of diabetic patients over the age of 40 years will fulfil the generally accepted risk threshold of 20% CVD risk over 10 years and should be offered statin therapy without further assessment [30]. Clearly, some diabetic patients will be at high CVD risk below the age of 40 years. In an attempt to address this issue, JBS 2 suggest that diabetic patients aged 18–39 years should be considered for statin therapy if there is evidence of small vessel disease with retinopathy or nephropathy, poor glycaemic control (HbA1c >9%), hypertension requiring drug therapy, total cholesterol >6 mmol/L, features of the metabolic syndrome or a family history of diabetes. Clearly these guidelines are not based on RCT evidence but attempt to identify those at high risk where early intervention is likely to be effective [30].

There is little information from RCTs to guide practice in patients with type 1 diabetes. HPS included 615 patients with type 1 diabetes. In this subgroup, there were 43 patients (13.7%) with first vascular events in the simvastatin group compared with 53 (17.5%) in the placebo group. The test for heterogeneity was not significant ($p = 0.9$), suggesting that the outcome in these patients is not likely to differ from the findings of the whole diabetic group [43]. The lifetime risk of CVD in type 1 diabetes is high and current guidelines do not distinguish the two in their recommendations [30].

So far goals of therapy have been discussed solely in terms of total or LDL-cholesterol. In diabetic dyslipidaemia, some potentially atherogenic cholesterol will be carried on particles other than LDL such as remnant particles. To take account of this, NCEP, ATP III provides additional guidance. When LDL-cholesterol is to goal and plasma triglycerides remain greater than 2.0 mmol/L, a secondary target is non-HDL-cholesterol (total cholesterol- HDL-cholesterol) and the goal for this measure is set at 0.8 mmol/L above the LDL goal [61]. In this situation the first line approach is to increase the statin dose. If the highest available dose of a particular compound is already employed a more potent statin, such as atorvastatin or rosuvastatin should be substituted. If the treatment goal is not reached then combination therapy needs to be considered as discussed later.

Choice of a particular statin will depend on several factors including efficacy, safety, concurrent medication, concurrent medical conditions, RCT evidence of benefit in reducing CVD events, baseline lipids, and, increasingly, cost, given the availability of generics [38]. All statins lower LDL effectively but they do differ in potency, the more potent statins being atorvastatin and rosuvastain [62,63]. All the available statins are safe drugs if used appropriately [64]. A major potential cause of serious side effects can be avoided by avoiding drug interactions. Simvastatin, lovastatin, and atorvastatin are metabolised through cytochrome p 450 (cyp) 3A4 so if these statins are given along with drugs that inhibit this pathway plasma levels will rise. Atorvastatin appears to be less susceptible to this interaction. Fluvastatin is metabolised through cyp 2C9 and rosuvastatin has approximately 10% of its metabolism through cyp 2C9 and 2C19. Pravastatin is not metabolised through the cytochrome system. An important further consideration with drugs metabolised through cyp 3A4 is grapefruit juice, and patients should know not to consume large amounts. RCTs of CVD prevention support all available statins apart from the most recent statin, rosuvastatin, but a major RCT is in progress with this drug and in a observational study using intravascular ultrasound its use was associated with regression of atherosclerosis in a large proportion of patients [65].

It is reassuring that given the potency of statins they are among the best tolerated of all drugs [64]. It might be assumed, given the mechanism of action, that there might be effects on other products of the cholesterol synthesis such as dolichols (required for glycoprotein synthesis) and ubiquinones (important in mitochondrial electron transport) but this does not appear to be a clinical problem. There are no clinical effects on steroid hormone synthesis or bile acid production.

The most common side effects are gastrointestinal disturbances, which generally remit if the drug is continued; weakness, headache, general aches, and pains are others. However, in the RCTs there was little to differentiate these symptoms between active and placebo groups.

The most important severe side effect is myopathy. Fortunately, this is vanishingly rare [64]. It is characterised by painful, tender muscles often with flu-like symptoms. The level of the muscle enzyme creatine phosphokinase (CPK) is at least 10-fold increased. The most important preventive measure is to warn the patient to stop the statin if these symptoms develop and to attend for a CPK estimation. Myopathy usually resolves on stopping the drug. Extremly rarely acute tubular necrosis can occur following rhabdomyolysis. The author does not measure CPK routinely except in complex patients at risk of drug interactions. It should be remembered that CPK levels vary enormously in patients not on drug as shown in the RCTs and that the normal range is higher in black patients. Other causes such as vigorous exercise and hypothyroidism should be excluded.

Serious liver abnormalities are also rare even when high doses are used. General advice is to reduce the dose if transaminases are greater than 3-fold increased (approximately 1 in 400). Many patients with diabetes will have abnormal liver function due to fatty liver and these patients should not be denied a statin.

It is important to warn women of child-bearing potential to use effective contraception and to stop the statin at least 6 weeks before conception.

The Statin-Intolerant Patient

Although among the best tolerated of all drugs some patients are intolerant of statins. The most common reason for discontinuation, in the author's experience, is muscle aches generally without elevation of CPK. Full blown myositis with muscle pain/tenderness and a CPK greater than 10-fold elevated is vanishingly rare if appropriate care is taken particularly in relation to drug interactions.

It is important to re-emphasize the importance of statin therapy to the patient and that the statin is unlikely to be at fault. However, sometimes it is necessary to reduce the dose and in some cases patients will not take the drug at all. If a small dose of statin is tolerated and LDL-cholesterol is not to goal, the addition of ezetimibe is useful providing up to a further 20% LDL-lowering. Ezetimibe is a potent, specific inhibitor of intestinal cholesterol absorption, which has been demonstrated to have its effect at a recently discovered critical mediator of cholesterol absorption, namely, Niemann-Pick C1-Like 1 protein which is situated on brush border of enterocytes [66]. Side effects of the combination are largely similar to the statin alone [67,68] Ezetimibe as sole agent is less useful producing a 15% LDL reduction although response will vary depending on the individuals ability to absorb cholesterol.

As described above, the outcome data with fibrates is mixed. Gemfibrozil is the fibrate with the best outcome data but should not be combined with a statin as it can increase plasma levels of all statins and therefore the risk of severe side effects. If the major abnormality is a high LDL-cholesterol, gemfibrozil will have little impact. Bezafibrate has a better impact on LDL as well as increasing HDL-cholesterol and decreasing triglyceride but the clinical benefits from RCTs relate only to post hoc analyses.

The bile acid sequestrants, cholestyramine and colestipol, reduce LDL-cholesterol by up to 30% and their use is supported by RCTs [69]. However, they are not well-tolerated chiefly because of gastro intestinal adverse effects. In patients already on multiple drug therapies timing of administration of resins is difficult as they can interfere with the absorption of other drugs. They need to be given at least 1 h before or at least 4 h after other medications.

Theoretically, nicotinic acid, which has a major effect on hepatic VLDL synthesis, is an ideal lipid-modifying agent in that it is able to correct the various components of diabetic dyslipidaemia; however, it is not commonly used because of poor tolerability [70]. There is no definitive RCT data to guide therapy but there are studies showing benefit on surrogate end points. Nicotinic acid is currently the best drug for increasing HDL-cholesterol; it is better tolerated in an extended-release preparation, particularly in terms of flushing. Furthermore, a compound that significantly blocks the flush is in clinical trial. It remains to be seen whether this will improve tolerability in the long term. At the present time, most physicians use extended-release nicotinic acid at doses of 1–1.5 g/day to lower triglycerides and increase HDL usually in combination with a statin. At low dose and in the extended release form, adverse effects on insulin sensitivity and glucose tolerance are much less marked. On its own, higher doses (4–6g/day) are required to reduce LDL effectively.

Treatment of Severe Hypertriglyceridaemia

Diabetic patients may develop severe hypertriglyceridaemia with fasting serum triglyceride concentrations over 10 mmol/L and sometimes in the 20–30 mmol/L range or higher. Triglyceride concentrations of this order result from a combination of exogenous and endogenous particles, namely chylomicrons and VLDL. Increased hepatic output from the liver together with post-prandial absorption of chylomicrons swamps the clearance pathway through the enzyme LPL. It is unusual for diabetes alone to result in such high triglyceride levels and there is usually an underlying lipid disorder such as familial combined hyperlipidaemia. Other secondary causes for example, hypothyroidism, high alcohol intake and renal disease should be excluded.

Severe hypertriglyceridaemia may be associated with recurrent attacks of abdominal pain and sometimes pancreatitis. This lipid abnormality may interfere with the assay for amylase in some laboratories. Hepatosplenomegaly due to accumulation of lipid-laden macrophages may occur. Rarely there may be memory disturbances and lack of concentration. Some patients develop spectacular skin eruptions, eruptive xanthomata, which appear as crops of raised pinkish, yellow spots over elbows, knees, and buttocks.

Massive hypertriglyceridaemia may interfere with the measurement of other analytes such as haemoglobin, bilirubin, and liver transaminases and, by decreasing water volume in plasma, can lead to artificially low sodium measurement.

Treatment is of some urgency given the risk of pancreatitis. It is important that the patient is counselled to follow a low total fat diet together with reductions in alcohol and refined carbohydrate. In addition, high doses of omega 3 fish oils are useful together with a fibrate or a nicotinic acid derivative. As diet and lifestyle measures progress it is often possible to stop the fibrate. If significant mixed lipaemia persists a statin is indicated.

Future Trends

The most important focus should be on translating findings from RCTs into clinical practice the. Audit data shows that many patients are not yet receiving optimal therapy to achieve LDL goals [71]. The next target in lipid management should be to increase HDL. However, this is the most heterogeneous of all the lipoproteins and increasing HDL in a particular way will need to be shown in RCTs to translate into CVD reduction. The potential impact in reducing residual risk is clear from HPS [43]. In this study those diabetic patients with low HDL showed the same proportional risk reduction as those with higher levels. However, those with low HDL on simvastatin had a larger residual risk of CVD events than those with higher HDL on placebo.

It has been an attractive option to use combination therapy of statin and fibrate when HDL remains low but there is no data from RCTs to support this approach. It is ironic that gemfibrozil with the best outcome data should not be used in this context given drug interactions. The results of the FIELD trial with fenofibrate as sole therapy were disappointing [59]; however, a combination trial with fenofibrate and statin in type 2 diabetes, the ACCORD study, is in progress.

Two important drugs in the management of glycaemia have important effects in increasing HDL. Pioglitazone increased HDL by almost 9% in the PROactive study [72]. In this secondary prevention trial pioglitazone was associated with a significant reduction in major CVD events in diabetic patients with symptomatic CVD although the primary end point, which included peripheral artery revascularisations, did not reach significance [54]. Pioglitazone was shown in the CHICAGO study [73] to reduce progression of carotid IMT compared with sulphonylurea and in this study HDL increased by 6%. A possible mechanism for the effects on HDL is the observed increase in adiponectin.

Rimonabant, an endocannabinoid receptor 1 (CB1) blocker has been shown to be effective in reducing weight in patients with type 2 diabetes with important effects on glycaemic control. In addition, HDL-cholesterol was increased by approximately 8% [74]. This compound also increases adiponectin.

Nicotinic acid has the most marked effect in increasing HDL. Several surrogate end point studies using coronary angiography or carotid intima medial thickening have pointed to potential benefit over and above that with statin alone [75]. A large morbidity and mortality trial has just started to examine the effects of an extended-release preparation combined with an inhibitor on the nicotinic acid-induced flush. This trial should demonstrate the tolerability of the combination compound together with the potential benefits, which may occur beyond statin therapy. The degree of potential adverse effects on glycaemia will also be observed.

References

1. Zimmet PZ, Alberti KGMM. The changing face of macrovascular disease in non-insulin-dependent diabetes mellitus: an epidemic in progress. Lancet. 1997;350(Suppl. 1):1–4.
2. Taskinen MR. Diabetic dyslipidaemia: from basic research to clinical practice. Diabetologia. 2003; 46:733–749.
3. Betteridge DJ. Dyslipidaemia and diabetes Pract Diabetes Int. 2001;18:201–208.
4. Assman E, Schulte H. The prospective cardiovascular Munster (PROCAM) study: prevalence of hyperlipidaemia in persons with hypertension and/or diabetes mellitus and the relationship to coronary heart disease. Am Heart J. 1988;116:1713–1724.
5. Isomaa B, Almgren P, Tuomi T, et al. Cardiovascular morbidity and mortality associated with the metabolic syndrome. Diabetes Care. 2001;24:683–689.
6. Lewis GF, Carpentier A, Adeli K, Giacca A. Disordered fat storage and mobilization in the pathogenesis of insulin resistance in type 2 diabetes. Endcr Rev. 2002;23:201–229.
7. Despres J-P. Abdominal obesity: the most prevalent cause of the metabolic syndrome and related cardiometabolic risk. Eur Heart J. 2006;8(Suppl. B) B4-B12.
8. Kadowaki T, Yamamuchi T. Adiponectin and adiponectin receptors. Endocr Rev. 2005;26: 439–451.
9. Chirieac DV, Chirieac LR, Corsetti JP, et al. Glucose-stimulated insulin secretion suppresses hepatic triglyceride-rich lipoprotein and apo B production. Am J Physiol Endocrinol Metabol. 2000;279: E1003-E1011.
10. Lin MCM, Gordon D, Wetterau JR. Microsomal triglyceride transfer protein (MTP) regulation in HEPG2 cells: insulin negatively regulates MTP gene expression. J Lipid Res. 1995;36:1073–1081.
11. Ginsberg HN, Illingworth DG. Postprandial dyslipidaemia; an atherogenic disorder common in patients with diabetes mellitus. Am J Cardiol. 2001;88(Suppl 9):9H-15H.
12. Lee S-J, Moye LA, Campos H, et al. Hypertriglyceridaemia but not diabetic status is associated with VLDL containing apolipoprotein CIII in patients with coronary heart disease. Atherosclerosis. 2003;167:293–302.
13. Ginsberg HN. Insulin resistance and cardiovascular disease. J Clin Invest. 2000;106:453–458.
14. Ceriello A, Tabga C, Tonutti L, et al. Evidence for an independent and cumulative effect of postprandial hypertriglyceridaemia and hyperglycaemia on endothelial dysfunction and oxidative stress generation. Effects of short and long-term simvastatin therapy. Circulation. 2002;106:1211–1218.
15. Lamarche B, Rashid S, Lewis GF, etal. HDL metabolism in hypertriglyceridaemic states: an overview. Clin Chem Acta.1999;286:145–161.
16. Toth PP. Adiponectin and high density lipoprotein: a metabolic association through thick and thin. Eur Heart J. 26:1579–1581.
17. Tan KC, Cooper MB, Ling KL, et al. Fasting and postprandial determinants for the occurrence of small dense LDL species in non-insulin-dependent diabetic patients with and without hypertriglyceridaemia: the involvement of insulin, insulin precursor species and insulin resistance. Atherosclerosis. 1995;113: 273–287.
18. Rainwater DL. Lipoprotein correlates of LDL particle size. Atherosclerosis. 2000;148:151–158.
19. Gray RS, Robbins DC, Wang W, et al. Relation of LDL size to insulin resistance syndrome and

coronary heart disease in American Indians. Arterioscler Thromb Vasc Biol. 1997;17:2713–2720.
20. Stamler J, Vaccaro O, Neaton JD, et al for the Multiple Risk Factor Intervention Trial Research Group. Diabetes, other risk factors and 12 year cardiovascular mortality for men screened in the Multiple Risk Factor Intervention Trial. Diabetes Care. 1993;16:434–444.
21. Turner RC, Millns H, Neil HAW for the United Kingdom Prospective Diabetes Study Group. Risk factors for coronary artery disease in non-insulin dependent diabetes mellitus: United Kingdom prospective diabetes study (UKPDS:23). BMJ. 1998;316:823–828.
22. Howard BV, Robbins DC, Sievers ML, et al. LDL cholesterol is a strong predictor of coronary artery disease in diabetic individuals with insulin resistance and low LDL. The Strong Heart Study. Arterioscler Thromb Vasc Biol. 2000;20:830–835.
23. Chapman MJ, Guerin M, Bruckert E. Atherogenic dense low density lipoproteins: pathophysiology and new therapeutic approaches. Eur Heart J. 1998;19:(Suppl. A)A24–A30.
24. Chait A, Wight TN. Interaction of native and modified low density lipoproteins with extracellular matrix. Curr Opin Lipidol. 2000;11:451–456.
25. Sniderman AD, Scantlebury T, Cianflone K. Hypertriglyceridaemic hyper apoB: the unappreciated atherogenic dyslipidaemia in type 2 diabetes mellitus. Ann Intern Med. 2001;135:447–459.
26. Steinbrecher UP, Witztum JL. Glycosylation of low density lipoproteins to an extent comparable to that seen in diabetes slows their catabolism. Diabetes. 1984;33:130–134.
27. Gordon DJ, Probstfield JL, Garrison RJ, et al. High-density lipoprotein cholesterol and cardiovascular disease. Four prospective American studies. Circulation. 1989;79:8–15.
28. Kreiger M. Scavenger receptor class B type 1 is a multi-ligand HDL receptor that influences diverse physiologic systems. J Clin Invest. 2001;108:793–797.
29. Schmitz G, Kaminski WE. ATP-binding cassette (ABC) transporter in atherosclerosis. Curr Atheroscler Rep. 2002;4:243–251.
30. JBS 2 Joint British Societies' guidelines on prevention of cardiovascular disease in clinical practice. Heart. 2005;91(Suppl. V):v1–v52.
31. Yusuf S, Hawken S, Ounpuu S, et al. on behalf of the INTERHEART Study Investigators. Effect of potentially modifiable risk factors associated with myocardial infarction in 52 countries (the INTERHEART study): a case control study. Lancet. 2004;364:937–952.
32. Hulley SB, Rosenman RH, Bawal RD, et al. Epidemiology as a guide to clinical decisions: the association between triglyceride and coronary heart disease. N Engl J Med. 1980;302:1383–1389.
33. Hokanson E, Austin MA. Plasma triglyceride is a risk factor for cardiovascular disease independent of high density lipoprotein cholesterol level; a meta-analysis of population-based prospective studies. J Cardiovascular Risk. 1996;3:213–219.
34. Assmann E, Sculte H. Relation of high density lipoprotein cholesterol and triglycerides to incidence of coronary artery disease (the PROCAM experience). Am J Cardiol. 1992;70:733–737.
35. Manninen V, Tenkanen H, Koskinen P, et al. Joint effects of triglycerides and LDL cholesterol and HDL cholesterol concentrations on coronary heart disease in the Helsinki Heart Study. Implications for treatment. Circulation. 1992;85:37–45.
36. Lehto S, Ronnemaa T, Haffner SM, et al. Dyslipidaemia and hyperglycaemia predict coronary heart disease in middle-aged patients with NIDDM. Diabetes. 1997;46:1354–1359.
37. Betteridge DJ, Morrell JM. Lipids and Coronary Heart Disease. Arnold, London. 2003.
38. Betteridge DJ, Khan M. Statins and Coronary Artery Disease. (2nd edition) Science Press. London. 2003.
39. Scandinavian Simvastatin Survival Study Group (4S) Randomised trial of cholesterol lowering in 4444 patients with coronary heart disease: the Scandinavian Simvastatin Survival Study. Lancet. 1994;344:1383–1389.
40. Pyorala K, Pedersen TR, Kjekshus J, et al. Cholesterol lowering with simvastatin improves prognosis of diabetic patients with coronary heart disease. A subgroup analysis of the Scandinavian Simvastatin Survival Study (4S). Diabetes Care. 1997;20:614–620.
41. Betteridge DJ. Benefits of lipid-lowering therapy in patients with type 2 diabetes Am J Med. 2005;118:(suppl 12A)10S–15S.
42. Haffner SM, Alexander CM, Cook TJ, et al. Reduced coronary events in simvastatin-trated patients with coronary heart disease and diabetes or impaired fasting glucose levels. Subgroup analysis in the Scandinavian Simvastatin Survival Study. Arch Int Med. 1999;159:2661–2667.
43. Heart Protection Study Collaborative Group. MRC/BHF Heart Protection Study of cholesterol lowering with simvastatin in 5963 people with diabetes: a randomized placebo-controlled trial. Lancet. 2003;361:2005–2016.
44. Athyros VG, Papagrorgious AA, Mercouris BR, et al. Treatment with atorvastatin to the National Cholesterol Education Program Goal versus

"usual"care in secondary coronary heart disease prevention. Curr Med Res Opin. 2002;18:220–228.
45. Cannon CP, Braunwald E, Mccabe CH, et al. Intensive versus moderate lipid-lowering with statins after acute coronary syndromes. N Engl J Med. 2004; 350:1495–1504.
46. LaRosa JC, Grundy SM, Waters D, et al. for the Treating to New Targets (TNT) Investigators. Intensive lipid lowering with atorvastatin in patients with stable coronary disease. N Engl J Med. 2005; 352:1452–1435.
47. Shepherd J, Barter P, Carmena R. et al. Effect of lowering LDL cholesterol substantially below recommended levels in patients with coronary heart disease: the Treating to New Targets (TNT) Study. Diabetes Care. 2006;29:1220–1226.
48. Deedwania P, Barter P, Carmena R, et al. Reduction of low density lipoprotein cholesterol in patients with coronary heart disease and metabolic syndrome: analysis of the Treating to New Targets study. Lancet. 2006;368:919–928.
49. Cannon CP, Steinberg BA, Murphy SA, et al. Meta-analysis of cardiovascular outcomes trials comparing intensive versus moderate statin therapy. JACC. 2006;48:438–455.
50. Colhoun HM. Betteridge DJ, Durrington PN, et al. on behalf of the CARDS investigators. Primary prevention of cardiovascular disease in type 2 diabetes in the Collaborative Atorvastatin Diabetes Study (CARDS): multicentre randomized placebo-controlled trial. Lancet. 2004;364:685–696.
51. Sever PS, Dahlof B, Poulter NR, et al. Prevention of coronary and stroke events with atorvastatin in hypertensive patients who have average or lower than average cholesterol concentrations in the Anglo Scandinavian Cardiac Outcomes Trial-Lipid-Lowering Arm (ASCOT-LLA): a multicentre randomized controlled trial. Lancet. 2003;361:1149–1158.
52. Hebert PR, Gaziano JM, Chan KS, Hennekens CH. Cholesterol lowering with statin drugs, risk of stroke and total mortality: an overview of randomized trials. JAMA. 1997;278:313–321.
53. The Stroke Prevention by Aggressive Reduction in Cholesterol Levels (SPARCL) Investigators. High-dose atorvastatin after stroke or transient ischaemic attack. N Engl J Med. 2006;355:549–559.
54. Staels B, Dallongeville J, Auwerx J, et al. Mechanism of action of fibrates on lipid and lipoprotein metabolism. Circulation. 1998;98:2088–2093.
55. Frick MH, Elo O, Haapa K, et al. The Helsinki Heart Study: primary prevention trila with gemfibrozil in middle-aged men with dyslipidaemia. Safety of treatment changes in risk factors and incidence of coronary heart disease. N. Engl J Med. 1987;317: 1237–1245.
56. Robins SJ, Rubins HB, Collins D, et al. for the Veterans Affairs HDL Intervention Trial (VAHIT). Gemfibrozil for the secondary prevention of coronary heart disease in men with low levels of high density lipoprotein cholesterol. N Engl J Med. 1999; 241:410–418.
57. Bezafibrate Infarction Prevention Study Group. Secondary prevention by raising HDL cholesterol and reducing triglycerides in patients with coronary artery disease: the Bezafibrate Infarction Prevention (BIP) study. Circulation. 2000;102:21–27.
58. Tenenbaum A, Motro M, Fisman EZ, et al. Bezafibrate for the secondary prevention of myocardial infarction in patients with metabolic syndrome. Arch Intern Med. 2005;165:1154–1160.
59. The FIELD Study Investigators. Effects of long-term fenofibrate therapy on cardiovascular events in 9795 people with type 2 diabetes mellitus (the FIELD study): randomized controlled trial Lancet. 2005;366:1849–1861.
60. Colhoun H. After FIELD: should fibrates be used to prevent cardiovascular disease in diabetes? Lancet. 2005;366:1829–1831.
61. Grundy SM, Cleeman JI, Merz CNB, et al. for the Coordinating Committee of the National Cholesterol Education Program. Implications of recent clinical trials for the National Cholesterol Education Program Adult Treatment Panel III Guidelines. Circulation. 2004;110:227–239.
62. Jones PH, Kafonek S, Laurota I et al. Comparative dose efficacy study of atorvastatin versus simvastatin, pravastatin, lovastatin, and fluvastatin in patients with hypercholesterolaemia (the CURVES study) Am J Cardio.l 1998;81:582–587.
63. Jones PH, Davidson MH, Stein EA, et al. Comparison of the efficacy and safety of rosuvastatin versus atorvastatin, simvastatin, and pravastatin across doses (STELLAR Trial) Am J Cardiol. 2003;92:152–160.
64. Kashani A, Phillips CO, Foody JM, et al. Statin use is associated with a low incidence of adverse events. Circulation. 2006;114:2788–2797.
65. Nissen SE, Nicholls Sj, Sipahi I, et al. Effects of very high intensity statin therapy on regression of coronary atherosclerosis. JAMA. 2006;295:1556–1565.
66. Garcia-Calvo M, Lisnock J, Bull HG, et al. The target of ezetimibe is Niemann-Pick C1-LikeMayo Clin Proc. (NPC1L1) PNAS. 2005;102:8132–8137.
67. Goldberg AC, Sapre A, Liu J, et al. Efficacy and safety of ezetimibe coadministered with simvastatin in patients with primary hypercholesterolaemia: a randomized, double-blind, placebo-controlled trial. Mayo Clin Proc. 2004;79:620–629.
68. Ballantyne CM, Houri J, Notarbartolo A, et al. Effect of ezetimibe coadministered with atorvastatin in 628

pateints with primary hypercholesterolaemia. A prospective, randomized, double-blind trial. Circulation. 2003;107:2409–2415.

69. Hunninghake DB. Bile acid sequestering agents (resins) In: Lipoproteins in Health and Disease. Edotors DJ Betteridge, DR Illingworth, J. Shepherd. Arnold, London. 1999. pp. 1133–1144.
70. Walldius G, Wahlberg G. Nicotinic acid and its derivatives In Lipoproteins in Health and Disease. Editors DJ Betteridge, DR Illingworth, J Shepherd Arnold, London. 1999. pp. 1181–1198.
71. Leiter LA, Betteridge DJ, Chacra AR, et al. on behalf of the AUDIT Study Steering Committee. AUDIT study. Evidence of global undertreatment of dyslipidaemia in patients with type 2 diabetes. Br J Diabetes Vasc Dis. 2006;6:31–41.
72. Dormandy JA, Charbonnel B, Eckland DJA, et al. Secondary prevention of macrovascular events in patients with type 2 diabetes in the PROactive Study (PROspective pioglitAzone Clinical Trial In macroVascular Events): a randomized controlled trial. Lancet. 2005;366:1279–1288.
73. Mazzone T, Meyer PM, Feinstein SB, et al. Effect of pioglitazone compared with glimepiride on carotid intima-media thickness in type 2 diabetes. JAMA. 2006;296:2572–2581.
74. Scheen AJ, Finer N, Hollander P, et al. Efficacy and tolerability of rimonabant in overweight or obese patients with type 2 diabetes: a randomized, controlled trial. Lancet. 2006 368;368:1660–1672.
75. Brown BG, Zhao X-Q, Chait A, et al. Simvastatin and niacin, antioxidant vitamins, or the combination for the prevention of coronary disease N Engl J Med. 2001;345:1583–1592.

17
Coronary Intervention and Ischemic Cardioprotection in Diabetic Patients

Torsten Toftegaard Nielsen

Keywords: Coronary angiography, percutaneous intervention (PCI), coronary bypass surgery (CABG), Testenosis, acute myocardial infarction, insulin-glucose infusion.

Diabetes mellitus, especially type 2, predisposes to cardiovascular mortality. The risk of coronary heart disease (CHD) mortality and mobidity is 2–4 times higher in diabetic patients than in non-diabetic subjects [1]. Although advances in both pharmacological and interventional treatment have resulted in a pronounced reduction in cardiovascular mortality of non-diabetic patients, diabetic patients have not gained the same benefit. After en acute myocardial infarction (MI) short- and long-term mortality in diabetic patients has remained twice of that in non-diabetics (Fig. 1) [2,3]. The global growth of the diabetic population [4] makes the choice of the optimal preventive and treatment modalities one of the most challenging issues facing both the diabetologist and the cardiologist today.

Macrovascular Disease and Cardiovascular Risk in Diabetes

Haffner and colleagues suggested that patients with diabetes alone had some risk of future heart attack as patients without diabetes who had suffered a myocardial infarction [5]. Although there is universal agreement on the excess of coronary risk in diabetic patients, recent data indicate that this statement should be modified depending on the presence or absence of macrovascular disease. There is growing evidence that the presence of atherosclerosis in itself represents a risk of cardiovascular disease (CVD) additional to that obtained from "traditional" risk factors as hypertension, dyslipidaemia, microalbuminuria, abdominal obesity, and so on, probably by including the yet inexplicable phenomenon of vascular (endothelial) susceptibility to atherosclerosis [6,7]. So far, visualization of atherosclerotic disease in the clinical stetting has, however, been limited because of the invasive nature of available techniques – first of all contrast x-ray coronary angiography. In a small coronary angiographic study of 750 patients, patients with diabetes and no signs of CHD had same low 3 years cardiovascular risk as those without diabetes and CHD, and a lower risk than patients with CHD. The well-documented high risk of having both diabetes and CHD compared with that of CHD alone was confirmed [8]. There are epidemiological studies of support for the view that CHD is a stronger predictor of the cardiovascular prognosis than diabetes alone. The Multiple Risk Factor Interventional Trialists (MRFIT) found that incident non-fatal CVD was a stronger predictor of 18-year mortality than incident diabetes in a population of 11,000 persons [9].

From the above it seems reasonable to advocate for early visualization of macrovascular disease, especially CAD, in diabetics with mild or moderate cardiac symptoms to identify both low- and high-risk patients. During recent years non-invasive techniques as multiple slice tomography scanning (MSTC) and magnetic resonance imaging (MRI) [10,11] have become available for visualization of macrovascular arterial disease. In addition, to show

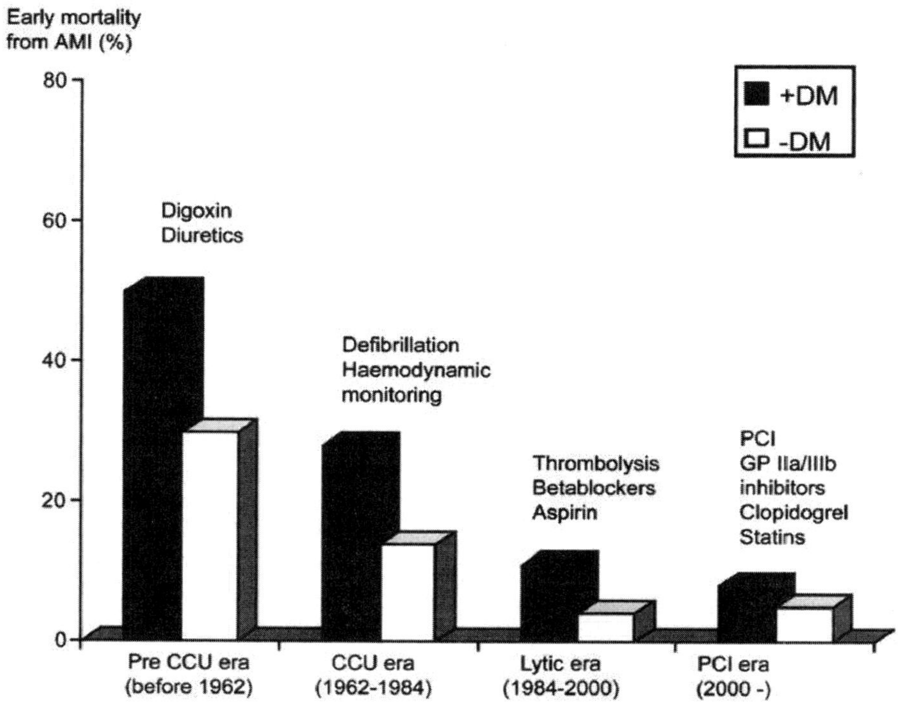

FIG. 1. Early mortality after acute myocardial infarction (AMI) in the pre-coronary care unit (CCU) era, the CCU era, the lytic era and in the percutaneous coronary intervention era (PCI). GP IIa/IIIb = glycoprotein IIa/IIIb inhibitor.

vascular disease indirectly by evaluating luminal narrowing – as by conventional invasive angiography – these techniques are able to or have the potential non-invasiveness to visualize the vessel wall disease directly by estimating the atherosclerotic plaque extent (burden), composition and activity [12]. We have reported a close association between plaque burden and impaired kidney function in type 1 diabetics using MRI imaging [13]. With the appearance of new generation scanners MSCT imaging most certainly in the near future will be available widespread in health communities. Clinical use and evaluation of non-invasive coronary artery imaging should focus on patients predisposed to atherosclerosis including those with diabetes.

How and to what extent introduction of large-scale angiographic evaluation of macrovascular disease in diabetic patient will change treatment modalities are unknown.

The American–Canadian Bypass Angioplasty Revascularization Investigation 2 Diabetes (BARI 2D) trial [3] includes angiographic screening for ischemic heart disease of 2,800 type 2 diabetic patients with mild or no cardiac symptoms, and randomizes patients with significant CAD to aggressive medical treatment or coronary revascularization with 5-year mortality as the primary end point. Further, the cardiovascular effect of improved metabolic and glycaemic control by provision of insulin or by amelioration of insulin resistance will be evaluated. Hopefully, the BARI 2 D trial will provide us with clinical insight and answers on how to prevent development of symptomatic IHD in diabetic patients by early treatment. In the meantime, it is in my view reasonable to offer patients with diabetes coronary angiography on rather wide and liberal indications.

Coronary Revascularization: Angioplasty versus Surgery – a Persistent Controversy?

During the last 2–3 decades invasive coronary revascularization of symptomatic CHD patients by angioplasty (percutaneous coronary intervention, PCI) or coronary bypass surgery (CABG) has been implemented worldwide in an almost exponential way. For the whole CHD population the invasive treatment approach has given a survival benefit [14]. What concerns the mode of revascularization, PCI versus surgery, only few would question PCI as treatment of choice in patients with 1 and 2 vessel disease without stenosis in the left descending artery (LAD), and CABG in patients with 3 vessel disease and extent vascular disease. Given the rapid technological improvement of PCI, the population with multivessel disease in which patients are eligible for both PCI and surgery has increased, and resulted in an augmented use of PCI relatively to that of CABG. This development in treatment strategy seems justified for the CHD population in general as no difference in either long-term survival, non-fatal MI or cerebrovascular accidents have been demonstrated in several randomized controlled trials comparing CABG and PCI in the 1980s and early 1990s [15–18], or later after introduction of coronary stenting [19]. The main drawback of PCI is a higher need for repeat revascularization than after CABG.

Particular emphasis has been placed on the mode of coronary revascularization in diabetics patients. Major worry was raised when a post hoc subgroup analysis of the first BARI in 1996 demonstrated a less favourable prognosis among diabetic patients with multivessel disease treated with PCI than those subjected to CABG [18]. The 5-year mortality was 19.4% among 184 diabetic patients assigned to CABG and 34.5% among 173 assigned to PCI ($p < 0.03$) [20]. The wide difference in mortality could be related to the use of arterial internal mammary grafts in the surgical group. Although not statistically significant, similar trends were observed in other smaller trials (Fig. 2). The BARI subgroup analysis gave the American National Heart Lung and Blood Institute reason to transmit an alert on PCI in diabetic patients in 1995. Since then, there has been a consistent controversy about PCI treatment of patients with diabetes. Unfortunately, it is at present not possible to dispel the worry as no randomized trial on PCI versus CABG in a diabetic population alone has been reported. However, there are several reasons to argue against a general alert on PCI in patients with diabetes.

First, it appears difficult to justify an extrapolation of data from the early 1990s to the clinical practice today. The studies were performed before the stent era and the adjunctive pharmacotherapy is now available. The alert on PCI of diabetic patients was based on small subgroup post hoc analyses of larger

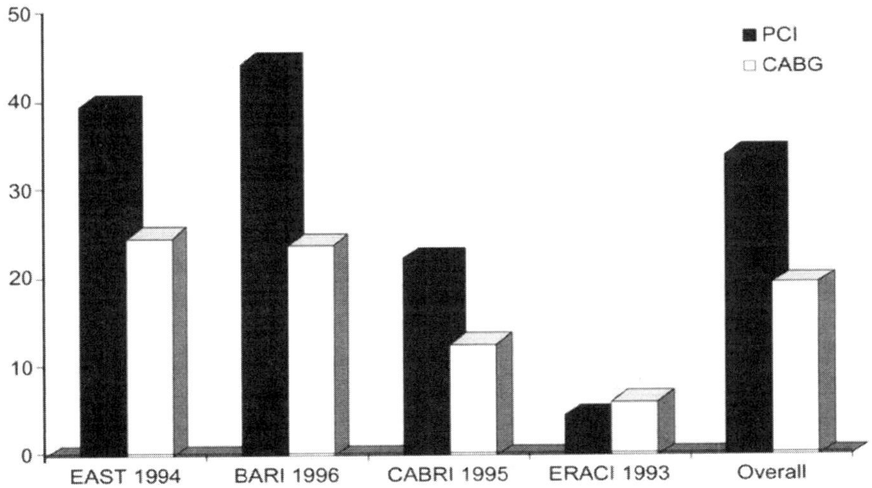

FIG. 2. Bar chart showing mortality rates in randomized trials of elective patients undergoing coronary bypass surgery and coronary angioplasty. EAST, Emory Angioplasty versus Surgery Trial; BARI, Bypass Angioplasty versus Surgical Trial; CABRI, Coronary Angioplasty versus Bypass Revascularization Investigation; ERACI, Argentine Randomized Study: Coronary Angioplasty versus Coronary Bypass Surgery in Multivessel disease.

studies. Further, registry studies including the BARI registry [20] have not been able to disclose the same difference in mortality outcome as the randomized trials. The ARTS trial (Arterial Revascularization Therapies Study) from 2001 compared CABG to multivessel PCI with stenting [19]. The study revealed no difference in the composite end point of death, MI and CVA after 1 and 5 years in 1,205 randomized patients, nor in the diabetic subgroup of 208 patients. The requirement for additional revascularization was higher after PCI than after CABG, for both patients with and without diabetes. The results suggest improvement in periprocedural complications compared with older trials, but only little change on the impact of restenosis, a major problem after PCI treatment of diabetic patients.

Restenosis after PCI in Diabetics

Restenosis after PCI is caused by three mechanisms: intimal hyperplasia, recoil and less frequently by constrictive remodelling. Since the first PCI registry results in 1984 [21], diabetes has been known to be a strong and non-procedure related predictor of restenosis. The predominant cause of restenosis in diabetics is exaggerated intimal hyperplasia. While recoil and constrictive restenosis can be prevented with bare metal stents (BMS), BMS did not solve the problem of restenosis in diabetic patients [22,23]. Polymer-based drug eluting stents (DES) with slow release of antiproliferative, anti-inflammatory drugs (sirolimus, paclitaxel) markedly reduce restenosis and late lumen loss. A meta-analysis of six recent trials has shown a significant 80% relative reduction in restenosis rate after DES compared with BMS in both diabetic patients (n = 697) and non-diabetics (n = 2,491), resulting in the highest absolute effect in diabetics [24]. Angiographically, the effect has been confirmed in a single randomized study of 204 diabetic patients. Restenosis rates after DES and BMS were 7.8% and 33.7%, respectively [25]. Whether these impressive angiographic results can be translated to improved short- and long-term clinical outcome remains to be proven. A randomized trial (n = 1,314, diabetics 24%) has reported a significant decrease in non-fatal MI and revascularization of the target vessel during a 1-year follow up after DES compared with BMS [26]. However, no long-term mortality effect of DES compared with BMS have been found in recent meta-analyses including thousands of patients [27,28]. Whether it is diabetes per se or the small vessel size and complexity of coronary disease in diabetics that predict restenosis remains controversial. Nevertheless, DESs significantly improve or eliminate a major limitation of conventional stenting/PCI in diabetic patients. Most recently, there has been concern about the risk of stent trombosis by using DES [29]. There is neither a substantial evidence of a higher risk in diabetics, nor is stent trombosis more common after DES than BMS. To achieve best clinical outcome following PCI with DES in diabetic patients future clinical trials, continued improvement in DES delivery and optimal adjunctive pharmacotherapy are needed. There is a lack of knowledge about the influence of metabolic control on restenosis rate. Glitazones may be drugs capable of decreasing restenosis in diabetic patients after stenting [30].

Coronary Revascularization of Diabetic Patients with Acute Myocardial Infarction

During recent years clinical trials have shown early or acute invasive coronary revascularization to be superior to medical stabilization or thrombolysis. The benefit has been demonstrated in patients with unstable angina or moderate infarction (non-ST elevation MI, non-STEMI) [31,32], as well as in patients with large ST elevation MI (STEMI) [33,34]. The short-term relative benefit in subgroups of diabetic patients concurrently has been found to be the same as in non-diabetic patients resulting in a larger absolute risk reduction because diabetics in all trials had considerable higher event rates post-MI than non-diabetics, in agreement with data from large registry studies [35].

In the Frisc II trial PCI or CABG treatment of 299 diabetic patients with unstable angina or non-STEMI tended to reduce the risk of death or MI after 1-year follow-up, 20.6% in invasive versus 29.9% in medically treated cases (RR:0.61, 95% CI: 0.36–1.04) equal to a 9.3% absolute risk reduction compared with 3.1% in 2,158 patients without diabetes [36]. Data from subgroup analyses of invasive coronary revascularization of non-STEMI diabetic patients from other trials are in agreement with the FRISCII results. Available data do not allow any estimation of the effect of PCI versus CABG in this group of diabetics. Randomized and long-term studies on larger diabetic population with unstable angina/non-STEMI are warranted.

In patients with acute STEMI, increasing evidence suggests mechanical revascularization by PCI within few hours after symptom onset, primary PCI (pPCI) to be superior to thrombolysis. A beneficial effect has been demonstrated in both patients admitted directly to invasive hospitals and patients transferred from local hospitals [33]. In a recent meta-analysis including a total of 6,763 STEMI patients from 22 randomized trials comparing pPCI with thrombolysis, 30-day mortality in 935 diabetic patients with symptom duration of 2 h or more was 6.2% after pPCI versus 12.4% after thrombolysis (RR:0.5, 95% CI: 0.3–0.7). Corresponding mortalities in 3.081 non-diabetic patients were 5.8% vs 8.2%. Again, because the event rate was increased in diabetics, their absolute mortality benefit exceeds that of non-diabetic patients. For diabetics the NNT was 17, the lowest among all subgroups studied, versus 43 in non-diabetics [34]. Long-term results of pPCI treatment of STEMI patients are scanty and almost lacking. Data from a few hundred of patients suggest the initial mortality benefit to be maintained over several years, especially in high-risk patients among which are diabetic patients [37,38]. Long-term studies on the clinical outcome after pPCI of diabetic STEMI patients are highly needed.

In a subgroup analysis of the DANAMI-2 trial [39] we found that the beneficial effect of pPCI compared with thrombolysis on the risk of clinical reinfarction was abolished in 113 diabetic patients but maintained in 1,455 non-diabetic patients after 3 years follow-up. We were unable to detect any mortality benefit. We found the same result in another and larger high-risk group of patients, those with anterior index MI. A significant short-term effect of pPCI on reinfarction incidence was lost during 3-year follow-up, which could be related to discontinuation of antiischemic and antithrombotic medical treatment [40].

In summary, it is not possible to totally dispel the concern of the early 1990s that the long-term clinical outcome of PCI treatment of diabetic patients may be poorer than that of CABG. By markedly reducing restenosis, DESs seem to eliminate a major limitation of conventional stenting/PCI in diabetic patients. However, it must be stressed that DESs compared with BMS do not reduce long-term mortality in non-diabetic CHD patients. Whether the same applies for diabetic patients remains to be studied. Further, continued improvement in DES delivery as well as optimal adjunctive pharmacotherapy will be required to achieve the best clinical outcome after PCI. CABG has limitations with a higher perioperative mortality and morbidity in patients with diabetes than in those without. CABG involves multiple organs and is associated with prolonged rehabilitation. Excessive co-morbidity may contraindicate CABG in diabetic patients. Selection of the best coronary revascularization modality in diabetic patients, or recommendation of non-invasive treatment, must rely on a careful individual patient evaluation.

Adjunctive Ischemic Cardioprotecion

Clinical outcome of invasive coronary treatment of CHD patients does not solely depend on the revascularization modality. In a long-term study of a low-risk trial population (n = 1,228), short-term outcome was driven by procedural complications and restenosis, whereas the outcome beyond 1 year after stenting was determined by disease progression outside the treated coronary lesions. Diabetes and multivessel disease were independently associated with an increased cardiovascular event rate [41].

Diabetics are characterized by hemostatic abnormalities involving platelet hyperreactivity and impaired fibrinolytic balance. Increased platelet adhesion and aggregation is associated with increased thromboxan A2 synthesis, decreased nitric oxide, decreased antioxidant levels and increased expression of activation-dependent adhesion molecules such as P-selectin and glycoprotein IIb/IIIa (GP IIb/IIIa) [42]. The latter has been considered an important mechanism behind the beneficial effect of the GPIIb/IIIa inhibitor abciximab in a subgroup analysis of 491 diabetic patients in the EPISTENT trial [43]. In a meta-analysis of six trials, GP IIb/IIIa inhibitors reduced 30-day mortality in diabetics compared with non-diabetic patients with non-STEMI [44]. The ISAR-SWEET study included 701 diabetic patients undergoing elective PCI without showing a beneficial effect of abciximab after pretreatment with clopidogrel. However, high-risk patients were excluded and only few insulin-requiring patients were included in that study [45]. Therefore, we still recommend using GP IIb/IIIa inhibitors in relation to interventional coronary treatment of diabetic patients. This should be given on top of antithrombotic treatment with aspirin and clopidogrel. Because there is growing evidence that withdrawal of clopidogrel may be of same importance for developing stent thrombosis as procedure-related factors, clopidogrel treatment should be continued for a minimum of 1 year.

Diabetes is associated with an increased chronic low-grade inflammatory state also affecting the coronary arteries [46]. In recent years there has been much attention on the possible effect of specific anti-inflammatory treatment of CHD. A large randomized trial studying the effect of an anti-C5 complement antibody (pexelizumab) in a little less than 6,000 patients with STEMI has been disappointing as no tendency of a benefit could be demonstrated [47]. At present the issue of anti-inflammatory treatment of chronic or acute CHD seems speculative.

Glycaemic Control

There is compelling evidence that tight glycaemic control reduces diabetic microangiopathy and neuropathy. Both the original randomized and observational data from the UK prospective diabetes study (UKDPS) documented a relation between hyperglycaemia and macrovascular disease, but weaker and less clear than that of microvascular complications [48,49]. The Diabetes Control and Complication Trial (DCCT) has provided indirect [50] and direct evidence [51] of a beneficial effect of intensive metabolic control (HbA_{1c}) on cardiovascular risk in type 1 diabetics. The results of the PROACTIVE trial reducing both insulin resistance and HbA_{1c} are in line with this [52]. However, no significant effect on total or cardiac mortality was found in these trials. A comprehensive discussion of the long-term effect of glycaemic control on macrovascular disease is beyond the scope of this chapter.

There is no unequivocal answer to whether optimal glucometabolic control influences clinical outcome after coronary revascularization of diabetic patients with stable and unstable coronary syndromes. Observational studies have reported poor glycaemic regulation to be associated with an increased need for additional target lesion revascularization and restenosis [53,54]. Coronary revascularization results in normalized epicardial flow, which however, not necessarily is followed by improved myocardial perfusion and cardiac function. The angiographic no-flow phenomenon denotes a post-PCI condition of impaired microcirculation despite non-stenotic coronary arteries. There is some evidence that hyperglycaemia predisposes to the no-flow condition in MI patients, more often in diabetic than non-diabetic patients [55,56].

In recent years large-scale randomized clinical trials dealing with the possible effect of acute insulin–glucose infusion followed by intensive insulin treatment in non-diabetic and diabetic MI patients have been published [57–59]. Overall the results have been conflicting or neutral. Despite important differences in the study designs regarding the delay of start of treatment, the reduction in glucose level, the mode of revascularization, pPCI or thrombolysis, and so on, there is agreement, that insulin per se as adjunctive treatment in acute MI has no effect [60]. This should not be interpreted as evidence that optimal long-term glycaemic control is of minor importance for the cardiovascular risk in diabetic patients – all available knowledge indicates the opposite. The lack of a clinical benefit of insulin in MI patients is in contrast to findings in a Belgian study of cardio-surgical intensive care unit (ICU) patients in whom insulin treatment targeting normal glucose level reduced short- and long-term mortality and morbidity [61]. There are obvious differences between MI patients and patients admitted to an ICU. In the ICU study, patients who stayed longer than 5 days almost completely accounted for the benefit, whereas hospital stay of MI patients usually is short. Further a close monitoring of the balance between amounts of glucose and insulin infused seems to be of importance. In a study of long-stay ICU patients without glucose level control, the amount of glucose infused was found to be an independent predictor of hospital mortality suggesting a toxic effect of glucose supply in excess [62]. Clinical algorithms to ensure a tight glucose control matching the metabolic need of the heart are a prerequisite to embark insulin treatment of MI patients. Such complex monitoring has not been developed, and the question how an insulin-mediated increase in glucose uptake may improve cardiac function is unsolved, why acute adjunctive insulin treatment in MI patients has no clinical role at present.

Despite the insufficient effect of insulin administration to MI patients, a large number of reports unanimously have shown an increased blood glucose at admission level to be a strong predictor of an adverse short- and long-term outcome in diabetic and non-diabetic patients [60,63]. The relationship may be complex as it has been reported to be U-shaped in a cohort of 4,000 patients [64]. Recently, both a high baseline glucose and failure of glucose level to decrease within 24 h were found to predict high mortality in non-diabetic, but not in diabetic patients [65]. Overall, there is substantial evidence that a disturbed glucose metabolism carries a high prognostic impact on cardiovascular events in MI patients, although the underlying mechanisms are far from elucidated and no specific treatment is available.

Need of a Strengthened Diagnostic Strategy of Diabetes in Acute Coronary Syndrome Patients

Among patients admitted to hospital for acute coronary syndrome (ACS), unstable angina or MI, about 20–25% have known diabetes [35]. The proportion of diabetic patients in the total ACS population may be twice as high [60,66]. A cardiovascular event, including ACS, often represents the first clinical "manifestation" in type 2 diabetic patients, and there is an obvious need for improving the diagnostic screening for diabetes in CHD patients with ACS. The optimal way to implement this is a matter of debate. The European Society of Cardiology and the European Association for the Study of Diabetes recommend all ACS patients to be evaluated by an oral glucose tolerance test (OGTT), based on studies showing 2 h post-load plasma glucose to be a stronger and more age-independent predictor of cardiovascular events than fasting glucose level and HbA_{1c} [60,67]. No randomized studies dealing with the clinical benefit of the recommended strategy have been reported. In the authors view, the personnel and economic costs of efforts to implement OGTT in preference to fasting glucose and HbA_{1c} should be balanced against the very high need and costs of improving secondary prevention in diabetic CHD patients. In a recent report on management of CHD patients with and without diabetes in 25 European countries, the acute management was found to be reasonable, while secondary prevention was concluded to be unacceptably poor [68]. Prevention guidelines on hypertension and dyslipidaemia treatment were only adhered in half of the patients with an inadequate and less aggressive management in patients with diabetes than in those without. While the need of a future strengthening of the diagnostic screening for diabetes in CHD patients is beyond any question, it is in my view more open whether patients totally will obtain more benefit from risk stratification by simple risk markers as fasting glucose level and HbA_{1c} than from a more extensive evaluation by OGTT. Anyhow, a stronger daily collaboration between diabetologists and cardiologists may be of highest importance.

Conclusion

Clinical evaluation and treatment of CVD in diabetic patients follow the same evidence-based indications as those used in patients without diabetes. Both short- and long-term cardiovascular event rate and complications in diabetics are constantly two- to threefold higher than in non-diabetics. The relative effect of both invasive and medical treatment is the same in diabetics and non-diabetics, resulting in a higher absolute treatment effect in diabetic patients. No available treatment is able to reduce clinical cardiovascular outcome in diabetic patients to that of non-diabetic patients. For these reasons, patients with diabetes had to be considered as high-risk patients with a documented need of aggressive treatment, as outlined in Table 1. Coronary angiography should be offered on liberal indications, and invasive coronary revascularization should be performed taking the individual complexity of the artery disease into consideration. DES should be used for coronary stenting together with long-lasting antithrombotic therapy. Recent

TABLE 1. Treatment options in diabetic patients with coronary artery disease.

Coronary revascularization
Coronary angiography on liberal indications
Stable patients: CABG in moderate favour of PCI (multivessel disease)
Acute coronary syndrome:
Non-STEMI: PCI or CABG on individual indication
STEMI: Primary PCI mode of revascularization
PCI with stent implantation: Drug-eluting stents should be used
PCI: Glycoprotein IIb/IIIa inhibitor indicated in diabetic patients
Aggressive secondary prevention by means of
Life style habits including smoking cessation, physical activity and food
Anti-platelet medication (aspirin/clopidogrel)
Blocking the renin–angiotensin system
Anti-hypertensive medication
Lipid-lowering medication
Blood glucose control

CABG: coronary bypass surgery, PCI: percutaneous intervention, STEMI: ST-segment elevation myocardial infarction.

health surveys stress the high need for a strengthened secondary prevention with multifactorial interventions including lifestyle changes, aggressive medical treatment of hypertension, dyslipidaemia and heart failure.

References

1. Pyorala K, Laakso M, Uusitupa M. Diabetes and atherosclerosis: an epidemiologic view. Diabetes Metab Rev 1987;3:463–524.
2. Laskey WK, Selzer F, Vlacvhos HA, Johnston J, Jacobs A, King SB III, Holmes DR, Douglas J, Block P, Wilensky R, Williams DO, Detre K. Comparison of in-hospital and one-year outcomes in patients with and without diabetes mellitus undergoing percutaneous catheter intervention (form the National Heart, Lung and Blood Institute Dynamic Registry). Am J Cardiol 2002;90:1062–1067.
3. Sobel BE, Frye R, Detre KM. Burgeoning dilemmas in the management of diabetes and cardiovascular disease. Rationale for the Bypass Angioplasty Revascularization Investigation 2 D (BARI 2D) trial. Circulation 2003;107:636–642.
4. Murray CJ, Lopez AD. Alternative projections of mortality and disability by cause 1990–2020: Global Burden of Disease Study. Lancet 1997;349:1498–1504.
5. Haffner SM, Lehto S, Ronnemaa T, Pyorala K, Laakso M. Mortality from coronary heart disease in subjects with type 2 diabetes and in nondiabetic subjects with and without prior myocardial infarction. N Eng J Med 1998;339:229–234.
6. Naghavi M, Falk E, Hecht HS, Jamieson MJ, Kaul S, Berman D, Fayad Z, Budoff MJ, Rumberger J, Naqvi TZ, Shaw LJ, Faergeman O, Cohn J, Bahr R, Koenig W, Demirovic J, Arking D, Herrera VL, Badimon J, Goldstein JA, Rudy Y, Airaksinen J, Schwartz RS, Riley WA, Mendes RA, Douglas P, Shah PK. From vulnerable plaque to vulnerable patient – part III: Executive summary of screening for heart attack prevention and education (SHAPE) task force report. Am J Cardiol 2006;98:2H–15H.
7. Falk E. Pathogenesis of atherosclerosis. J Am Coll Cardiol 2006:47:C7–C12.
8. Saely CH, Aczel S, Marte T, Langer P, Drexel H. Cardiovascular complications in type 2 diabetes mellitus depend on the coronary angiographic state rather than on the diabetic state. Diabetologia 2004;47:145–146.
9. Eberly LE, Cohen JD, Prineas R, Yang L. Multiple Risk Factor Intervention Trial Research Group. Impact of incident diabetes and incident nonfatal cardiovascular disease on 18-year mortality. Diabetes Care 2003;26:848–854.
10. Clouse ME, Chen J, Krumholz HM. Noninvasive screening for coronary artery disease with computed tomography is useful. Circulation 2006;113:125–146.
11. Kim WY, Danias PG, Stuber M, Flamm SD, Plein S, Nagel E, Langerak SE, Weber OM, Pedersen EM, Schmidt M, Botnar RM, Manning WJ. Coronary magnetic resonance angiography for detection of coronary stenosis. N Engl J Med 2001;345:1863–1869.
12. Purushothaman KR, Sanz J, Zias E, Fuster V, Moreno PR. Atherosclerosis neovascularisation and imaging. Curr Mol Med 2006;6:549–556.
13. Kim WY, Astrup AS, Stuber M, Tarnow L, Falk E, Botnar RM, Simonson C, Pietraszek L, Hansen PR,

Manning WJ, Andersen NT, Parving HH. Subclinical coronary and aortic atherosclerosis detected by magnetic resonance imaging in type 1 diabetes with and without diabetic nephropathy. Circulation 2007;115:180–187.
14. Johnsen SP, Videbaek J, Pedersen L, Steffensen R, Videbaek R, Niemann T, Nielsen TT, Sørensen HT. Survival trends among Danish patients undergoing coronary angiography for known or suspected ischemic heart disease: a population based follow up study, 1992–2000. Heart 2006;92:27–31.
15. Rodriguez A, Boullon F, Perez-Balino N, Paviotti C, Liprandi MI, Palacios IF. Argentina randomized trial of percutaneous transluminal coronary angioplasty versus coronary artery bypass surgery in multivessel disease (ERACI); in-hospital results and 1-year follow-up. J Am Coll Cardiol 1993;22:1060–1067.
16. King SB III, Lembo NJ, Weintraub WS, Kosonski AS, Barnhart HX, Kutner MH, Alazraki NP, Guyton RA, Zhao XQ. A randomized trial comparing coronary angioplasty with coronary bypass surgery. Emory Angioplasty versus Surgery Trial (EAST). N Engl J Med 1994;331:1044–1050.
17. First-year results of CABRI (Coronary Angioplasty versus Revascularization Investigation). CABRI Trial Participants. Lancet 1995;346:1179–1184.
18. The Bypass Angioplasty Revascularization Investigation (BARI)Investigators. Comparison of coronary bypass surgery with angioplasty in patients with multivessel disease. N Engl J Med 1996;335:217–225.
19. Serruys PW, Unger F, Sousa JE, Jatene A, Bonnier HJ. Schonberger JP, Buller N, Bonser R, van den Brand MJB, van Herwerden LA, Morel MA, van Hout BA, – The Arterial Revascularization Therapies Study Group. Comparison of coronary bypass surgery and stenting for the treatment of multivessel disease. N Engl J Med 2001;344:1117–1124.
20. Detre KM, Guo P, Holubkov R, Califf RM, Sopko G, Bach R, Brooks MM, Bourassa MG, Shemin RJ, Rosen AD, Krone RJ, Frye RL, Feit F. Coronary revascularization in diabetic patients: A comparison of the randomized and observational components of the bypass angioplasty revascularization investigation (BARI). Circulation 1999;99:633–640.
21. Holmes DR Jr, Vlietstra RE, Smith HC, Vetrovec, GW, Kent KM, Cowley HJ, Faxon DP, Gruentzig AR, Kelsey SF, Detre KM. Restenosis after percutaneous transluminal coronary angioplasty (PTCA): a report from the PTCA Registry of the National Heart, Lung and Blood Institute. Am J Cardiol 1984;53:77C–81C.
22. Mak KH, Faxon DP. Clinical studies on coronary revascularization in patients with type 2 diabetes. Eur Heart J 2003;24:1087–1103.
23. Meheran R, Dangas GD, Kobayashi Y, Lansky AJ, Mintz GS, Aymong ED, Fahy M, Moses JW, Stone GW, Leon MB. Short- and long-term results after multivessel stenting in diabetic patients. Am J. Coll Cardiol 2004;43:1348–1154.
24. Scheen AJ, Warzée F, Legard VMG. Drug-eluting stents: meta-analysis in diabetic patients. Eur Heart J 2004;25:2167–2176.
25. Sabaté M, Jiménez-Quevedo PJ, Angioolillo DJ, Gómez-Hospital JA, Alfonso F, Hernández-Antolin R, Goicolea J, Bañuelos C, Escaned J, Moreno R, Fernández C, Fernández-Abilés F, Macaya C. Randomized comparison of sirolimus-eluting stent versus standard stent for percutaneous coronary revascularization in diabetic patients (Diabetes Trial). Circulation 2005;112:2175–2183.
26. Stone GW, Ellis SG, Cox DA, Hermiller J, O'Shaughnessy C, Mann JT, Turco M, Caputo R, Bergin P, Greenberg J, Popma JJ, Russel ME. One-year clinical results with the slow-release, polymer based, paclitaxel-eluting taxus stent. The taxus-IV trial. Circulation 2004;109:1942–1947.
27. Nordmann AJ, Briel M, Bucher HC. Mortality in randomized controlled trials comparing drug-eluting vs bare metal stents in coronary artery disease: a meta-analysis. Eur Heart J 2006:27:2784–2814.
28. Kastrai A, Mehelli J, Pache J, Kaiser C, Valgimigli M, Kelbæk H, Menichelli M, Sabaté M, Suttorp MJ, Baumgart D, Seyfarth M, Pfisterer ME, Schörnig A. Analysis of 14 trials comparing sirolimus-eluting stents with bare-metal stents. N Engl J Med 2007;356;1030–1039.
29. Maisel WH. Unanswered questions – Drug-eluting stents and the risk of late thrombosis. N Engl J Med 2007;356:981–984.
30. Takagi T, Akasaka T, Yamamuro A, Honda Y, Hozumi T, Morioka S, Yoshida K. Troglitazone reduces neointimal tissue proliferation after coronary stent implantation in patients with non-insulin dependent diabetes mellitus. J Am Coll Cardiol 2000;36:1529–1535.
31. Fragmin and Fast Revascularisation during instability in Coronary artery disease (FRISCII) investigators. Invasive compared with non-invasive treatment, in unstable coronary-artery disease:FRISCII prospective randomised multicenter study. Lancet 1999; 354:708–715.
32. Fox KA, Pool-Wilson PA, Henderson RA, Clayton TC, Chamberlain Da, Show TR, et al. Interventional versus conservative treatment for patients with unstable angina or non-ST-elevation myocardial infarction; the British Heart Foundation RITA 3 randomised trial. Randomized Intervention Trial of unstable Angina. Lancet 2002;360:743–751.

33. Andersen HR, Nielsen TT, Rasmussen K, Thuesen L, Kelbaek H, Thayssen P, Abildgaard U, Pedersen F, Madsen JK, Grande P, Villadsen AB, Krusell LR, Haghfelt T, Lomholt P, Husted SE, Vigholt E, Kjaergaard HK, Mortensen LS. DANAMI-2 investigators. A comparison of coronary angioplasty with fibrinolytic therapy in acute myocardial infarction. N Engl J Med 2003;349:733–742.
34. Boersma E, and the (PCAT)-2 trialists collaborative group. Does time matter? A pooled analysis of randomized clinical trials comparing primary percutaneous coronary intervention and in-hospital fibrinolysis in acute myocardial infarction patients. Eur Heart J 2006;27:779–788.
35. Franklin K, Goldberg RJ, Spencer F, Klein W, Budaj A, Brieger D, Marre M, Steg PG, Gowda N, Gore JM. GRACE investigators. Implications of diabetes in patients with acute coronary syndromes. The global Registry of Acute Coronary Events. Arch Intern Med 2004;164:1457–1463.
36. Norhammer A, Malmberg K, Diderholm E, Lagerqvist B, Lindahl B, Rydén L, Wallentin L. Diabetes mellitus: The major risk factor in unstable coronary artery disease even after consideration of the extent of coronary artery disease and benefits of revascularization. J Am Coll Cardiol 2004;43:585–591.
37. Henriques JPS, Zijlstra F, van't Hof AWJ, de Boer MJ, Dambrink JHE, Gosselink ATM, Hoorntje JCA, Ottervang JP, Suryapranata H. Primary percutaneous coronary intervention versus thrombolytic treatment: long term follow up according to infarct location. Heart 2006;92:75–79.
38. Hsu LF, Mak KH, Lau KW, Sim LL, Chan C, Koh TH, Chiah SC, Kam R, Ding ZP, Teo WS, Lim YL. Clinical outcomes of patients with diabetes mellitus and acute myocardial infarction treated with primary angioplasty or fibrinolysis. Heart 200;88:260–265.
39. Madsen MM, Busk M, Søndergaard HM, Bottcher M, Mortensen LS, Andersen HR, Nielsen TT. DANAMI-2 investigators. Does diabetes mellitus abolish the beneficial effect of primary coronary angioplasty on long-term risk of reinfarction after acute ST-segment elevation myocardial infarction compared with fibrinolysis? Am J Cardiol 2005;96:1469–1475.
40. Busk M, Mortensen LS, Thuesen L, Andersen HR, Rasmussen K, Madsen JK, Nielsen TT. Reinfarction after anterior ST-elevation myocardial infarction: initial benefit of primary angioplasty compared to fibrinolysis is lost during long-term follow up. Circulation 2005;112(Suppl. II):569.
41. Cutlip DE, Chhabra AG, Baim DS, Chauhan MS, Marulkar S, Massaro J, Bakhai A, Cohen DJ, Kuntz RE, Ho KK. Beyond restenosis. Five-year clinical outcome from second-generation coronary stent trials. Circulation 2004;110:1226–230.
42. Colwell JA, Nesto RW. The platelet in diabetes: focus on prevention of ischemic event. Diabetes care 2003;26:2181–2188.
43. Marso SP, Lincoff M, Elklis SG, Bhatt DL, Tanguay JF, Kleiman NS, Hammoud T, Booth JE, Sapp SK, Topol EJ. Optimizing the percutaneous interventional outcomes for patients with diabetes. Results from the Epistent Diabetic Substudy. Circulation 1999;100:2477–2484.
44. Roffi M, Chew DP, Mukherjee D, Bhatt DL, White JA, Heeschen C, Hamm CW, Moliterno DJ, Califf RM, White HD, Kleiman NS, Theroux P, Topol EJ. Platelet glycoprotein IIb/IIIa inhibitors reduce mortality in diabetic patients with non-ST-segment-elevation acute coronary syndromes. Circulation 2001;104:2767–2771.
45. Mehilli J, Kastrati A, Schuhlen H, Dibra A, Dotzer F, von Beckerath N, Bollwein H, Pache J, Dirschinger J, Berger PP, Schömig A. ISAR-SWEET Study Investigators. Randomized clinical trial of abciximab in diabetic patients undergoing elective percutaneous coronary intervention after treatment with a high loading dose of clopidogrel. Circulation 2004;110:3627–3635.
46. Biondi-Zoccai GG, Abbate A, Liuzzo G, Biasucci LN. Atherothrombosis, inflammation, and diabetes. J Am Coll Cardiol 2003;41:1071–1077.
47. The APEX AMI investigators. Pexelizumab for acute ST-elevation myocardial infarction in patients undergoing primary percutaneous coronary intervention. A randomized controlled trial. JAMA 2007;297:43–51.
48. UKPDS Group. Intensive blood glucose control with sulphonylureas or insulin compared with conventional treatment and risk of complications in patients with type 2 diabetes (UKPDS 33). Lancet 1998;352:837–853.
49. Stratton IM, Adler AI, Neil AW, Matthews DR, Manley SE, Cull CA, Hadden D, Turner RC, Holman RR, UKPDS Group. Association of glycaemia with macrovascular and microvascular complications of type 2 diabetes (UKPDS 35):prospective observational study. BMJ 2000;321:405–412.
50. DDCT/EDIC Study Research Group. Intensive diabetes therapy and carotid intima-media thickness in type 1 diabetes mellitus. N Engl J Med 2003;348:2294–2303.
51. DDCT/EDIC Study Research Group. Intensive diabetes treatment and cardiovascular disease in patients with type 1 diabetes. N Engl J Med 2005;353:2643–2653.
52. Proactive investigators. Secondary prevention of macrovascular events in patients with type 2 diabetes in the PROactive Study(PROspective pioglitAzone Clinical Trial In macroVascular Events): A randomized controlled trial. Lancet 2005;366:1279–1289.

53. Corpus RA, George PB, House JA, Dixon SR, Ajluni SC, Devlin WH, Timmis GC, Balasubramaniam M, O'Neill WW. Optimal glycemic control is associated with a lower rate of target vessel revascularization in treated type II diabetic patients undergoing elective percutaneous coronary intervention. J Am Coll Cardiol 2004;43:8–14.
54. Mazeika P, Prasad N, Bui S, Seidelin PH. Predictors of angiographic restenosis after coronary intervention in patients with diabetes mellitus. Am Heart J 2003;145:1013–1021.
55. Iwakura K, Ito H, Ikushima M, Kawano S, Okamura A, Asano K, Kuroda T, Tanaka K, Masuyama T, Hori M, Fujii K. Association between hyperglycemia and the no-flow phenomenon in patients with acute myocardial infarction. J Am Coll Cardiol 2003;41:1–7.
56. Timmer JR, van der Horst ICC, de Luca G, Ottervanger JP, Hoorntje JCA, de Boer MJ, Suryapranata H, Dambrink JHE, Gosselink M, Zijlstra F, van't Hof AWJ. Comparison of myocardial perfusion after successful primary percutaneous coronary intervention in patients with ST-elevation myocardial infarction with and without diabetes mellitus. Am J Cardiol 2005;95:1375–1377.
57. van der Horst ICC, Zijlstra F, van't Hof AWJ, Doggen CJM, de Boer MJ, Suryapranata H, Hoorntje JCA, Dambrink JHE, Gans ROB, Bilo HJG. Glucose-insulin potassium infusion in patients treated with primary angioplasty for acute myocardial infarction. The glucose-insulin-potassium study: a randomized study. J Am Coll Cardiol 2003;42:784–791.
58. Malmberg K, Rydén L, Wedel H, Birkeland K, Bootsma A, Dickstein K, Efendric S, Fisher M, Hamsten A, Herlitz J, Hildebrandt P, Macleod K, Laakso M, Torp-Pedersen C, Waldenström A. Intense metabolic control by means of insulin in patients with diabetes mellitus and acute myocardial infarction (DIGAMI 2): effects on mortality and morbidity. Eur Heart J 2005;26:650–661.
59. The CREATE-ECLA Trial Group Investigators. Effect of glucose-insulin-potassium infusion on mortality in patients with acute ST-segment elevation myocardial infarction. The Create-Ecla randomized controlled trial. JAMA 2005;293:437–446.
60. The task force on diabetes and cardiovascular diseases of the European Society of cardiologi (ESC) and of the European Association for the Study of Diabetes (EASD).Guidelines on diabetes, pre-diabetes, and cardiovascular Diseases: executive summary. Eur Heart J 2007;28:88–136.
61. van den Bergie G, Wouters P, Weekes F, Verwaest C, Bruyninckx F, Schetz M, Vlasselaers D, Ferdinande P, Lauwers P, Bouillon R. Intensive insulin treatment in critically ill patients. N Engl J Med 2001;345:1359–1367.
62. van der Voort PHJ, Feenstra RA, Bakkert AJ, de Heide L, Boerma C, van der Horst ICC. Intravenous glucose intake independently related to intensive care unit and hospital mortality: an argument for glucose toxicity in critically ill patients. Clinical Endocrinol 2006;64:141–145.
63. Malmberg K, Norhammer A, Wedel H, Rydén L. Glycometabolic state at admission: important risk marker of mortality in conventionally treated patients with diabetes mellitus and acute myocardial infarction: long-term results from the Diabetes and Insulin-Glucose infusion in Acute Myocardial Infarction (DIGAMI) Study. Circulation 1999;99:2626–2632.
64. Pinto DS, Skolnick AH, Kirtane AJ, Murphy SA, Barron HV, Giugliano RP, Cannon CP, Braunwald E, Gibson CM (TIMI study group). U-shaped relationship of blood glucose with adverse outcomes among patients with ST- segment elevation myocardial infarction. J Am Coll Cardiol 2005;46:178–180.
65. Goyal A, Mahaffey KW, Garg J, Nicolau JC, Hochman JS, Weaver WD, Therous P, Oliveira GBF, Todaro TG, Mojcik CF, Armstrong PW, Ganger CB. Prognostic significance of the change in glucose level in the first 24 h after acute myocardial infarction: results from the CARDINAL study. Eur Heart J 2006;27:1289–1297.
66. Norhammer A, Tenerz Aa, Nilsson G, Hamsten A, Efrendíc S, Rydén L, Malmberg K. Glucose metabolism in patients with acute myocardial infarction and no previous diagnosis of diabetes mellitus: a prospective study. Lancet 2002;359:2140–2144.
67. The DECODE Study Group Consequences of the new diagnostic criteria for Diabetes in older men and women. DECODE Study (Diabetes epidemiology: Collaborative Analysis of Diagnostic Criteria in Europe). Diabetes Care 1999;22:1667–671.
68. Anselimo M, Bartnik M, Malmberg K, Rydén L. Management of coronary artery disease in patients with and without diabetes mellitus. Acute management reasonable but secondary prevention unacceptable poor: a report from the Euro Heart Survey on Diabetes and the heart. Eur J Cardiovasc Prev Rehabil 2007;14:28–36.

Section: Diabetic Complications and Side-effects

18 ACE-I and ARB and Blood Pressure Lowering, Including Effect on Renal Disease. Treatment of Advanced Diabetic Renal Disease

Per Løgstrup Poulsen and Johan V. Poulsen

Keywords: Diabetic nephropathy, renal disease, hypertension, blood pressure, antihypertensive treatment, ACE-1, ARB, dual blockade.

Introduction

Hypertension is the main risk factor for renal as well as atherosclerotic disease in diabetes, and the quest for strict blood pressure (BP) control has continuously evolved over the last three decades. It was first described 30 years ago that the decline in glomerular filtration rate (GFR) correlated with systemic BP in patients with overt diabetic nephropathy [1]. This was in contrast to the prevailing concept that a certain level of BP elevation was essential for the preservation of renal as well as organ perfusion in general [2]. In the subsequent 30 years, however, data of numerous studies have confirmed that BP elevation is a major determinant in the progression toward end-stage renal failure [3–7]. This early observation [1] formed part of the basis for the concept of antihypertensive treatment in patients with diabetic nephropathy, one of the most clinically significant interventions in modern diabetology, documented to preserve GFR [8–11] and reduce mortality [12–15].

In this chapter, we will focus on clinical aspects of intervention in the renin–angiotensin system (RAS). Treatment with angiotensin-converting enzyme inhibitors (ACE-I) or angiotensin II receptor blockers (ARB), in relation to other antihypertensive regimes (the concept of BP-independent renoprotection), whether ACE-I or ARB, should be first-line therapy and the combination of ACE-I and ARB (dual blockade).

Hypertension in Diabetes

In patients with type 1 diabetes, hypertension is usually associated with underlying diabetic nephropathy and typically becomes manifest when patients develop microalbuminuria. In contrast, in patients with type 2 diabetes, hypertension is present at the time of diagnosis of diabetes in over one-third of patients, often coexisting with dyslipedimia, central obesity, and increased susceptibility to cardiovascular disease [16].

Cardiovascular disease accounts for a large proportion of the excess mortality related to diabetes [17,18]. In relation to incidence of myocardial infarction, recent data indicate that the presence of diabetes confers an equivalent risk to ageing 15 years [19].

In a prospective study, we examined the long-term prognostic significance of BP along with other risk factors for all-cause mortality in type 1 diabetes. In 1977, a representative sample of 272 adult type 1 diabetic patients was identified through outpatient clinics and GPs. The main endpoint was mortality after 25 years. Follow-up was almost complete (98.8%). After 25 years, all-cause mortality was 37% (99/269) for the whole group. Figure 1 illustrates the cumulative survival in patients

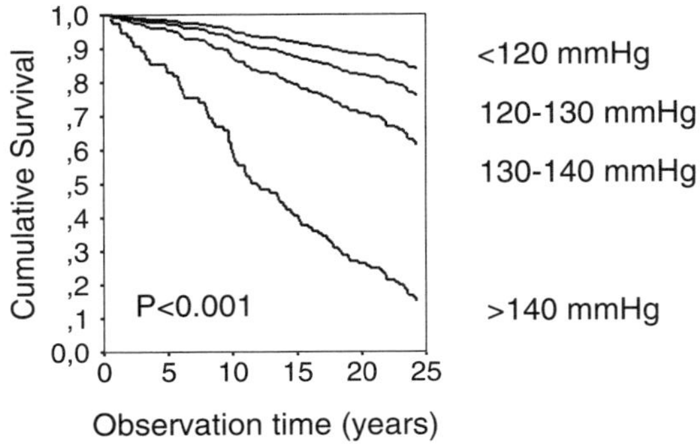

FIG. 1. Cumulative survival over 25 years in 269 patients with type 1 diabetes divided into quartiles of systolic blood pressure.

divided into quartiles of systolic BP. In a Cox multiple regression analysis, pulse pressure, along with abnormally increased urinary albumin concentration, glycemic control, and smoking, all potentially modifiable risk factors, were identified as important predictors of increased mortality in type 1 diabetes.

Antihypertensive treatment has improved renal prognosis and survival in diabetic nephropathy [15], and recent guidelines agree (JN-VII) on the need for early, aggressive reduction of BP, with a goal of <130/80 mmHg in patients with diabetes [20]. An important question relates to the optimal BP and the component of the elevated BP that affects the risk. In a recent post hoc analysis of the IDNT trial, cardiovascular events were increased in patients with BP below 120/85 mmHg [21]. Obviously, these data revived the discussion as to whether there is a J effect [22,23]. Such an effect was not observed in the subset of patients with diabetes in the HOT trial [24], but in this study the lowest achieved BP did not go below 141/81 mmHg. Clearly, it is important to consider the concept of reverse causality, that is that low BP could be the consequence of baseline morbidities rather than a cause of cardiovascular events. Determining an optimal BP level is a very difficult task, and at present a target BP of approximately 120/80–85 mmHg would seem reasonable, and indeed difficult to achieve in many patients.

Intervention in the RAS System: Additive Renoprotective Effect Independent of Blood Pressure?

Many guidelines endorse the view that inhibition of the RAS should be first-line antihypertensive therapy in patients with diabetic nephropathy [20,25,26]. The background is the concept of an additive renoprotective effect beyond reduction of BP alone. As indicated in Table 1, various study designs have be employed in the assessment of a possible renoprotective effect. As indicated, a number of studies claim BP-independent protection of kidney function. However, the concept of additive renoprotective effect has recently been challenged on several occasions. In a post hoc analysis from the large ALLHAT study [27], no difference in incidence of end-stage renal disease (ESRD) or a 50% or greater reduction in GFR was observed for patients taking lisinopril compared with those taking chlorthalidone, either for the total group or for participants with diabetes at baseline. It is important to stress that ALLHAT was not a renal study (no data on albuminuria) but perhaps more important that the design of ALLHAT renders firm interpretations regarding conventional renoprotective regimens difficult: ACE-I and diuretics were compared in separate active arms (often combined with older

TABLE 1. Evaluation of specific BP-independent renoprotective effects: Possible strategies.

Design	Example	Comments
ACE/ARB versus placebo in "normotensive" patients	Lewis 1993 Mathiesen 1991	Inevitably associated with BP differences, which in some studies may fully explain differences in renal endpoints
ACE/ARB versus placebo titration of open-label drug to reach BP target	RENAAL 2001 MICRO-HOPE 2000	Often also BP differences, multivariate statistical analysis employed to claim BP independence
ACE/ARB versus alternative antihypertensive drug + titration in each treatment arm of open-label drugs to reach blood pressure target	IDNT 2001	The best design, despite identical BP significantly better renal outcome in the irbesartan arm compared with the amlodipine arm

antihypertensive drugs). Thus, the commonly used combination of ACE-I and diuretics could not be evaluated [28]. Another point of concern is the use of a low dose of ACE-I (lisinopril 10 mg) [29].

Another study challenging a specific renoprotective effect of ACE-I or ARB is the meta-analysis by Casas et al. [30] stating that "The benefits of ACE-I or ARB on renal outcomes probably result from a BP effect ... additional renoprotective actions beyond lowering BP remain unproven" and in addition "These findings have implications for the use of ACE-I or ARB in patients with diabetes and renal disease" – in other words claiming a need for revision of the guidelines mentioned here. As the analyses are dominated by the ALLHAT trial, the same points of criticism apply to this study [31]. Notably, a BP-independent antiproteinuric effect of ACE-I and ARB is documented in the meta-analysis. This is of interest as "on-treatment" reduction of albuminuria recently has emerged as an important prognostic factor in relation to both renal and cardiovascular risks [32–35]. Thus, it is important not only to screen for microalbuminuria but also to monitor the regression in albuminuria during treatment. In patients with persisting high levels of albuminuria, intensified treatment should be considered, despite apparently acceptable BP values.

Finally, a population-based study by Suissa et al. [36] analyzed data from diabetic patients treated with antihypertensive drugs in the Province of Saskatchewan, Canada, between 1982 and 1986. The study was based on a registry of medication prescription. The rate ratio of end-stage renal failure with the use of ACE-I was found to be 0.8 (ns) during the first 3 years of follow-up, but increased to 4.2 (95% confidence interval 2.0–9.0) after 3 years, suggesting that the use of ACE-I apparently does not decrease the long-term risk of ESRD in diabetes, but might on the contrary actually increase the risk for ESRD, thus contributing to the increasing incidence of diabetes-related ESRD. A major drawback is the lack of information on the indication for the medication, making "confounding by indication" a potential problem although information on the use of ACE-I in diabetic nephropathy still was scarce between 1982 and 1986. Other concerns include lack of information regarding risk factors for development of diabetic nephropathy and absence of information regarding the cause of renal failure. Furthermore, there was no information regarding doses of ACE inhibition.

In conclusion, BP reduction independent from the class of drugs used is essential in conserving renal function. Detection of specific BP-independent renoprotective effects of ACE-I or ARB is difficult from a design point of view. There is, however, at least one well-designed randomized double-blind clinical trial clearly suggesting BP independence [37]. The main evidence for renoprotective action of RAS blockade is perhaps provided by its well-documented antiproteinuric action, which cannot completely be attributed to the reduction in BP. Proteinuria reduction during therapy is the single most important factor predicting both the renal and the cardiovascular prognosis in diabetic patients, and ACE-I and ARB are well-tolerated, effective drugs in both respects.

ACE-I or ARB: Does it Matter?

As mentioned earlier, treatment with both ACE-I and ARB carries strong documentation for the beneficial effects in diabetic nephropathy. In type 1 diabetes, the documentation is strongest for ACE-I [38–41], whereas in type 2 diabetes the best evidence is for ARB [37,42–44]. However, an important question is whether one class of drugs is superior both in relation to preventing development and progression of nephropathy and cardiovascular disease. This question was addressed in the DETAIL study. In this long-term (5-year) double-blind study in a mixed population of micro- and macroalbuminuric patients with type 2 diabetes, the effect of an ACE-I (enalapril) was compared with an ARB (telmisartan). The main endpoint was fall in GFR, and after 5 years the fall from baseline was similar in the two groups (15 mL/min in the ACE-I-treated patients compared with 17 mL/min in the ARB group). BP reduction was similar in the two groups and no cases of ESRD and only very few CV events were observed, probably illustrating the beneficial effects of RAS intervention in general as well as other interventions (e.g., lipid-lowering) in this patient population. The inclusion of both macro- and microalbuminuric patients (the latter with a presumed low rate of GFR reduction) and lack of GFR determinations in a considerable number of patients could have led to a diminished discriminatory power [45], but nevertheless, this study does not point toward a specific advantage of ARB compared with ACE-I in patients with type 2 diabetes. Similarly, in a 1-year double-blind trial in 92 hypertensive type 2 diabetics with early nephropathy, treatment with either losartan or enalapril was associated with the same reduction in albuminuria and the same rate of decline in GFR [46].

In a recent randomized, nonblinded study in 68 nondiabetic patients, the renoprotective effects of ACE-I (benazepril 1.25–5 mg daily or trandolapril 0.5–4 mg daily) and ARB (candesartan 2–8 mg daily or losartan 25–100 mg daily) were compared over a 5-year period. After 4 years, the decline in GFR in patients treated with ARB was significantly greater than that seen in patients treated with an ACE-I ($p < 0.05$). Furthermore, the rate of introduction of dialysis therapy was also significantly greater in the ARB-treated patients (52.7% in ACE-I and 81.2% in ARB group at year 5. $p < 0.01$) [47]. It should however be noted that, although not statistically significant, baseline GFR was lower and proteinuria higher in the ARB group. Obviously, it is also important to consider the reliability of data derived from nonblinded studies. Patients with diabetic nephropathy are, as earlier mentioned. characterized by a high risk of ischemic heart disease and also congestive heart failure [48]; so, in addition to renoprotection, it is important to consider potential differential effects of ACE-I and ARB in this context. Recently, controversy has emerged whether ARB is less effective in preventing myocardial infarction or may even increase the risk of myocardial infarction in comparison with ACE-I and calcium antagonists [49,50]. These aspects are further discussed by Toftegård in Chapter 17.

To summarize, both ACE-I and ARB have documented positive effects in relation to reduction of cardiovascular events. Regarding renal endpoints, the documentation is strongest for ACE-I in type 1 diabetes and for ARB in type 2 diabetes, but emerging data suggest that ACE-I is effective also in type 2 diabetes. The actual choice may, in addition to other factors, depend on economic considerations and side effects.

Dual Blockade

As mentioned earlier, hypertension and proteinuria are the main risk factors for renal disease progression. Although there is clear evidence that pharmacological blockade of the RAS with ACE-I or ARB reduces proteinuria and slows down the progression of diabetic renal disease, it is however important to realize that progression is far from stopped in all patients. The presence of inadequately controlled hypertension and persistent proteinuria despite ACE-I or ARB treatment portends a poor prognosis.

A possible explanation for the lack of effect may be the phenomenon of ACE escape, whereby levels of angiotensin II and aldosterone return to pretreatment levels despite continued use of an ACE-I, possibly due to increased chymase activity and increased angiotensin II formation [51].

Dual blockade of the RAS is based on a principle of obtaining more efficient blockade of the effects of angiotensin II, by combining ACE-I and ARB. ARB produces a complete blockade of the RAS and stimulates the vasodilating and nonproliferative actions of AII via the AT-2 receptor. Furthermore, ACE-I, but not ARB, inhibit the metabolism of kinins, which increases the level of bradykinin, a potent vasodilator.

Interestingly, the addition of ARB but not beta-blockers to antihypertensive medications, which may include ACE-I and/or calcium channel blockers, results in an improvement in resistance artery remodeling in diabetic hypertensive patients [52].

In relation to diabetic nephropathy, evaluation of the potential beneficial effects of dual-blockade therapy is a work in rapid progress, as indicated in Table 2. Although the studies show some divergence, the majority of data demonstrate significant reductions in either BP or albuminuria or in both factors. It should however be noted that the studies in general are small with short follow-up. As the optimal doses of both types of drug remain to be determined, it is also relevant to consider whether the same effect can be obtained by optimizing the dose of ACE-I or ARB in monotherapy [53–55].

No long-term endpoint studies in patients with diabetic nephropathy have yet been published but in nondiabetic nephropathy data from two studies are now available. In the COOPERATE trial 263 Japanese patients with nondiabetic renal disease (calculated GFR: 20–70 mL/min) were randomly assigned ARB (losartan, 100 mg daily), ACE-I (trandolapril, 3 mg daily) or a combination of both drugs at equivalent doses. After 3 years, significantly fewer patients [10 (11%) of 85] in the dual-blockade group had reached the combined primary endpoint of time to doubling of serum creatinine or ESRD

TABLE 2. Dual blockade in diabetic nephropathy: Effects on blood pressure and proteinuria.

Study	Intervention	n	Duration	Endpoint	Results
Hebert et al. [73]	Losartan 50 mg/ACE-I	7	1 week	Blood pressure Proteinuria	Significant reduction No significant effect
Rossing et al. [74]	Candesartan 8 mg/ACE-I	18	9 weeks	Blood pressure Proteinuria	Significant reduction Significant reduction
Rossing et al. [75]	Candesartan 16 mg/ACE-I	20	8 weeks	Blood pressure Proteinuria	No significant reduction Significant reduction
Jacobsen et al. [76]	Irbesartan 300 mg/ACE-I	21	8 weeks	Blood pressure Proteinuria	Significant reduction Significant difference
Jacobsen et al. [77]	Irbesartan 300 mg /enalapril 40 mg	24	8 weeks	Blood pressure Proteinuria	Significant reduction Significant difference
CALM [78]	Candesartan 16 mg /lisinopril 20 mg	199	12 weeks	Blood pressure Proteinuria	Significant reduction No significant difference
CALM 2 [79]	Candesartan 16 mg + lisinopril 20 mg versus lisinopril 40 mg	75	12 months	Blood pressure Proteinuria	No significant difference No significant difference
Sengul et al. [80]	Lisinopril 20 mg/ telmisartan 80 mg	219	28 weeks	Blood pressure Proteinuria	Significant reduction Significant difference
Tutuncu et al. [81]	Enalapril 5 mg/ losartan, 50 mg	34	12 month	Blood pressure Proteinuria	No significant difference No significant difference
Matos et al. [82]	Perindopril 8 mg/ irbesartan 300 mg	20	16 weeks	Blood pressure Proteinuria	No significant difference No significant difference
Fujisawa et al. [83]	Imidapril 10 mg or candesartan 8 mg versus imidapril 5 mg + candesartan 4 mg	27	3 months	Blood pressure Proteinuria	No significant difference Significant difference
Song et al. [84]	Candesartan 4–8 mg/ ramipril 5–7.5 mg	18	16 weeks	Blood pressure Proteinuria	No significant difference No significant difference

compared with 20 (23%) of 85 on trandolapril alone, and 20 (23%) of 86 on losartan alone. A potential drawback of this study is underdosing of the ACE-I [56]. Likewise, in a very recent open-label study also form Japan, 90 patients receiving ACE-I for hypertension and nondiabetic renal insufficiency were randomized to receive candesartan plus ACE-I or continue with ACE-I monotherapy only [57]. During 3.1 years of follow-up, the authors found significant reductions in urine protein excretion compared with the ACE-I-treated control group, despite similar BP levels. Furthermore, after 3 years, the serum creatinine level was significantly lower with candesartan plus ACE-I than with ACE-I only. It should be stressed that this is a nonblinded study, and as also acknowledged by the authors, a substantial proportion of patients received submaximal doses of ACE-I.

The safety of combined ACE-I and ARB therapy is an important issue that was evaluated in recent meta-analysis in patients with chronic proteinuric renal disease [58]. Dual blockade resulted in a significant but small increase in serum potassium levels of 0.11 mmol/L (95% confidence interval: 0.05–0.17 mmol/L) and a nonsignificant decrease in glomerular filtration. Addition of an ARB resulted in a further decrease in proteinuria in both patients with diabetic and nondiabetic renal disease.

Although it is beyond the scope of this chapter, a more recently addressed question is whether intervention in the RAS system by adding a mineralocorticoid receptor antagonist is associated with beneficial effects. Several small, short-term studies have been published [59–64] but clearly further documentation is needed before a possible clinical role of this intervention can be assessed. Hyperkalemia is a major concern, but in a recent study by Epstein et al. [65], where coadministration of eplerenone and ACE-I over 12 weeks resulted in significant reduction in albuminuria, no significant increases in hyperkalemia was observed.

In summary, several short-term studies suggest that dual blockade reduces both BP and albuminuria in patients with diabetes but long-term clinical trials are needed to further establish the role of dual blockade in renal protection in diabetic nephropathy. The combination of ACE-I and ARB therapy in patients with diabetic renal disease is seldom associated with clinically meaningful changes in serum potassium levels or GFRs. Despite the apparent safety of dual RAS blockade in this regard, it is important to emphasize that initiating treatment with, or increasing the doses of, either drug should be followed by serum potassium and creatinine monitoring.

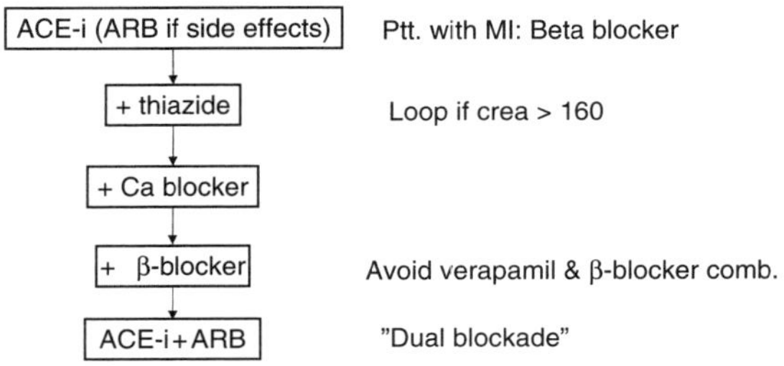

FIG. 2. Treatment flowchart for diabetic patients with hypertension and/or microalbuminuria.0

Conclusions

BP reduction and reduction of proteinuria during therapy are the most important factors predicting cardiovascular as well as renal prognosis, independent from the class of drugs used. The best evidence for a BP-independent renoprotective action of blocking the RAS is provided by its well-documented antiproteinuric action. This is important as regression of proteinuria during antihypertensive treatment now has emerged as an important prognostic factor. There are ample data to support the effect of ACE-I or ARB in combination with diuretics both in relation to nephro- and cardioprotection, although documentation of the latter may be best for ACE-I. This is perhaps reflecting that ACE-I have been longest on the stage. The optimal doses of both types of drug remain to be determined. In many short-term studies combining ACE-I with ARB (dual blockade), further reduction of albuminuria and BP is observed, but long-term endpoint studies in diabetic patients are lacking. Dual blockade appears to be relatively safe, but monitoring of potassium and creatinine is important. An example of a treatment flowchart is given in Fig. 2.

Treatment of Advanced Diabetic Renal Disease

Despite the improvement in controlling diabetes and preventing the onset and progression of diabetic nephropathy outlined in this book, diabetes is the leading cause of ESRD in the world.

In Denmark, the number of incident diabetic patients with ESRD, who are started on chronic renal replacement therapy (RRT), has stabilized around 32 patients per million population per year [66] corresponding to approximately 25% of all incident patients with ESRD. In United States, the occurrence of diabetes among incident ESRD patients has exceeded 50% corresponding to more than 150 patients per million population per year [67].

For diabetic patients with chronic kidney disease (CKD) stages I–II (Creatinine clearance between normal and 60 mL/min/1.73 m^2), stage-independent actions such as control of cardiovascular risk factors (hypertension, hyperlipidemia, and smoking), avoidance of drug toxicity and diagnostic injury, control of progression, and reduction of proteinuria are essential.

For patients with CKD stage III (creatinine clearance between 30 and 60 mL/min/1.73 m^2) important actions are prevention, identification, and treatment of potential complications such as renal anemia, malnutrition, and disturbances in mineral metabolism. Treatment of these complications is beyond the scope of this book but should generally follow national, regional, or international guidelines [68–71].

For patients with CKD stage IV (creatinine clearance between 15–30 mL/min/1.73 m^2) important actions are preparation of RRT and continuous control of complications. Preparation of RRT includes predialysis education of patients and relatives, dialysis modality selection, and eventually preparation for preempty renal transplantation from a living or a cadaveric donor.

For patients with CKD stage V (dialysis or creatinine clearance <15 mL/min/1.73 m^2) the most important actions are preempty renal transplantation or timely creation of dialysis access and timely initiation of dialysis.

Timely referral of patients suffering from progressive CKD to the nephrologist has a positive influence on patients' outcome in terms of mortality, morbidity, dialysis modality selection in favor of peritoneal dialysis, dialysis access outcome, dialysis technique failure, renal transplant eligibility, and total cost at initiation of dialysis [72].

Joint Care of Patients with Diabetic Renal Disease in Stages III–V

In many countries, patients with diabetic renal disease in stages I–III are primarily treated by diabetologists. As indicated earlier, there are however already in stage III important aspects regarding anemia, mineral metabolism, dialysis modality selection, and potential family kidney donation that must also be considered. On the other hand, patients in stages IV–V are primarily seen by nephrologists. The continued screening for and treatment of other diabetic complications as well as optimal glycemic control is however still of utmost importance. Thus, ideally, control and treatment of the diabetic patient with CKD stages III–V should be performed by a well-organized multidisciplinary team of dedicated endocrinologists, nephrologists, nurses, dieticians, social workers, and others.

References

1. Mogensen, CE: Progression of nephropathy in long-term diabetics with proteinuria and effect of initial anti-hypertensive treatment. *Scand. J. Clin. Lab. Invest*. 36:383–388, 1976.
2. Mogensen, CE: Diabetic renal disease: the quest for normotension–and beyond. *Diabet. Med*. 12:756–769, 1995.
3. Hasslacher, C, Stech, W, Wahl, P, Ritz, E: Blood pressure and metabolic control as risk factors for nephropathy in type 1 (insulin-dependent) diabetes. *Diabetologia* 28:6–11, 1985.
4. Berglund, J, Lins, LE, Lins, PE: Metabolic and blood pressure monitoring in diabetic renal failure. *Acta Med. Scand*. 218:401–408, 1985.
5. Parving, H-H, Hommel, E, Mathiesen, E, Skott, P, Edsberg, B, Bahnsen, M, Lauritzen, M, Hougaard, P, Lauritzen, E: Prevalence of microalbuminuria, arterial hypertension, retinopathy and neuropathy in patients with insulin dependent diabetes. *Br. Med. J. (Clin. Res. Ed.)* 296:156–160, 1988.
6. Rossing, P, Hommel, E, Smidt, UM, Parving, H-H: Impact of arterial blood pressure and albuminuria on the progression of diabetic nephropathy in IDDM patients. *Diabetes* 42:715–719, 1993.
7. Hovind, P, Rossing, P, Tarnow, L, Smidt, UM, Parving, H-H: Progression of diabetic nephropathy. *Kidney Int*. 59:702–709, 2001.
8. Mogensen, CE: Long-term antihypertensive treatment inhibiting progression of diabetic nephropathy. *Br. Med. J. (Clin. Res. Ed.)* 285:685–688, 1982.
9. Parving, HH, Andersen, AR, Smidt, UM, Svendsen, PA: Early aggressive antihypertensive treatment reduces rate of decline in kidney function in diabetic nephropathy. *Lancet* 1:1175–1179, 1983.
10. Anderson, S, Brenner, BM: Influence of antihypertensive therapy on development and progression of diabetic glomerulopathy. *Diabetes Care* 11:846–849, 1988.
11. Parving, H-H, Smidt, UM, Hommel, E, Mathiesen, ER, Rossing, P, Nielsen, F, Gall, MA: Effective antihypertensive treatment postpones renal insufficiency in diabetic nephropathy. *Am. J. Kidney Dis*. 22:188–195, 1993.
12. Parving, HH, Hommel, E: Prognosis in diabetic nephropathy [see comments]. *BMJ* 299:230–233, 1989.
13. Mathiesen, ER, Borch Johnsen, K, Jensen, DV, Deckert, T: Improved survival in patients with diabetic nephropathy. *Diabetologia* 32:884–886, 1989.
14. Hasslacher, C, Borgholte, G, Ritz, E, Wahl, P: Impact of hypertension on prognosis in IDDM. *Diabete Metab*. 15:338–342, 1989.
15. Astrup, AS, Tarnow, L, Rossing, P, Pietraszek, L, Riis, HP, Parving, HH: Improved prognosis in type 1 diabetic patients with nephropathy: a prospective follow-up study. *Kidney Int*. 68:1250–1257, 2005.
16. Adler, AI, Stratton, IM, Neil, HA, Yudkin, JS, Matthews, DR, Cull, CA, Wright, AD, Turner, RC, Holman, RR: Association of systolic blood pressure with macrovascular and microvascular complications of type 2 diabetes (UKPDS 36): prospective observational study. *BMJ* 321:412–419, 2000.
17. Haffner, SM, Lehto, S, Ronnemaa, T, Pyorala, K, Laakso, M: Mortality from coronary heart disease in subjects with type 2 diabetes and in nondiabetic subjects with and without prior myocardial infarction. *N. Engl. J. Med*. 339:229–234, 1998.
18. Juutilainen, A, Lehto, S, Ronnemaa, T, Pyorala, K, Laakso, M: Type 2 diabetes as a "coronary heart disease equivalent": an 18-year prospective population-based study in Finnish subjects. *Diabetes Care* 28:2901–2907, 2005.
19. Booth, GL, Kapral, MK, Fung, K, Tu, JV: Relation between age and cardiovascular disease in men and women with diabetes compared with non-diabetic

people: a population-based retrospective cohort study. *Lancet* 368:29–36, 2006.
20. Chobanian, AV, Bakris, GL, Black, HR, Cushman, WC, Green, LA, Izzo, JL, Jr., Jones, DW, Materson, BJ, Oparil, S, Wright, JT, Jr., Roccella, EJ: The seventh report of the Joint National Committee on prevention, detection, evaluation, and treatment of high blood pressure: the JNC 7 report. *JAMA* 289:2560–2572, 2003.
21. Berl, T, Hunsicker, LG, Lewis, JB, Pfeffer, MA, Porush, JG, Rouleau, JL, Drury, PL, Esmatjes, E, Hricik, D, Pohl, M, Raz, I, Vanhille, P, Wiegmann, TB, Wolfe, BM, Locatelli, F, Goldhaber, SZ, Lewis, EJ: Impact of achieved blood pressure on cardiovascular outcomes in the Irbesartan Diabetic Nephropathy Trial. *J. Am. Soc. Nephrol.* 16:2170–2179, 2005.
22. Cruickshank, JM: Antihypertensive treatment and the J-curve. *Cardiovasc. Drugs Ther.* 14:373–379, 2000.
23. Hansson, L: Antihypertensive treatment: does the J-curve exist? *Cardiovasc. Drugs Ther.* 14:367–372, 2000.
24. Hansson, L, Zanchetti, A, Carruthers, SG, Dahlof, B, Elmfeldt, D, Julius, S, Menard, J, Rahn, KH, Wedel, H, Westerling, S: Effects of intensive blood-pressure lowering and low-dose aspirin in patients with hypertension: principal results of the Hypertension Optimal Treatment (HOT) randomised trial. HOT Study Group [see comments]. *Lancet* 351:1755–1762, 1998.
25. Williams, B, Poulter, NR, Brown, MJ, Davis, M, McInnes, GT, Potter, JF, Sever, PS, McG, TS: Guidelines for management of hypertension: report of the fourth working party of the British Hypertension Society, 2004-BHS IV. *J. Hum. Hypertens.* 18:139–185, 2004.
26. American Diabetes Association: Standards of medical care in diabetes. *Diabetes Care* 28 Suppl 1: S4–S36, 2005.
27. Rahman, M, Pressel, S, Davis, BR, Nwachuku, C, Wright, JT, Jr., Whelton, PK, Barzilay, J, Batuman, V, Eckfeldt, JH, Farber, M, Henriquez, M, Kopyt, N, Louis, GT, Saklayen, M, Stanford, C, Walworth, C, Ward, H, Wiegmann, T: Renal outcomes in high-risk hypertensive patients treated with an angiotensin-converting enzyme inhibitor or a calcium channel blocker vs a diuretic: a report from the Antihypertensive and Lipid-Lowering Treatment to Prevent Heart Attack Trial (ALLHAT). *Arch. Intern. Med.* 165:936–946, 2005.
28. Levey, AS, Uhlig, K: Which antihypertensive agents in chronic kidney disease? *Ann. Intern. Med.* 144:213–215, 2006.
29. Hollenberg, NK: Omission of drug dose information. *Arch. Intern. Med.* 166:368–369, 2006.
30. Casas, JP, Chua, W, Loukogeorgakis, S, Vallance, P, Smeeth, L, Hingorani, AD, MacAllister, RJ: Effect of inhibitors of the renin-angiotensin system and other antihypertensive drugs on renal outcomes: systematic review and meta-analysis. *Lancet* 366:2026–2033, 2005.
31. Rossing, P, Parving, HH, de Zeeuw, D: Renoprotection by blocking the RAAS in diabetic nephropathy–fact or fiction? *Nephrol. Dial. Transplant.* 21:2354–2357, 2006.
32. Hovind, P, Rossing, P, Tarnow, L, Toft, H, Parving, J, Parving, HH: Remission of nephrotic-range albuminuria in type 1 diabetic patients. *Diabetes Care* 24:1972–1977, 2001.
33. Hovind, P, Tarnow, L, Rossing, P, Carstensen, B, Parving, HH: Improved survival in patients obtaining remission of nephrotic range albuminuria in diabetic nephropathy. *Kidney Int.* 66:1180–1186, 2004.
34. Ibsen, H, Olsen, MH, Wachtell, K, Borch-Johnsen, K, Lindholm, LH, Mogensen, CE, Dahlof, B, Snapinn, SM, Wan, Y, Lyle, PA: Does albuminuria predict cardiovascular outcomes on treatment with losartan versus atenolol in patients with diabetes, hypertension, and left ventricular hypertrophy? The LIFE study. *Diabetes Care* 29:595–600, 2006.
35. de Zeeuw, D, Remuzzi, G, Parving, HH, Keane, WF, Zhang, Z, Shahinfar, S, Snapinn, S, Cooper, ME, Mitch, WE, Brenner, BM: Albuminuria, a therapeutic target for cardiovascular protection in type 2 diabetic patients with nephropathy. *Circulation* 110:921–927, 2004.
36. Suissa, S, Hutchinson, T, Brophy, JM, Kezouh, A: ACE-inhibitor use and the long-term risk of renal failure in diabetes. *Kidney Int.* 69:913–919, 2006.
37. Lewis, EJ, Hunsicker, LG, Clarke, WR, Berl, T, Pohl, MA, Lewis, JB, Ritz, E, Atkins, RC, Rohde, R, Raz, I: Renoprotective effect of the angiotensin-receptor antagonist irbesartan in patients with nephropathy due to type 2 diabetes. *N. Engl. J. Med.* 20;345:851–860, 2001.
38. Lewis, EJ, Hunsicker, LG, Bain, RP, Rohde, RD: The effect of angiotensin-converting-enzyme inhibition on diabetic nephropathy. The Collaborative Study Group [see comments] [published erratum appears in *N. Engl. J. Med.* Jan 13;330(2):152, 1993]. *N. Engl. J. Med.* 329:1456–1462, 1993.
39. The ACE Inhibitors in Diabetic Nephropathy Trialist Group: Should all patients with type 1 diabetes mellitus and microalbuminuria receive Angiotensin-Converting Enzyme Inhibitors? A meta-analysis of individual patient data. *Ann. Intern. Med.* 134:340–379, 2001.
40. Mogensen, CE, Keane, WF, Bennett, PH, Jerums, G, Parving, HH, Passa, P, Steffes, MW, Striker, GE, Viberti, GC: Prevention of diabetic renal disease with special reference to microalbuminuria [see comments]. *Lancet* 346:1080–1084, 1995.

41. Cooper, ME: Pathogenesis, prevention, and treatment of diabetic nephropathy. *Lancet* 352:213–219, 1998.
42. Ruggenenti, P, Fassi, A, Ilieva, AP, Bruno, S, Iliev, IP, Brusegan, V, Rubis, N, Gherardi, G, Arnoldi, F, Ganeva, M, Ene-Iordache, B, Gaspari, F, Perna, A, Bossi, A, Trevisan, R, Dodesini, AR, Remuzzi, G: Preventing microalbuminuria in type 2 diabetes. *N. Engl. J. Med.* 351:1941–1951, 2004.
43. Parving, HH, Lehnert, H, Brochner-Mortensen, J, Gomis, R, Andersen, S, Arner, P: The effect of irbesartan on the development of diabetic nephropathy in patients with type 2 diabetes. *N. Engl. J. Med.* 20;345:870–878, 2001.
44. Brenner, BM, Cooper, ME, de Zeeuw, D, Keane, WF, Mitch, WE, Parving, HH, Remuzzi, G, Snapinn, SM, Zhang, Z, Shahinfar, S: Effects of losartan on renal and cardiovascular outcomes in patients with type 2 diabetes and nephropathy. *N. Engl. J. Med.* 20;345:861–869, 2001.
45. Parving, HH, Hovind, P, Rossing, P: Telmisartan vs. enalapril in type 2 diabetes. *N. Engl. J. Med.* 352:835–836, 2005.
46. Lacourciere, Y, Belanger, A, Godin, C, Halle, JP, Ross, S, Wright, N, Marion, J: Long-term comparison of losartan and enalapril on kidney function in hypertensive type 2 diabetics with early nephropathy. *Kidney Int.* 58:762–769, 2000.
47. Shoda, J, Kanno, Y, Suzuki, H: A five-year comparison of the renal protective effects of angiotensin-converting enzyme inhibitors and angiotensin receptor blockers in patients with non-diabetic nephropathy. *Intern. Med.* 45:193–198, 2006.
48. Nichols, GA, Gullion, CM, Koro, CE, Ephross, SA, Brown, JB: The incidence of congestive heart failure in type 2 diabetes: an update. *Diabetes Care* 27:1879–1884, 2004.
49. Verma, S, Strauss, M: Angiotensin receptor blockers and myocardial infarction. *BMJ* 329:1248–1249, 2004.
50. Strippoli, GF, Craig, M, Deeks, JJ, Schena, FP, Craig, JC: Effects of angiotensin converting enzyme inhibitors and angiotensin II receptor antagonists on mortality and renal outcomes in diabetic nephropathy: systematic review. *BMJ* 329:828, 2004.
51. Ihara, M, Urata, H, Kinoshita, A, Suzumiya, J, Sasaguri, M, Kikuchi, M, Ideishi, M, Arakawa, K: Increased chymase-dependent angiotensin II formation in human atherosclerotic aorta. *Hypertension* 33:1399–1405, 1999.
52. Savoia, C, Touyz, RM, Endemann, DH, Pu, Q, Ko, EA, De Ciuceis, C, Schiffrin, EL: Angiotensin receptor blocker added to previous antihypertensive agents on arteries of diabetic hypertensive patients. *Hypertension* 48:271–277, 2006.
53. Andersen, NH, Poulsen, PL, Knudsen, ST, Poulsen, SH, Eiskjaer, H, Hansen, KW, Helleberg, K, Mogensen, CE: Long-term dual blockade with candesartan and lisinopril in hypertensive patients with diabetes: the CALM II study. *Diabetes Care* 28:273–277, 2005.
54. Rossing, K, Schjoedt, KJ, Jensen, BR, Boomsma, F, Parving, HH: Enhanced renoprotective effects of ultrahigh doses of irbesartan in patients with type 2 diabetes and microalbuminuria. *Kidney Int.* 68:1190–1198, 2005.
55. Schmieder, RE, Klingbeil, AU, Fleischmann, EH, Veelken, R, Delles, C: Additional antiproteinuric effect of ultrahigh dose candesartan: a double-blind, randomized, prospective study. *J. Am. Soc. Nephrol.* 16:3038–3045, 2005.
56. Nakao, N, Kimura, G: Submaximal dose of trandolapril in the COOPERATE trial? *Kidney Int.* 64:1921–1922, 2003.
57. Kanno, Y, Takenaka, T, Nakamura, T, and Suzuki, H. Add-on angiotensin receptor blocker in patients who have proteinuric chronic kidney diseases and are treated with angiotensin-converting enzyme inhibitors. *Clin. J. Am. Soc. Nephrol.* 1:730–737, 2006.
58. MacKinnon, M, Shurraw, S, Akbari, A, Knoll, GA, Jaffey, J, Clark, HD: Combination therapy with an angiotensin receptor blocker and an ACE inhibitor in proteinuric renal disease: a systematic review of the efficacy and safety data. *Am. J. Kidney Dis.* 48:8–20, 2006.
59. Rossing, K, Schjoedt, KJ, Smidt, UM, Boomsma, F, Parving, HH: Beneficial effects of adding spironolactone to recommended antihypertensive treatment in diabetic nephropathy: a randomized, double-masked, cross-over study. *Diabetes Care* 28:2106–2112, 2005.
60. Sato, A, Hayashi, K, Naruse, M, Saruta, T: Effectiveness of aldosterone blockade in patients with diabetic nephropathy. *Hypertension* 41:64–68, 2003.
61. van den Meiracker, AH, Baggen, RG, Pauli, S, Lindemans, A, Vulto, AG, Poldermans, D, Boomsma, F: Spironolactone in type 2 diabetic nephropathy: Effects on proteinuria, blood pressure and renal function. *J. Hypertens.* 24:2285–2292, 2006.
62. Schjoedt, KJ, Rossing, K, Juhl, TR, Boomsma, F, Tarnow, L, Rossing, P, Parving, HH: Beneficial impact of spironolactone on nephrotic range albuminuria in diabetic nephropathy. *Kidney Int.* 70:536–542, 2006.
63. Rachmani, R, Slavachevsky, I, Amit, M, Levi, Z, Kedar, Y, Berla, M, Ravid, M: The effect of spironolactone, cilazapril and their combination on albuminuria in patients with hypertension and diabetic nephropathy is independent of blood pressure reduction: a randomized controlled study. *Diabet. Med.* 21:471–475, 2004.
64. van den Meiracker AH, Baggen, RGA, Pauli S, Lindemans A, Vulto AG, Poldermans D, Boomsma

F: Spironolactone in type 2 diabetic nephropathy: Effects on proteinuria, blood pressure and renal function. *J. Hypertens.* 24:2285–2292, 2006.
65. Epstein M, Williams GH, Weinberger M, Lewin A, Krause S, Mukherjee R, Patni R, Beckerman B.: Selective aldosterone blockade with eplerenone reduces albuminuria in patients with type 2 diabetes. *Clin. J. Am. Soc. Nephrol.* 1:940–951, 2006.
66. Danish National Registry Report on Dialysis and Transplantation in Denmark, 2005. www.Nephrology.dk
67. U.S. Renal Data System, USRDS 2006 Annual Data Report: Atlas of End-Stage Renal Disease in the United States, National Institutes of Health, National Institute of Diabetes and Digestive and Kidney Diseases, Bethesda, MD, 2006.
68. National Kidney Foundation: KDOQI Clinical Practice Guidelines and Clinical Practice Recommendations for diabetes and chronic kidney disease. *Am. J. Kidney Dis.* 49;2:S12–S154, 2007.
69. Moe S, Drueke T, Cunningham J, Goodman W, Martin K, Olgaard K et al.: Definition, evaluation, and classification of renal osteodystrophy:: A position statement from Kidney Disease: Improving Global Outcomes (KDIGO). *Kidney Int.* 69;11:1945–1953, 2006.
70. National Kidney Foundation. K/DOQI clinical practice guidelines for bone metabolism and disease in chronic kidney disease. *Am. J. Kidney Dis.* 42:1–201, 2003.
71. National Kidney Foundation. KDOQI Clinical Practice Guidelines and Clinical Practice Recommendations for Anemia in Chronic Kidney Disease. *Am. J. Kidney Dis.* 47:S1–S146, 2006.
72. Lameire N, Wauters J-P, Teruel JLG, Bissen WV, Vanholder R. An update on the referral pattern of patients with end-stage renal disease. *Kidney Int.* 61:S27–S34, 2002.
73. Hebert, LA, Falkenhain, ME, Nahman, NS, Jr., Cosio, FG, O'Dorisio, TM: Combination ACE inhibitor and angiotensin II receptor antagonist therapy in diabetic nephropathy. *Am. J. Nephrol.* 19:1–6, 1999.
74. Rossing, K, Christensen, PK, Jensen, BR, Parving, HH: Dual blockade of the renin-angiotensin system in diabetic nephropathy: a randomized double-blind crossover study. *Diabetes Care* 25:95–100, 2002.
75. Rossing, K, Jacobsen, P, Pietraszek, L, Parving, HH: Renoprotective effects of adding angiotensin II receptor blocker to maximal recommended doses of ACE inhibitor in diabetic nephropathy: a randomized double-blind crossover trial. *Diabetes Care* 26:2268–2274, 2003.
76. Jacobsen, P, Andersen, S, Rossing, K, Hansen, BV, Parving, HH: Dual blockade of the renin-angiotensin system in type 1 patients with diabetic nephropathy. *Nephrol. Dial. Transplant.* 17:1019–1024, 2002.
77. Jacobsen, P, Andersen, S, Rossing, K, Jensen, BR, Parving, HH: Dual blockade of the renin-angiotensin system versus maximal recommended dose of ACE inhibition in diabetic nephropathy. *Kidney Int.* 63:1874–1880, 2003.
78. Mogensen, CE, Neldam, S, Tikkanen, I, Oren, S, Viskoper, R, Watts, RW, Cooper, ME: Randomised controlled trial of dual blockade of renin-angiotensin system in patients with hypertension, microalbuminuria, and non-insulin dependent diabetes: the candesartan and lisinopril microalbuminuria (CALM) study. *BMJ* 321:1440–1444, 2000.
79. Andersen, NH, Poulsen, PL, Knudsen, ST, Poulsen, SH, Eiskjaer, H, Hansen, KW, Helleberg, K, Mogensen, CE: Long-term dual blockade with candesartan and lisinopril in hypertensive patients with diabetes: the CALM II study. *Diabetes Care* 28:273–277, 2005.
80. Sengul, AM, Altuntas, Y, Kurklu, A, Aydin, L: Beneficial effect of lisinopril plus telmisartan in patients with type 2 diabetes, microalbuminuria and hypertension. *Diabetes Res. Clin. Pract.* 71:210–219, 2006.
81. Tutuncu, NB, Gurlek, A, Gedik, O: Efficacy of ACE inhibitors and ATII receptor blockers in patients with microalbuminuria: a prospective study. *Acta Diabetol.* 38:157–161, 2001.
82. Matos, JP, de Lourdes, RM, Ismerim, VL, Boasquevisque, EM, Genelhu, V, Francischetti, EA: Effects of dual blockade of the renin angiotensin system in hypertensive type 2 diabetic patients with nephropathy. *Clin. Nephrol.* 64:180–189, 2005.
83. Fujisawa, T, Ikegami, H, Ono, M, Nishino, M, Noso, S, Kawabata, Y, Ogihara, T: Combination of half doses of angiotensin type 1 receptor antagonist and angiotensin-converting enzyme inhibitor in diabetic nephropathy. *Am. J. Hypertens.* 18:13–17, 2005.
84. Song, JH, Lee, SW, Suh, JH, Kim, ES, Hong, SB, Kim, KA, Kim, MJ: The effects of dual blockade of the renin-angiotensin system on urinary protein and transforming growth factor-beta excretion in 2 groups of patients with IgA and diabetic nephropathy. *Clin. Nephrol.* 60:318–326, 2003.

19
Aspirin and Antiplatelet Drugs in the Prevention of Cardiovascular Complications of Diabetes

Alberto Zanchetti

Keywords: Aspirin, antiplatelet drugs, myocardial infarction, stroke, bleeding.

Introduction

Type-2 diabetes mellitus is known to increase dramatically the risk of cardiovascular death, as shown, among several other studies, in the large cohort of 340,000 men screened in the Multiple Risk Factor Intervention Trial [1]. Useful information has also been provided by the Hypertension Optimal Treatment (HOT) study [2], with analyses comparing cardiovascular outcomes in 1,503 diabetic hypertensives and 17,230 non-diabetic hypertensives, all subjected to intense antihypertensive treatment: incidences of myocardial infarction, stroke, all major cardiovascular events, cardiovascular and all-cause mortalities were much higher in diabetics than in non-diabetics with relative risk of 1.45–2.13 even after adjusting for all other baseline risk factors (Fig. 1). Calculations from a recent meta-analysis of antihypertensive treatment trials [3] in 34,148 diabetics and 107,605 non-diabetics showed incidence of major cardiovascular events was 60% greater and that of cardiovascular mortality 85% greater in diabetics (Fig. 2). It is therefore reasonable to recommend that patients with diabetes be considered as "coronary heart disease risk equivalents" [4], although they may be more properly defined as "cardiovascular disease equivalents."

A considerable body of evidence has accumulated about the benefits of antiplatelet therapy, in most cases aspirin, in patients with a previous cardiovascular event (previous myocardial infarction, acute myocardial infarction, previous stroke or transient ischemic attack). The 2002 collaborative meta-analysis of the Antithrombotic Trialists' Collaboration has calculated a reduction between 22% and 25% of all cardiovascular events in patients receiving antiplatelet therapy [5]. This meta-analysis involved as many as 287 studies and 135,000 patients at high risk, and in view of the high risk represented by diabetes it is somewhat surprising that only 9 studies involving few more than 5,000 patients were specifically on diabetes. Other data on the effects of aspirin in diabetic patients are available from subgroup analyses of a few trials of antiplatelet therapy in individuals free of previous cardiovascular events (so-called "primary prevention" trials), but not all these trials have separately analysed outcomes in diabetics. Surprisingly, some of the antiplatelet therapy studies on diabetics have given insufficient attention to the possible harmful effects of antiplatelet activity, namely excessive bleeding, thus making clinical conclusions even more difficult.

Effects of Antiplatelet Therapy on Cardiovascular Outcomes in Diabetes

The Early Treatment Diabetic Retinopathy Study and Other Studies Included in the Antithrombotic Trialists' Collaboration Meta-analysis

The 2002 Antithrombotic Trialists' Collaboration meta-analysis [5] includes 9 studies on 5,126 diabetic subjects, showing an overall incidence of cardiovascular

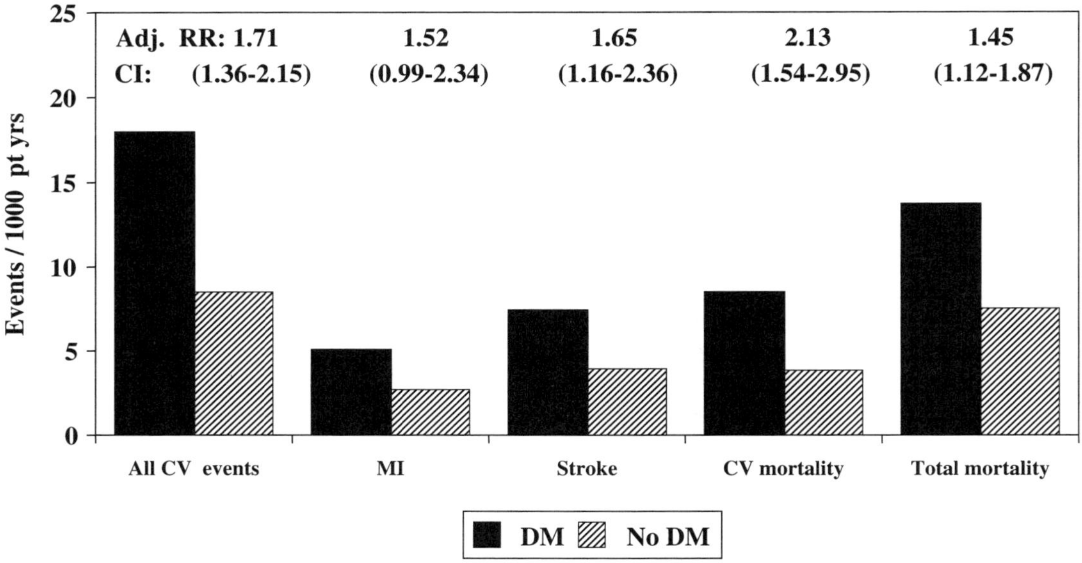

FIG. 1. Incidence of various types of cardiovascular (CV) events in diabetic (DM) and non-diabetic (no DM) patients within the intensely treated cohort of the Hypertension Optimal Treatment (HOT) Study. Event incidence per 1000 patient years (pt yrs). On top of the histograms adjusted relative risk (Adj. RR) and 95% confidence intervals (CI) of diabetics vs non-diabetics. MI:myocardial infarction. (Redrawn from ref. 2).

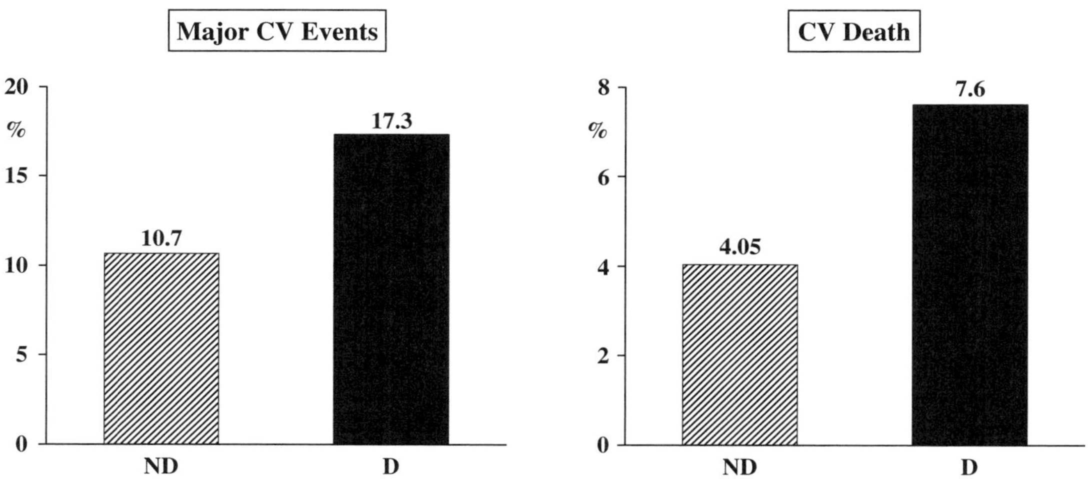

FIG. 2. Percent incidence of major cardiovascular (CV) events and of CV death among 107,605 patients without diabetes mellitus (ND) and 34,148 patients with diabetes mellitus (D) in studies included in the Blood Pressure Lowering Treatment Trialists' Collaboration (calculated from data in ref. 3).

events in subjects allocated to antiplatelet agents of 15.7% versus an incidence of 16.7% in controls, with a non-significant reduction of 7%. This small benefit should be compared with the 22% benefit shown in the entire meta-analysis, although statistical tests do not indicate any dishomogeneity. Most of the 9 trials, however, are small studies including very few subjects (see [6]) and much of the information comes from the ETDRS (Early Treatment Diabetic Retinopathy Study) study [7], in which 3,711 people with diabetes and, generally, no history of myocardial infarction or stroke were included. This is the only relatively large trial that has specifically allocated diabetic patients, and therefore deserves to be reported with some more detail.

In ETDRS 3,711 diabetic patients were allocated randomly and double-blindly to either aspirin or placebo, and followed up for at least 5 years. Thirty per cent of the patients were considered to have type 1 diabetes mellitus (and therefore this study also provides information on this type of diabetes), 31% type 2 diabetes, and in 39% type 1 or 2 could not be determined definitely. The dose of aspirin was of 650 mg once per day, that is, a dose that would be considered relatively large according to present standards. Table 1 illustrates the relative risk estimate for various types of outcomes. For all types of outcomes, except stroke, the relative risk estimate was slightly and non-significantly lower than 1, that is, in favor of patients receiving aspirin; the largest difference in favor of aspirin was found for the occurrence of fatal and non-fatal myocardial infarction. The relative risk was slightly in favor of placebo, but not significantly so, as fatal and non-fatal strokes were concerned. Separate examination of patients according to the type of diabetes showed a trend toward greater benefits of aspirin in type 1 than in type 2 diabetes, but in no case the difference was statistically significant. It may be worth mentioning that the primary objective of ETDRS, development of high-risk proliferative retinopathy, was not influenced by aspirin [8].

The British Male Doctors Trial

This 6-year randomized trial (British Male Doctors Trial – BMD [9]) was conducted among 5,139 apparently healthy male doctors, who were randomly allocated (2:1) to either aspirin 500 mg daily or no aspirin (the study was open, without placebo). Though total mortality was 10% lower in the treated than in the control group, this difference was not statistically significant and chiefly involved diseases other than stroke or myocardial infarction. Only 101 of the randomized subjects (2.0%) had a history of diabetes at the time of recruitment, and no specific data have been reported in this small group of patients; therefore, this study cannot contribute information on the effects of aspirin in diabetes.

The Physicians' Health Study

This study (Physicians' Health Study – PHS [10]) was a randomized, double-blind, placebo-controlled trial investigating the effects of low-dose aspirin (325 mg every other day) in 22,071 healthy male physicians in the USA. During a follow-up of 5 years there was a highly significant 44% reduction in the incidence of myocardial infarction, a slight non-significant increase in stroke (22%), and no reduction in cardiovascular mortality in subjects allocated to aspirin.

There were only 533 subjects (2.4%) with a diagnosis of diabetes mellitus at baseline. In these subjects the risk of myocardial infarction was markedly reduced by aspirin (relative risk 0.39),

TABLE 1. Five-year life table rates and estimates of relative risk in the ETDRS.

	5-Year life table rates			
	Aspirin (N = 1,856)	Placebo (N = 1,855)	Relative risk estimate (99% CI)	Adjusted relative risk estimate (99% CI)
Death–all causes	12.1	14.9	0.91 (0.75–1.11)	0.91 (0.75–1.11)
Cardiovascular death	9.3	11.2	0.87 (0.70–1.10)	0.87 (0.69–1.09)
Fatal or non-fatal myocardial infarction	9.1	12.3	0.83 (0.66–1.04)	0.82 (0.65–1.03)
Fatal or non-fatal stroke	4.5	3.8	1.17 (0.79–1.28)	1.17 (0.79–1.74)
Cardiovascular death, non-fatal myocardial infarction, or stroke	14.0	16.6	0.91 (0.75–1.10)	0.90 (0.74–1.09)
All deaths, non-fatal myocardial infarction or stroke	16.5	20.0	0.93 (0.78–1.10)	0.92 (0.77–1.09)

Redrawn from ref. 7.

whereas in the much larger cohort of non-diabetics the relative risk was 0.60. A test of interaction was negative, and therefore there was no evidence of a greater effect of aspirin among diabetics. The group of diabetics was very small, however, and this trial is not very informative concerning the issue of aspirin effects in diabetics.

The Thrombosis Prevention Trial

This British trial (Thrombosis Prevention Trial – TPT) [11] allocated 5,499 men with increased risk of coronary heart disease to either aspirin 75 mg daily or placebo, observing a 20% reduction of all coronary heart disease events (p = 0.04), almost entirely due to a 32% reduction in non-fatal events (p = 0.004). Diabetes was not one of the factors upon which baseline risk was calculated, and this probably explains why subsequent subgroup analyses of the trial results did not report separate data on diabetics [12]. Thus, TPT does not provide any information on the effects of aspirin in diabetic patients.

The Hypertension Optimal Treatment Study

The Hypertension Optimal Treatment–HOT Study [13] has been a large randomized trial that included 18,790 hypertensives (52.7% males) receiving intense antihypertensive therapy (91.5% with diastolic blood pressure ≤90 mmHg during 3.8 years of follow-up). One of the major objectives of this randomized, double-blind trial was to find out whether the addition of low-dose aspirin (75 mg once daily) to antihypertensive treatment reduced the rate of major cardiovascular events in comparison with addition of a placebo. The principal results of the HOT Study showed that patients randomized to aspirin had a reduced rate of major cardiovascular events by 15% (p = 0.03) and of myocardial infarction by 36% (p = 0.002), with no change in stroke, in comparison with patients receiving placebo. There were 1,501 hypertensive patients with diabetes mellitus (8%) among the HOT Study cohort, and the effects of aspirin on several outcomes were separately analyzed in diabetics and non-diabetic hypertensives, as well as in other subgroups of patients [14].

Table 2 and 3 compare the effects of aspirin in diabetics and in non-diabetics in the HOT study. The relative risk for major cardiovascular events was 0.87 in diabetics and 0.85 in non-diabetics and that for myocardial infarction 0.61 and 0.65, respectively. Both effects of aspirin were statistically significant in non-diabetics, although they were not significant in diabetics due to the smaller size of the sample. Aspirin had no substantial

TABLE 2. Events in patients with diabetes mellitus at baseline in relation to acetylsalicylic acid (ASA) (n = 752) and placebo (n = 749) in the Hypertension Optimal Treatment (HOT) Study (unpublished data).

Events	No. of events	Events/1,000 patients years	p-value	Relative risk	95% Confidence interval
Major cardiovascular events[a]					
ASA	47	17.0			
Placebo	54	19.6	0.47	0.87	0.59–1.28
All myocardial infarction[a]					
ASA	11	3.9			
Placebo	18	6.4	0.20	0.61	0.29–1.29
All stroke					
ASA	20	7.2			
Placebo	22	7.9	0.77	0.91	0.50–1.67
Cardiovascular mortality					
ASA	23	8.2			
Placebo	26	9.2	0.70	0.89	0.51–1.57
Total mortality					
ASA	40	14.2			
Placebo	36	12.7	0.62	1.12	0.72–1.76

[a]Silent MI excluded.

TABLE 3. Events in patients with no diabetes mellitus at baseline in relation to acetylsalicylic acid (ASA) ($n = 8647$) and placebo ($n = 8642$) in the HOT Study (unpublished data).

Events	No. of events	Events/1,000 patients years	*p*-value	Relative risk	95% Confidence interval
Major cardiovascular events[a]					
ASA	268	8.3			
Placebo	314	9.7	0.047	0.85	0.72–1.00
All myocardial infarction[a]					
ASA	71	2.2			
Placebo	109	3.4	0.004	0.65	0.48–0.87
All stroke					
ASA	126	3.9			
Placebo	126	3.9	0.97	1.00	0.78–1.27
Cardiovascular mortality					
ASA	110	3.2			
Placebo	114	3.5	0.76	0.96	0.74–1.25
Total mortality					
ASA	244	7.4			
Placebo	269	8.2	0.25	0.90	0.76–1.07

[a]Silent MI excluded.

effects on stroke and mortality either in diabetics or in non-diabetics. Interaction tests failed to show significant difference in aspirin effects between diabetics and non-diabetics [14].

Primary Prevention Project

The PPP (Primary Prevention Project) study [15] was a randomized, controlled (no placebo), open trial investigating low-dose aspirin (100 mg daily) in 4,495 subjects (42.5% males) with one or more cardiovascular risk factors. Follow-up was 3.6 years. Aspirin was found to lower the frequency of all the end points, being statistically significant for cardiovascular death (relative risk 0.56), and total cardiovascular events (relative risk 0.77), with non-significant reduction in myocardial infarction (relative risk 0.69) and stroke (risk reduction 0.67). Seven hundred and forty-two diabetics (17%) were included in the study but no separate information on this subgroup is provided in the original publication.

Women's Health Study

This very large trial (Women's Health Study – WHS) [16] randomized 39,876 women aged 45 years or older with no history of cardiovascular disease (and at a low overall cardiovascular risk) to very low dose aspirin (100 mg every other day) or placebo. During the long follow-up of 10.1 years, aspirin was associated with a non-significant reduction in major cardiovascular events (relative risk 0.91), no change in myocardial infarction (relative risk 1.02), and a significant reduction in stroke (relative risk 0.83, $p = 0.04$). One thousand twenty-seven (2.6%) of the subjects had diabetes mellitus at baseline. In these subjects aspirin was associated with a relative risk of major cardiovascular events of 0.9 (NS), a relative risk of stroke of 0.46 ($p = 0.01$), and a relative risk of myocardial infarction of 1.48 (NS). In non-diabetic subjects, relative risks were 0.9, 0.87 and 0.96, respectively (all NS).

Overall Cardiovascular Effects of Aspirin in Diabetic Patients

Figure 3 summarizes the major findings from the four trials that reported data on diabetics, the PHS giving information on myocardial infarctions only. Data from all trials consistently indicate a small but never significant benefit of aspirin for all major cardiovascular events. ETDRS, PHS, and HOT all indicate a trend toward a greater

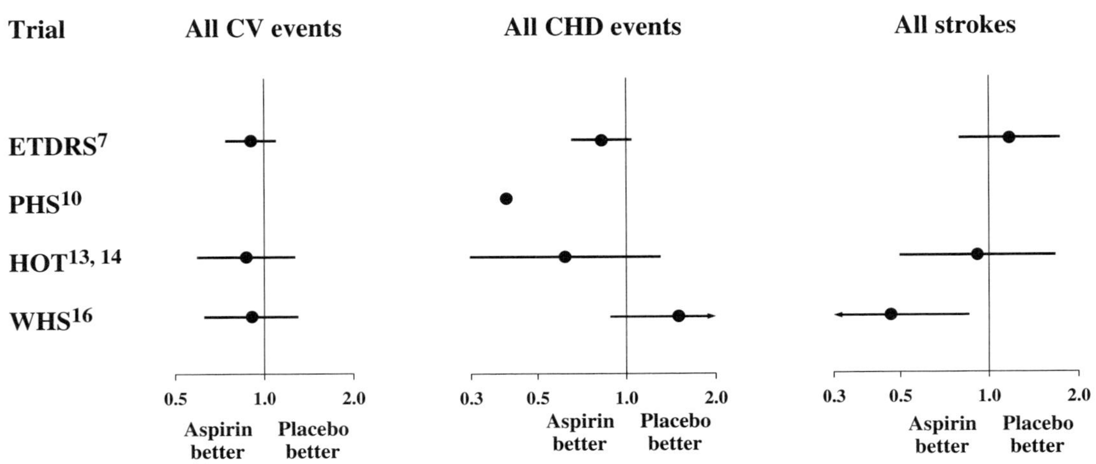

FIG. 3. Hazard ratios of aspirin versus placebo for all cardiovascular (CV) events, all coronary (CHD) events, and all strokes in diabetic patients included in four randomized trials. ETDRS: Early Treatment Diabetic Retinopathy Study; PHS: Physicians' Health Study; HOT: Hypertension Optimal Treatment Study; WHS: Women's Health Study. References are indicated by numbers accompanying the acronyms.

benefit for coronary events, whereas the WHS shows the reverse trend toward a benefit of placebo. As strokes are concerned, ETDRS and HOT show no significant benefit of either treatment, whereas WHS indicates a significant benefit of aspirin. In none of the three trials that investigated both diabetics and non-diabetics was there evidence that aspirin had different effects in the two groups of patients.

Effects of Antiplatelet Therapy on Intracranial and Major Extracranial Bleedings

The potential benefits of antiplatelet therapy in the prevention of cardiovascular events must be compared with the possible harmful effects on bleedings. Unfortunately, information on aspirin-associated bleedings in diabetics is scanty. The EDRS, the only trial entirely including diabetics, only uses hemoglobin less than 100 g/L or hematocrit less than 0.30 as signs of possible bleeding (2% in both groups) [7] and reports no excess of vitreous/preretinal hemorrhages ascribable to aspirin [17]. The PHS [10] and WHS [16] do not report bleedings separately for diabetics. In the overall PHS cohort, there was an increased risk of hemorrhagic stroke of borderline significance. The relative risk of major bleeding requiring transfusion was 1.71 ($p = 0.02$) and of minor bleeding episodes 1.32 [10] ($p < 0.00001$). In the WHS there was a non-significant increase in the risk of hemorrhagic stroke (relative risk 1.24, $p = 0.31$) and a 40% increase ($p = 0.02$) in gastrointestinal bleeding requiring transfusion [16].

HOT is the only trial having analyzed benefits and bleedings separately for diabetics and non-diabetics. Findings are reported in Table 4. The benefit (aspirin vs. placebo) both in terms of major cardiovascular events and of myocardial infarction was greater in diabetics than in non-diabetics, but major bleedings were possibly less among diabetics. The net result (benefit vs. harm) was of 2.5 events spared in diabetics, whereas benefit and harm almost exactly balanced in non-diabetics. A better quantitative evaluation of the benefits and harms of aspirin administration was obtained by calculating the Number Needed to Treat corrected for Unqualified Success (NNT_{us}, the number of patients who need to be treated with aspirin in order to prevent a cardiovascular event without a treatment-induced bleed) and the Number Needed to Treat corrected for Unmitigated Failure (NNT_{uf}, the number of patients who need to be treated in order to have a treatment-induced bleed in a patient in whom ASA has failed to provide protection from a cardiovascular event) [18]. The NNT_{us} was definitely smaller in diabetics

TABLE 4. Benefits and harms of aspirin versus placebo administration in diabetic patients in the HOT Study.

	Diabetics (n = 1,501)	Non-diabetics (n = 17,230)
Major CV events (per 1,000 patients years)	−2.6	−1.4
All myocardial infarction (per 1,000 patients years)	−2.5	−1.2
All major bleedings (per 1,000 patients years)	0	+1.5
NNT_{us} (for 3.8 years)	101	188
NNT_{uf} (for 3.8 years)	–	21,222

CV, cardiovascular; NNT_{us}, number needed to treat for unqualified success; NNT_{uf}, number needed to treat for unmitigated failure.
Data from refs 13 and 14 and unpublished data.

than non-diabetics, while harm, as assessed by NNT_{uf}, was mild in non-diabetics and even milder (in reality unassessable) in diabetics.

Conclusions and Summary

Despite the fact that antiplatelet therapy is widely recommended in patients at high cardiovascular risk, and evidence of benefits greater than harms is overwhelming for subjects who have already suffered a cardiovascular event [5], evidence concerning diabetes is more scanty than desirable, and good information on the balance between benefit (reduction in cardiovascular events, mostly myocardial infarction) and harm (mostly gastrointestinal bleedings but, more rarely, hemorrhagic stroke) is limited to data from the HOT Study. Thus, it is to be recommended that further specific trials in diabetic patients, especially those without a history of a cardiovascular accident, be undertaken to clarify a still confused issue.

Until more data are available, diabetic patients with a previous cardiovascular event should be prescribed antiplatelet therapy, mostly by a small dose of aspirin, unless they are known to be prone to gastrointestinal bleeding (or other types of bleeding). Diabetic patients without a history of cardiovascular events should be carefully evaluated for the risk of gastrointestinal bleeding, and their overall cardiovascular risk calculated. Those diabetic subjects whose cardiovascular risk is higher and bleeding risk low are reasonable candidates to antiplatelet therapy, after their blood pressure is normalized (to reduce the risk of cerebral hemorrhage). Available evidence is insufficient and should be widened, but for the time being diabetic patients should not be considered as indiscriminate candidates to antiplatelet therapy, as suggested by proposers of multiple administration (including aspirin) to subjects at any increased cardiovascular risk.

References

1. Stamler J, Vaccaro O, Neaton JD, et al. Diabetes, other risk factors, and 12-year cardiovascular mortality for men screened in the Multiple Risk Factor Intervention Trial. Diabetes Care 1993;16:434–444.
2. Zanchetti A, Hansson L, Dahlöf B, et al. Effects of individual risk factors on the incidence of cardiovascular events in the treated hypertensive patients of the Hypertension Optimal Treatment Study. J Hypertens 2001;19:1149–59.
3. Blood Pressure Lowering Treatment Trialists' Collaboration. Effects of different blood-pressure lowering regimens on major cardiovascular events in individuals with and without diabetes mellitus. Arch Intern Med 2005;165:1410–1419.
4. Expert Panel on Detection, Evaluation, and Treatment of High Blood Cholesterol in Adults (Adult Treatment Panel III). Executive Summary of the Third Report of the National Cholesterol Education Program (NCEP). JAMA 2001;285:2486–2497.
5. Antithrombotic Trialists' Collaboration. Collaborative meta-analysis of randomised trials of antiplatelet therapy for prevention of death, myocardial infarction, and stroke in high risk patients. BMJ 2002;324:71–86.
6. Antiplatelet Trialists' Collaboration. Collaborative overview of randomised trials of antiplatelet therapy I: Prevention of death, myocardial infarction, and stroke by prolonged antiplatelet therapy in various categories of patients. BMJ 1994;308:81–106.
7. Early Treatment Diabetic Retinopathy Study Report 14. Aspirin effects on mortality and morbidity in patients with diabetes mellitus. JAMA 1992;268:1292–1300.
8. Early Treatment Diabetic Retinopathy Study (ETDRS) Research Group: Effects of aspirin treatment on

diabetic retinopathy: ETDRS report number 8. Ophthalmology.1991;98(Suppl.):757–765.
9. Peto R. Gray R, Collins R, et al. Randomised trial of prophylactic daily aspirin in British male doctors. BMJ 1988;296:313–316.
10. Steering Committee of the Physicians' Health Study Research Group. Final Report on the aspirin component of the ongoing Physicians' Health Study. N Engl J Med. 1989;321:129–135.
11. The Medical Research Council's General Practice Research Framework. Thrombosis Prevention Trial: randomised trial of low-intensity oral anticoagulant with warfarin and low-dose aspirin in the primary prevention of ischaemic heart disease in men at increased risk. Lancet 1998;351:233–241.
12. Meade TW, Brennan PJ on behalf of the MRC General Practice Research Framework. Determination of who may derive most benefit from aspirin in primary prevention: subgroup results from a randomised controlled trial. BMJ 2000;321:13–17.
13. Hansson L, Zanchetti A, Carruthers SG et al for the HOT Study Group. Effects of intensive blood pressure lowering and low-dose aspirin in patients with hypertension: principal results of the Hypertension Optimal Treatment (HOT) randomised trial. Lancet 1998;351:1755–1762.
14. Zanchetti A, Hansson L, Dahlöf B, et al. Benefit and harm of low-dose aspirin in well-treated hypertensives at different baseline cardiovascular risk. J Hypertens 2002;20:2301–2307.
15. Collaborative Group of the Primary Prevention Project (PPP). Low-dose aspirin and vitamin E in people at cardiovascular risk: a randomised trial in general practice. Lancet 2001;357:89–95.
16. Ridker PJ, Cook NR, Lee IM. et al. A randomized trial of low-dose aspirin in the primary prevention of cardiovascular disease in women. N Eng J Med 2005;352:1293–1304.
17. Chew EY, Klein ML, Murphy RP, et al.Early Treatment Diabetic Retinopathy Study Research Group. Effects of aspirin on vitreous/preretinal hemorrhage in patients with diabetes mellitus. Arch Ophthalmol 1995;113:52–55.
18. Schulzer M, Mancini GBJ. "Unqualified success" and "unmitigated failure": number-needed-to-treat-related concepts for assessing treatment efficacy in the presence of treatment-induced adverse effects. Int J Epidemiol 1996;25:704–712.

20
Glycosylation Inhibitors, PKC Inhibitors and Related Interventions Against Complications

Aino Soro-Paavonen and Mark Cooper

Keywords: Hyperglycaemia, advanced glycation end-product, protein kinase C, diabetic complications, receptor for advanced glycation end-product.

Introduction

Chronic hyperglycaemia predisposes the diabetic patient to a markedly increased risk of end-organ complications in the eyes, kidneys, peripheral nerves and the vasculature. The most effective way to reduce the risk of diabetic complications is intensive insulin treatment leading to optimal glycaemic control [1,2]. However, excellent control of hyperglycaemia is achieved in less than 25% of type 1 diabetic patients [3]. Glucose-mediated vascular damage has been reported to occur via four major mechanisms including activation of the intracellular signal transductor, protein kinase C (PKC), increased polyol pathway accumulation, enhanced hexosamine pathway flux and increased formation of advanced glycation end-products (AGEs) [4]. All these processes are activated by mitochondrial superoxide production [4].

The Role of Advanced Glycation in the Development of Diabetic Complications

Glucose, acting as the initial substrate, generates early glycation products, termed Schiff bases, which then form more stable Amadori products. These Amadori products over months to years undergo further arrangements to yield AGEs. However, a more rapid method of AGE formation occurs via glycolytic intermediates such as 3-deoxyglucosone (3-DG) and methylglyoxal (MGO), also known as α-dicarbonyls or oxoaldehydes [5]. The AGEs become cross-linked and involve links between lysine and arginine residues of the target amino acids. A range of AGEs are from these pathways including hydroimidazolones, *N*-ε-(carboxyethyl)lysine, a homologue of carboxymethyl lysine (CML), and methylglyoxal lysine dimer (MOLD). The AGE-related cross-links are resistant to enzymatic degradation and are therefore very stable [5]. The rate of AGE formation is dependent on the sugar concentration, extent of oxidative stress and time of exposure [6].

Evidence from associational clinical studies and from animal experiments with exogenous AGE infusions support the concept that AGEs are directly involved in the development of diabetic complications [7–9]. AGEs mediate their effects both directly and via receptor-dependent mechanisms. AGEs change the structural integrity of proteins, disturbing their cellular function, thus having severe consequences on the affected organs [10]. AGEs accumulate on proteins including collagen, fibronectin, tubulin, haemoglobin, albumin and apolipoproteins [4,5]. AGEs affect the structural integrity of extracellular matrix (ECM) components causing the cross-linking of matrix molecules and the disruption of matrix–matrix and matrix–cell interactions. The AGE-related collagen cross-links decrease tissue elasticity causing diminished arterial and myocardial compliance and increased vascular stiffness [11]. In addition, AGEs quench nitric oxide (NO) and generate reactive oxygen species (ROS) by stimulating NAPDH oxidase activity [12,13]. The receptor-dependent effects of AGEs occur via binding to proteins including the receptor for AGEs (RAGE), AGE-R1 (p60), AGE-R2 (p90), AGE-R3 (galectin-3), macrophage scavenger receptor ScR-11 and CD-36 [14]. AGE-R1 and AGE-R3 are potentially involved in the clearance of AGEs, whereas binding to RAGE augments inflammation [14,15]. RAGE, a signal transduction receptor belonging to the immunoglobulin superfamily, is expressed on endothelial cells, monocyte/macrophages, platelets and renal mesangial cells and podocytes [15]. The AGE–RAGE interaction activates NADPH oxidase and triggers secondary messenger pathways such as the mitogen-activated protein kinases (MAPKs), p21^{ras}, extracellular signal-regulated kinase (ERKs) p38 and PKC, causing activation and translocation of nuclear transcription factor-κB (NF-κB) [16]. NF-κB upregulates the production of growth factors and cytokines, including transforming growth factor-β1 (TGF-β1), connective tissue growth factor (CTGF), platelet-derived growth factor (PDGF), tumor necrosis factor-α (TNF-α), interleukin-1 (IL-1) and IL-6 [17–20]. This signalling ultimately leads to inflammation and tissue damage. Typically, AGE accumulation and enhanced expression of AGE receptors can be observed at sites of complications such as the kidney, retina and the vasculature [21].

A variety of pharmacological interventions have been targeted to reduce advanced glycation and thereby AGE accumulation, via either attenuation of total AGE load or via chemical modification of existing AGEs to inactive forms. Aminoguanidine [22], pyridoxamine [9,23], benfotiamine [24], OPB-9195, ALT-946 and metformin reduce AGE accumulation by inhibiting AGE formation, whereas ALT-711, also known as alagebrium chloride, and its prototype, *N*-phenacylthiazolium bromide (PTB), act as AGE cross-link breakers [25,26]. AGE-reducing interventions have been proven to protect against the development of diabetic complications in experimental models with some compounds now proceeding to clinical development. The schematic presentations of the glycation process and target sites of different anti-AGE agents are presented in Fig. 1. The findings on individual compounds are discussed here.

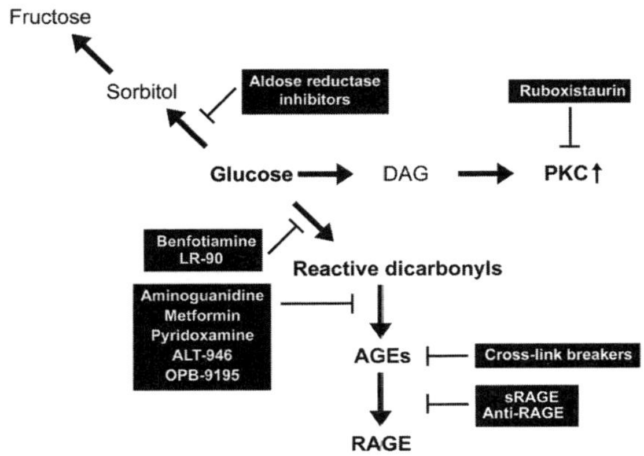

FIG. 1. Pathways of the glycosylation process during intracellular hyperglycaemia and target sites of AGE inhibitors, aldose reductase inhibitors, PKC inhibitors and RAGE-blocking agents. AGE, advanced glycation end-product; DAG, diacylglycerol; PKC, protein kinase C; RAGE, receptor for advanced glycation end-product.

Inhibition of Age Formation

Aminoguanidine

The initial inhibitor studied that reduces the formation of AGEs is aminoguanidine sulphate (AG), a nucleophilic hydrazine compound. AG reacts with Amadori-derived fragmentation products and scavenges the reactive dicarbonyl AGE precursors like MGO, malondialdehyde (MDA) and 4-hydroxy-2-nonenal (HNE) [27]. Nevertheless, one potential mechanism of AG action is postulated to be normalization of PKC activity [28]. Rosca et al. [29] recently demonstrated that aminoguanidine improves mitochondrial respiration and complex III activity and decreases oxidative damage to mitochondrial proteins. AG treatment inhibits renal AGE accumulation and decreases albuminuria in experimental diabetes [30–32]. Some studies have also shown this treatment to be beneficial against diabetic retinopathy [33] and peripheral nerve dysfunction [34] in diabetic rats, whereas others have remained negative [35], or the effects have been modest compared with those seen with insulin treatment [36]. AG, also known as pimagedine, was used in the "A Clinical Trial in Overt Nephropathy of Type 1 diabetes" (ACTION) trial, the first placebo-controlled, double-blind clinical study on renoprotective effects of AG [37]. Proteinuria and progression of the retinal damage were significantly reduced by pimagedine, but the primary end-point, delay of time to doubling of the serum creatinine levels, was not achieved. Despite preventing AGE formation, AG also inhibits nitric oxide synthase (NOS) [38], causes neurotoxicity due to the trapping of pyridoxal, produces hydrogen peroxide and even causes DNA damage via hydroxyl radical and hydrogen peroxide [39]. In the ACTION trial, 3 patients out of 225 receiving AG developed glomerulonephritis with increased levels of myeloperoxidase (MPO) and antineutrophil (ANCA) antibodies [37]. Due to its toxic effects and failure to achieve the primary end-point in the ACTION study, it is unlikely that AG will proceed to be used in the treatment or prevention of diabetic end-organ complications in the near future.

Other Inhibitors of AGE Formation

Metformin (dimethylbiguanide) is a widely used oral anti-hyperglycaemic drug in the management of type 2 diabetes [2]. Interestingly, it has structural similarities with AG, and it binds to the α-dicarbonyls, MGO and 3-DG [40]. Recent studies on the pharmacological effects of metformin have shown that it inhibits PKC-β2 activity [41] and protects pancreatic islet cells from apoptosis via a reduction in oxidative stress [42]. The novel thiazolidine derivative, OPB-9195, inhibits AGEs potentially via trapping the reactive dicarbonyl groups, key intermediates in AGE formation [43]. In diabetic rats, OPB-9195 has been shown to decrease circulating AGE levels, attenuate urinary albumin excretion and decrease kidney CML deposition. It also suppresses the renal expression of various growth factors including TGF-β1 and vascular endothelial growth factor (VEGF) as well as type I and type IV collagen [43]. ALT-946 inhibits AGE formation with minimal effects on NO synthesis [44]. This agent also appears to have less toxic effects than AG, although it has not been studied in as much detail. ALT-946 reduces kidney AGE accumulation and albuminuria in diabetic Sprague–Dawley rats [44] and in hypertensive, diabetic transgenic (mRen-2)27 rats [45]. A new AGE inhibitor, LR-90, reduces in vivo AGE accumulation, AGE–protein cross-linking and protein oxidation [46]. In diabetic rats, it had beneficial effects against structural kidney abnormalities such as glomerulosclerosis, tubular degeneration and collagen deposition [46]. The authors proposed that LR-90 inhibits the autooxidation pathways during the formation of reactive carbonyl sugars. No clinical studies have been conducted or are currently in progress with the novel AGE inhibitors discussed here.

Pyridoxamine

Pyridoxamine, a vitamin B6 derivative, inhibits the formation of AGEs (CML and CEL) as well as the formation of advanced lipoxidation end-products (ALEs) [47]. It scavenges reactive carbonyl intermediates in AGE/ALE formation and inhibits the formation of AGEs from Amadori compounds [48]. In vitro, pyridoxamine protects renal glomerular cells, including podocytes and mesangial cells, against MGO-induced changes in cell adhesion [49]. In diabetic rats, pyridoxamine treatment had potent antioxidant effects and decreased albuminuria, plasma creatinine and hyperlipidaemia without changing plasma glucose levels [23,50]. Interestingly, in rats with an enhanced renin–angiotensin system (RAS) activation as a result of angiotensin II infusion, pyridoxamine decreased serum AGE levels and renal AGE/ALE deposition [9]. It also prevented renal hypertrophy and decreased salt retention [9]. Pyridoxamine has also been shown to attenuate retinal ECM gene expression and limit laminin protein upregulation in diabetic rats [51]. In a rodent model of type II diabetic nephropathy, the db/db mouse, pyridoxamine treatment decreased the progression of albuminuria and glomerular lesions, and when combined to the ACE inhibitor enalapril, pyridoxamine reduced both mortality and the progression of diabetic nephropathy [52]. The safety and tolerability of the commercial vitamin B6 form, pyridoxine hydrochloride (Pyridorin), is currently being studied in Phase 2 clinical trials. These studies will evaluate the use of pyridoxamine in preventing the progression of diabetic nephropathy. As yet, no published data on these studies are available.

Benfotiamine

Benfotiamine, a lipid-soluble thiamine (vitamin B1) derivative, prevents the increase in the intracellular hexosamine pathway and polyol pathway activation during hyperglycaemia [53]. It decreases hyperglycaemia-induced intracellular AGE formation and reduces PKC activity [24]. Thiamine therapy has been shown to prevent vascular accumulation of AGEs [54], development of microalbuminuria and proteinuria [55] and to prevent the progression of retinopathy [24] in diabetic rodents. Winkler et al. [56] showed that benfotiamine has a benefit in patients with diabetic neuropathy. The BEDIB study, Benfotiamine in the treatment of diabetic polyneuropathy, confirmed these earlier results [57]. Benfotiamine has also been shown to improve nerve conduction velocity in patients with diabetic polyneuropathy [58]. Interestingly, benfotiamine improved endothelial function in type II diabetic patients when tested in a postprandial state after an AGE-rich meal [59]. Currently ongoing Phase II clinical trials will reveal whether benfotiamine influences the progression of microvascular complications in diabetic patients.

AGE Cross-Link Breakers

Thiazolium compounds such as PTB and its derivative alagebrium chloride (ALT-711; 3-phenyacyl-4,5-dimethylthiazolium chloride) cleave covalent AGE-derived protein cross-links [25,60]. The removal of established AGE cross-links in diabetic rats with ALT-711 has been shown to reverse the diabetes-induced increase in large artery stiffness [61], to increase collagen solubility, reduce vascular [25] and cardiac AGE accumulation [62] and to prevent the diabetes-associated increases in the AGE receptors, RAGE and AGE-R3 [26]. ALT-711 treatment prevents the progression of diabetic nephropathy in diabetic rats, reducing arterial pressure, renal hypertrophy and albuminuria [26]. In addition, ALT-711 attenuates renal accumulation of AGEs, fibronectin and laminin, and reduces the expression of VEGF, possibly via decreasing PKC-α activation [63]. Forbes et al. [64] have also shown a significant reduction in diabetes-accelerated atherosclerosis with ALT-711 treatment in diabetic apolipoprotein E knockout mice. Subsequent studies in rodents with experimental diabetes have confirmed the beneficial effects of ALT-711 therapy on cardiovascular and renal functions [65,66]. In a clinical setting, ALT-711 has been shown to reduce pulse pressure and to improve vascular compliance in patients with systolic hypertension [67]. Subsequently, safety and efficacy of the ALT-711 treatment has been tested in patients with diastolic heart failure and cardiovascular disease (data source: www.clinicaltrials.gov), although these studies have not been published. At present, no clinical data are available on the effects of ALT-711 in the prevention of diabetic micro- or macrovascular complications. Ongoing Phase 2 clinical studies are examining whether ALT-711 treatment improves cardiac compliance and diastolic function in aged individuals (data source: www.alteon.com).

Blockade of the AGE–RAGE Interaction

The RAGE is an immunoglobulin superfamily receptor that binds to a diverse set of ligands including AGEs, S100/calgranulins, amphoterin (high mobility group box-1, HMGB1) and amyloid-β peptide [68]. Activation of RAGE on critical target cells such as endothelial cells, mononuclear phagocytes, lymphocytes, vascular smooth muscle cells and neurons [69] triggers the intracellular messenger NF-κB, leading to an inflammatory response and tissue damage [70,71]. RAGE has a secretory splice isoform, soluble RAGE (sRAGE), which lacks the transmembrane domain and neutralizes circulating ligands, thus functioning as a decoy receptor. In fact, blockade of AGE–RAGE binding by sRAGE inhibited the progression of atherosclerotic changes and nephropathy in diabetic mice [72,73]. Furthermore, treatment with either sRAGE or a neutralizing antibody to RAGE decreased arterial neointimal expansion in both hyperglycaemic and euglycaemic animals [74]. Treatment with sRAGE and anti-RAGE antibodies suppressed NF-κB activation and inflammatory cytokine expression [70]. Importantly, mice with a deletion of *RAGE* have less diabetes-associated albuminuria and glomerulosclerosis [73,74]. Promising results with RAGE antagonism in animal models have encouraged the development RAGE-neutralizing compounds for clinical use. Cross-sectional studies have found both decreased [75] and increased [76] plasma levels of sRAGE in diabetic patients. Low sRAGE levels have also been associated with increased cardiovascular risk [75,77]. The RAGE-modulating agent, TTP488, is currently being studied in Phase 2 clinical trials in patients with Alzheimer's disease and in patients with diabetic nephropathy. Another compound, TTP4000, is soon to commence Phase

1 clinical trials (data source: http://www.clinicaltrials.gov and http://www.ttpharma.com).

Aldose Reductase Inhibitors

During hyperglycaemia, aldose reductase is the reducing enzyme in the reaction in which glucose is reduced to sorbitol [78]. This is the first and rate-limiting step of the polyol pathway, giving rise to intracellular sorbitol accumulation, osmotic stress and oxidative stress. Chemicals that inhibit aldose reductase have proved effective in the prevention of tissue injury in diabetic animals [79]. The aldose reductase inhibitor, sorbinil, was among the first compounds to be studied in clinical setting, but was found to be problematic due to hypersensitivity reactions and lack of effectiveness in the prevention of diabetic retinopathy or neuropathy [80]. The novel aldose reductase inhibitor, epalrestat, has been shown to decrease intracellular CML and 3-DG levels in diabetic patients [81]. Furthermore, fidarestat, epalrestat and ranirestat [82] have been tested in patients with diabetic neuropathy, with improvement in nerve function. Ranirestat is currently being studied in a Phase 3 clinical trial in patients with diabetic sensorimotor polyneuropathy.

Inhibition of the Protein Kinase C Activation

PKC enzymes phosphorylate serine or threonine residues on intracellular proteins and operate as signal transduction systems for many cytokines and hormones [83]. Mammalian cells express up to 12 different PKC isoforms, of which the conventional isoforms, PKC-α, ß1, ß2 and γ have binding domains for both diacylglycerol (DAG) and phorbol esters as well as for Ca^{2+}. Persistent hyperglycaemia in diabetes increases the formation of DAG from glycolytic intermediates, which then activate PKC [84]. Hyperglycaemia also causes indirect PKC activation through increasing AGE-induced oxidative stress [63], and through increasing polyol and hexosamine pathway flux [85,86]. PKC is expressed in a wide range of tissues, each isoform being transcribed by a separate gene and therefore having their own specific regulation. Studies in diabetic rats have shown that the endothelial and smooth muscle cells express the isoforms α, ß1, ß2 and δ [87], whereas the isoforms PKC-α, ß1, ß2 and ε are expressed in the retina [88], and the isoforms PKC-α and ß1 in renal glomeruli [63,84]. A number of studies in rodent models and in diabetic patients have demonstrated chronic PKC activation in diabetic vascular tissues. Rask-Madsen and King [83] have recently reviewed the mechanisms by which PKC promotes the development of vascular complications in diabetes. PKC stimulates ROS production via activation of NADPH oxidase in vascular tissues [89] and mesangial cells [90]. PKC activation has also been shown to impair endothelium-dependent vasodilatation [91] and to inhibit NO production in endothelial cells via phosphorylation of the endothelial nitric oxide synthase (eNOS) [92].

The key abnormalities observed in the diabetic kidney include thickening of capillary basement membranes and matrix expansion. PKC-α and PKC-ß1/2 signalling have been shown to trigger VEGF, leading to enhanced endothelial cell permeability and increased mesangial cell matrix synthesis [63,93]. PKC activation causes upregulation in the expression of collagen IV and accumulation of fibronectin and laminin in the kidney [63,90]. Increased PKCβ activation has also been shown to upregulate VEGF in the retina, causing increased vascular permeability and neovascularization [94]. Conversely, PKC activation has been associated with retinal vasoconstriction, possibly via impaired NO availability or increased ET-1 expression [95]. In addition, PKC-mediated increased vascular resistance in the microcirculation contributes to the development of diabetic neuropathy [96].

Ruboxistaurin

Inhibition of the DAG–PKC pathway has been widely studied in rodent models as a therapeutic tool against diabetic complications with some evidence also existing in the clinical context. As general inhibition of PKC, without isoform specificity, would impair normal organ physiology and vital functions, a highly selective inhibitor for the PKC-β1/2 isoforms, ruboxistaurin mesylate (LY333531), has been developed. Ruboxistaurin acts as a catalytic domain inhibitor, targeting the ATP-binding site in the PKC protein structure. Ishii et al. [93] first showed that administration of ruboxistaurin to diabetic rats inhibited PKC-β activity and retarded the development of vascular complications in the kidney and eyes in a dose-dependent manner. Later intervention studies in animals have confirmed that ruboxistaurin attenuates manifestations of diabetic retinopathy [97], nephropathy [84] and neuropathy [98] with no observed toxic effects. The first multicenter randomized clinical trial with ruboxistaurin, the Protein Kinase C beta Inhibitor Diabetic Retinopathy Study (PKC-DRS), reported prevention of moderate visual loss in patients with type 1 or 2 diabetes with ruboxistaurin therapy [99], but no clear effect was observed against progression of diabetic retinopathy. Nevertheless, subsequent studies have shown that ruboxistaurin reduces retinal leakage in patients with diabetic macular edema [100] and normalizes the retinal circulation [101]. Recently, Aiello et al. [102] showed that ruboxistaurin reduces vision loss in patients with nonproliferative diabetic retinopathy. Some data also exist on the attenuation of the progression of diabetic neuropathy and nephropathy [103,104] and on the improvement of endothelial function by ruboxistaurin [105]. Up to now, 11 placebo-controlled, double-masked clinical intervention studies with orally administered ruboxistaurin have been completed [106]. Ruboxistaurin appears to be well tolerated and does not cause significant adverse events. Currently ongoing clinical trials will evaluate whether ruboxistaurin provides further improvement for macular edema, renal function and peripheral haemodynamic function in patients with type 1 diabetes (http://www.clinicaltrials.gov). Unfortunately, at this stage, the clinical data do not appear to be adequate for the Food and Drug Administration (FDA) to approve registration of the drug and another 3-year Phase 3 clinical trial has been requested (data source: http://www.lifesciencesworld.com/news).

Conclusions

The data from experimental and clinical settings imply that inhibitors of advanced glycation could emerge as a potential new way to prevent diabetic complications. However, the novel therapeutic tools will always need to be administered as add-on therapies, together with intensive glucose monitoring and effective treatment of hypertension. Interestingly, a well-established hypoglycaemic agent metformin has proven to also act as an AGE inhibitor. Most likely, the novel inhibitors of AGEs and PKC will have widespread effects, many of which are not yet fully determined. At present, no data are available on the effects of RAGE blockade in diabetic patients, but clinical trials are currently under way and awaited with great anticipation.

References

1. The Diabetes Control and Complications Trial Research Group. The effect of intensive treatment of diabetes on the development and progression of long-term complications in insulin-dependent diabetes mellitus. N Engl J Med 1993;329:977–86.
2. UK Prospective Diabetes Study (UKPDS) Group. Intensive blood-glucose control with sulphonylureas or insulin compared with conventional treatment and risk of complications in patients with type 2 diabetes (UKPDS 33). Lancet 1998;352:837–853.
3. Fagerudd J, Forsblom C, Pettersson-Fernholm K, Groop PH. Implementation of guidelines for the prevention of diabetic nephropathy. Diabetes Care 2004;27:803–804.
4. Brownlee M. Biochemistry and molecular cell biology of diabetic complications. Nature 2001; 414:813–820.
5. Thornalley PJ, Langborg A, Minhas HS. Formation of glyoxal, methylglyoxal and 3-deoxyglucosone in the glycation of proteins by glucose. Biochem J 1999;344:109–116.
6. Fu MX, Wells-Knecht KJ, Blackledge JA, Lyons TJ, Thorpe SR, Baynes JW. Glycation, glycoxidation, and cross-linking of collagen by glucose. Kinetics, mechanisms, and inhibition of late stages of the Maillard reaction. Diabetes 1994; 43:676–683.
7. Monnier VM, Bautista O, Kenny D, et al. Skin collagen glycation, glycoxidation, and crosslinking are lower in subjects with long-term intensive versus conventional therapy of type 1 diabetes: relevance of glycated collagen products versus HbA1c as markers of diabetic complications. DCCT Skin Collagen Ancillary Study Group. Diabetes Control and Complications Trial. Diabetes 1999;48:870–880.
8. Vlassara H, Fuh H, Makita Z, Krungkrai S, Cerami A, Bucala R. Exogenous advanced glycosylation end products induce complex vascular dysfunction in normal animals: A model for diabetic and aging complications. Proc Natl Acad Sci U S A 1992; 89:12043–12047.
9. Thomas MC, Tikellis C, Burns WM, et al. Interactions between renin angiotensin system and advanced glycation in the kidney. J Am Soc Nephrol 2005;17:17.

10. Brownlee M. Advanced protein glycosylation in diabetes and aging. Annu Rev Med 1995;46:223–234.
11. Aronson D. Cross-linking of glycated collagen in the pathogenesis of arterial and myocardial stiffening of aging and diabetes. J Hypertens 2003;21:3–12.
12. Hogan M, Cerami A, Bucala R. Advanced glycosylation endproducts block the antiproliferative effect of nitric oxide. Role in the vascular and renal complications of diabetes mellitus. J Clin Invest 1992; 90:1110–1115.
13. Nishikawa T, Edelstein D, Du XL, et al. Normalizing mitochondrial superoxide production blocks three pathways of hyperglycaemic damage. Nature 2000;404:787–790.
14. Vlassara H. The AGE-receptor in the pathogenesis of diabetic complications. Diabetes Metab Res Rev 2001;17:436–443.
15. Kislinger T, Tanji N, Wendt T, et al. Receptor for advanced glycation end products mediates inflammation and enhanced expression of tissue factor in vasculature of diabetic apolipoprotein E-null mice. Arterioscler Thromb Vasc Biol 2001;21:905–910.
16. Goldin A, Beckman JA, Schmidt AM, Creager MA. Advanced glycation end products: sparking the development of diabetic vascular injury. Circulation 2006;114:597–605.
17. Miyata T, Inagi R, Iida Y, et al. Involvement of beta 2-microglobulin modified with advanced glycation end products in the pathogenesis of hemodialysis-associated amyloidosis. Induction of human monocyte chemotaxis and macrophage secretion of tumor necrosis factor-alpha and interleukin-1. J Clin Invest 1994;93:521–528.
18. Rumble JR, Cooper ME, Soulis T, et al. Vascular hypertrophy in experimental diabetes. Role of advanced glycation end products. J Clin Invest 1997;99:1016–1027.
19. Kelly DJ, Gilbert RE, Cox AJ, Soulis T, Jerums G, Cooper ME. Aminoguanidine ameliorates overexpression of prosclerotic growth factors and collagen deposition in experimental diabetic nephropathy. J Am Soc Nephrol 2001;12:2098–2107.
20. Twigg SM, Chen MM, Joly AH, et al. Advanced glycosylation end products up-regulate connective tissue growth factor (insulin-like growth factor-binding protein-related protein 2) in human fibroblasts: a potential mechanism for expansion of extracellular matrix in diabetes mellitus. Endocrinology 2001;142:1760–1769.
21. Soulis T, Thallas V, Youssef S, et al. Advanced glycation end products and their receptors co-localise in rat organs susceptible to diabetic microvascular injury. Diabetologia 1997;40:619–628.
22. Soulis T, Cooper ME, Sastra S, et al. Relative contributions of advanced glycation and nitric oxide synthase inhibition to aminoguanidine-mediated renoprotection in diabetic rats. Diabetologia 1997; 40:1141–1151.
23. Degenhardt TP, Alderson NL, Arrington DD, et al. Pyridoxamine inhibits early renal disease and dyslipidemia in the streptozotocin-diabetic rat. Kidney Int 2002;61:939–950.
24. Hammes HP, Du X, Edelstein D, et al. Benfotiamine blocks three major pathways of hyperglycemic damage and prevents experimental diabetic retinopathy. Nat Med 2003;9:294–299.
25. Cooper ME, Thallas V, Forbes J, et al. The cross-link breaker, N-phenacylthiazolium bromide prevents vascular advanced glycation end-product accumulation. Diabetologia 2000;43:660–664.
26. Forbes JM, Thallas V, Thomas MC, et al. The breakdown of preexisting advanced glycation end products is associated with reduced renal fibrosis in experimental diabetes. Faseb J 2003;17:1762–1764.
27. Edelstein D, Brownlee M. Mechanistic studies of advanced glycosylation end product inhibition by aminoguanidine. Diabetes 1992;41:26–29.
28. Osicka TM, Yu Y, Panagiotopoulos S, et al. Prevention of albuminuria by aminoguanidine or ramipril in streptozotocin-induced diabetic rats is associated with the normalization of glomerular protein kinase C. Diabetes 2000;49:87–93.
29. Rosca MG, Mustata TG, Kinter MT, et al. Glycation of mitochondrial proteins from diabetic rat kidney is associated with excess superoxide formation. Am J Physiol Renal Physiol 2005; 289:F420–F430.
30. Soulis-Liparota T, Cooper M, Papazoglou D, Clarke B, Jerums G. Retardation by aminoguanidine of development of albuminuria, mesangial expansion, and tissue fluorescence in streptozocin-induced diabetic rat. Diabetes 1991;40:1328–1334.
31. Edelstein D, Brownlee M. Aminoguanidine ameliorates albuminuria in diabetic hypertensive rats. Diabetologia 1992;35:96–97.
32. Lassila M, Seah KK, Allen TJ, et al. Accelerated nephropathy in diabetic apolipoprotein e-knockout mouse: role of advanced glycation end products. J Am Soc Nephrol 2004;15:2125–2138.
33. Kern TS, Tang J, Mizutani M, et al. Response of capillary cell death to aminoguanidine predicts the development of retinopathy: comparison of diabetes and galactosemia. Invest Ophthalmol Vis Sci 2000; 41:3972–3978.
34. Cameron NE, Cotter MA, Dines K, Love A. Effects of aminoguanidine on peripheral nerve function and polyol pathway metabolites in streptozotocin-diabetic rats. Diabetologia 1992;35:946–950.
35. Birrell AM, Heffernan SJ, Ansselin AD, et al. Functional and structural abnormalities in the nerves of type I diabetic baboons: aminoguanidine

treatment does not improve nerve function. Diabetologia 2000;43:110–116.
36. Wada R, Sugo M, Nakano M, Yagihashi S. Only limited effects of aminoguanidine treatment on peripheral nerve function, (Na+,K+)-ATPase activity and thrombomodulin expression in streptozotocin-induced diabetic rats. Diabetologia 1999;42:743–747.
37. Bolton WK, Cattran DC, Williams ME, et al. Randomized trial of an inhibitor of formation of advanced glycation end products in diabetic nephropathy. Am J Nephrol 2004;24:32–40.
38. Tilton RG, Chang K, Hasan KS, et al. Prevention of diabetic vascular dysfunction by guanidines. Inhibition of nitric oxide synthase versus advanced glycation end-product formation. Diabetes 1993; 42:221–232.
39. Suji G, Sivakami S. DNA damage by free radical production by aminoguanidine. Ann N Y Acad Sci 2006;1067:191–199.
40. Beisswenger P, Ruggiero-Lopez D. Metformin inhibition of glycation processes. Diabetes Metab 2003; 29:6S95–6S103.
41. Gallo A, Ceolotto G, Pinton P, et al. Metformin prevents glucose-induced protein kinase C-beta2 activation in human umbilical vein endothelial cells through an antioxidant mechanism. Diabetes 2005; 54:1123–1131.
42. Marchetti P, Del Guerra S, Marselli L, et al. Pancreatic islets from type 2 diabetic patients have functional defects and increased apoptosis that are ameliorated by metformin. J Clin Endocrinol Metab 2004;89:5535–5541.
43. Tsuchida K, Makita Z, Yamagishi S, et al. Suppression of transforming growth factor beta and vascular endothelial growth factor in diabetic nephropathy in rats by a novel advanced glycation end product inhibitor, OPB-9195. Diabetologia 1999;42:579–588.
44. Forbes JM, Soulis T, Thallas V, et al. Renoprotective effects of a novel inhibitor of advanced glycation. Diabetologia 2001;44:108–114.
45. Wilkinson-Berka JL, Kelly DJ, Koerner SM, et al. ALT-946 and aminoguanidine, inhibitors of advanced glycation, improve severe nephropathy in the diabetic transgenic (mREN-2)27 rat. Diabetes 2002;51:3283–3289.
46. Figarola JL, Scott S, Loera S, et al. LR-90 a new advanced glycation endproduct inhibitor prevents progression of diabetic nephropathy in streptozotocin-diabetic rats. Diabetologia 2003;46:1140–1152.
47. Onorato JM, Jenkins AJ, Thorpe SR, Baynes JW. Pyridoxamine, an inhibitor of advanced glycation reactions, also inhibits advanced lipoxidation reactions. Mechanism of action of pyridoxamine. J Biol Chem 2000;275:21177–21184.
48. Voziyan PA, Metz TO, Baynes JW, Hudson BG. A post-Amadori inhibitor pyridoxamine also inhibits chemical modification of proteins by scavenging carbonyl intermediates of carbohydrate and lipid degradation. J Biol Chem 2002;277:3397–3403.
49. Pedchenko VK, Chetyrkin SV, Chuang P, et al. Mechanism of perturbation of integrin-mediated cell-matrix interactions by reactive carbonyl compounds and its implication for pathogenesis of diabetic nephropathy. Diabetes 2005;54:2952–2960.
50. Alderson NL, Chachich ME, Frizzell N, et al. Effect of antioxidants and ACE inhibition on chemical modification of proteins and progression of nephropathy in the streptozotocin diabetic rat. Diabetologia 2004;47:1385–1395.
51. Stitt A, Gardiner TA, Alderson NL, et al. The AGE inhibitor pyridoxamine inhibits development of retinopathy in experimental diabetes. Diabetes 2002;51:2826–2832.
52. Zheng F, Zeng YJ, Plati AR, et al. Combined AGE inhibition and ACEi decreases the progression of established diabetic nephropathy in B6 db/db mice. Kidney Int 2006;70:507–514.
53. Berrone E, Beltramo E, Solimine C, Ape AU, Porta M. Regulation of intracellular glucose and polyol pathway by thiamine and benfotiamine in vascular cells cultured in high glucose. J Biol Chem 2006; 281:9307–9313.
54. Gadau S, Emanueli C, Van Linthout S, et al. Benfotiamine accelerates the healing of ischaemic diabetic limbs in mice through protein kinase B/Akt-mediated potentiation of angiogenesis and inhibition of apoptosis. Diabetologia 2006;49:405–420.
55. Babaei-Jadidi R, Karachalias N, Ahmed N, Battah S, Thornalley PJ. Prevention of incipient diabetic nephropathy by high-dose thiamine and benfotiamine. Diabetes 2003;52:2110–2120.
56. Winkler G, Pal B, Nagybeganyi E, Ory I, Porochnavec M, Kempler P. Effectiveness of different benfotiamine dosage regimens in the treatment of painful diabetic neuropathy. Arzneimittelforschung 1999;49:220–224.
57. Haupt E, Ledermann H, Kopcke W. Benfotiamine in the treatment of diabetic polyneuropathy–a three-week randomized, controlled pilot study (BEDIP study). Int J Clin Pharmacol Ther 2005; 43:71–77.
58. Stracke H, Lindemann A, Federlin K. A benfotiamine-vitamin B combination in treatment of diabetic polyneuropathy. Exp Clin Endocrinol Diabetes 1996;104:311–316.
59. Stirban A, Negrean M, Stratmann B, et al. Benfotiamine prevents macro- and microvascular endothelial dysfunction and oxidative stress following

a meal rich in advanced glycation end products in individuals with type 2 diabetes. Diabetes Care 2006;29:2064–2071.
60. Vasan S, Zhang X, Kapurniotu A, et al. An agent cleaving glucose-derived protein crosslinks in vitro and in vivo. Nature 1996;382:275–278.
61. Wolffenbuttel BH, Boulanger CM, Crijns FR, et al. Breakers of advanced glycation end products restore large artery properties in experimental diabetes. Proc Natl Acad Sci U S A 1998;95:4630–4634.
62. Candido R, Forbes JM, Thomas MC, et al. A breaker of advanced glycation end products attenuates diabetes-induced myocardial structural changes. Circ Res 2003;92:785–792.
63. Thallas-Bonke V, Lindschau C, Rizkalla B, et al. Attenuation of extracellular matrix accumulation in diabetic nephropathy by the advanced glycation end product cross-link breaker ALT-711 via a protein kinase C-alpha-dependent pathway. Diabetes 2004; 53:2921–2930.
64. Forbes JM, Yee LT, Thallas V, et al. Advanced glycation end product interventions reduce diabetes-accelerated atherosclerosis. Diabetes 2004; 53:1813–1823.
65. Susic D, Varagic J, Ahn J, Frohlich ED. Cardiovascular and renal effects of a collagen cross-link breaker (ALT 711) in adult and aged spontaneously hypertensive rats. Am J Hypertens 2004;17:328–333.
66. Peppa M, Brem H, Cai W, et al. Prevention and Reversal of Diabetic Nephropathy in db/db Mice Treated with Alagebrium (ALT-711). Am J Nephrol 2006;26:430–436.
67. Kass DA, Shapiro EP, Kawaguchi M, et al. Improved arterial compliance by a novel advanced glycation end-product crosslink breaker. Circulation 2001;104:1464–1470.
68. Schmidt AM, Yan SD, Yan SF, Stern DM. The multiligand receptor RAGE as a progression factor amplifying immune and inflammatory responses. J Clin Invest 2001;108:949–955.
69. Schmidt AM, Yan SD, Brett J, Mora R, Nowygrod R, Stern D. Regulation of human mononuclear phagocyte migration by cell surface-binding proteins for advanced glycation end products. J Clin Invest 1993;91:2155–2168.
70. Hofmann MA, Drury S, Fu C, et al. RAGE mediates a novel proinflammatory axis: a central cell surface receptor for S100/calgranulin polypeptides. Cell 1999;97:889–901.
71. Kislinger T, Fu C, Huber B, et al. N(epsilon)-(carboxymethyl)lysine adducts of proteins are ligands for receptor for advanced glycation end products that activate cell signaling pathways and modulate gene expression. J Biol Chem 1999;274:31740–31749.
72. Park L, Raman KG, Lee KJ, et al. Suppression of accelerated diabetic atherosclerosis by the soluble receptor for advanced glycation endproducts. Nat Med 1998;4:1025–1031.
73. Wendt TM, Tanji N, Guo J, et al. RAGE drives the development of glomerulosclerosis and implicates podocyte activation in the pathogenesis of diabetic nephropathy. Am J Pathol 2003; 162:1123–1137.
74. Sakaguchi T, Yan SF, Yan SD, et al. Central role of RAGE-dependent neointimal expansion in arterial restenosis. J Clin Invest 2003;111:959–972.
75. Basta G, Sironi AM, Lazzerini G, et al. Circulating soluble receptor for advanced glycation end products is inversely associated with glycemic control and S100A12 protein. J Clin Endocrinol Metab 2006;91:4628–4634.
76. Tan KC, Shiu SW, Chow WS, Leng L, Bucala R, Betteridge DJ. Association between serum levels of soluble receptor for advanced glycation end products and circulating advanced glycation end products in type 2 diabetes. Diabetologia 2006;49:2756–2762.
77. Geroldi D, Falcone C, Emanuele E, et al. Decreased plasma levels of soluble receptor for advanced glycation end-products in patients with essential hypertension. J Hypertens 2005;23:1725–1729.
78. Srivastava SK, Ramana KV, Bhatnagar A. Role of aldose reductase and oxidative damage in diabetes and the consequent potential for therapeutic options. Endocr Rev 2005;26:380–392.
79. Sun W, Oates PJ, Coutcher JB, Gerhardinger C, Lorenzi M. A selective aldose reductase inhibitor of a new structural class prevents or reverses early retinal abnormalities in experimental diabetic retinopathy. Diabetes 2006;55:2757–2762.
80. Sorbinil Retinopathy Trial Research Group. The sorbinil retinopathy trial: neuropathy results. Neurology 1993;43:1141–1149.
81. Hamada Y, Nakamura J, Naruse K, et al. Epalrestat, an aldose reductase inhibitor, reduces the levels of Nepsilon-(carboxymethyl)lysine protein adducts and their precursors in erythrocytes from diabetic patients. Diabetes Care 2000;23:1539–1544.
82. Bril V, Buchanan RA. Long-term effects of ranirestat (AS-3201) on peripheral nerve function in patients with diabetic sensorimotor polyneuropathy. Diabetes Care 2006;29:68–72.
83. Rask-Madsen C, King GL. Proatherosclerotic mechanisms involving protein kinase C in diabetes and insulin resistance. Arterioscler Thromb Vasc Biol 2005;25:487–496.
84. Koya D, Jirousek MR, Lin YW, Ishii H, Kuboki K, King GL. Characterization of protein kinase C beta isoform activation on the gene expression of transforming growth factor-beta, extracellular matrix

components, and prostanoids in the glomeruli of diabetic rats. J Clin Invest 1997;100:115–126.

85. Kapor-Drezgic J, Zhou X, Babazono T, Dlugosz JA, Hohman T, Whiteside C. Effect of high glucose on mesangial cell protein kinase C-delta and -epsilon is polyol pathway-dependent. J Am Soc Nephrol 1999;10:1193–1203.
86. Goldberg HJ, Whiteside CI, Fantus IG. The hexosamine pathway regulates the plasminogen activator inhibitor-1 gene promoter and Sp1 transcriptional activation through protein kinase C-beta I and -delta. J Biol Chem 2002;277:33833–33841.
87. Kang N, Alexander G, Park JK, et al. Differential expression of protein kinase C isoforms in streptozotocin-induced diabetic rats. Kidney Int 1999; 56:1737–1750.
88. Shiba T, Inoguchi T, Sportsman JR, Heath WF, Bursell S, King GL. Correlation of diacylglycerol level and protein kinase C activity in rat retina to retinal circulation. Am J Physiol 1993;265:E783–E793.
89. Inoguchi T, Sonta T, Tsubouchi H, et al. Protein kinase C-dependent increase in reactive oxygen species (ROS) production in vascular tissues of diabetes: role of vascular NAD(P)H oxidase. J Am Soc Nephrol 2003;14:S227–S232.
90. Xia L, Wang H, Goldberg HJ, Munk S, Fantus IG, Whiteside CI. Mesangial cell NADPH oxidase upregulation in high glucose is protein kinase C dependent and required for collagen IV expression. Am J Physiol Renal Physiol 2006;290: F345–F356.
91. Tesfamariam B, Brown ML, Cohen RA. Elevated glucose impairs endothelium-dependent relaxation by activating protein kinase C. J Clin Invest 1991; 87:1643–1648.
92. Michell BJ, Chen Z, Tiganis T, et al. Coordinated control of endothelial nitric-oxide synthase phosphorylation by protein kinase C and the cAMP-dependent protein kinase. J Biol Chem 2001; 276:17625–17628.
93. Ishii H, Jirousek MR, Koya D, et al. Amelioration of vascular dysfunctions in diabetic rats by an oral PKC beta inhibitor. Science 1996;272:728–731.
94. Suzuma K, Takahara N, Suzuma I, et al. Characterization of protein kinase C beta isoform's action on retinoblastoma protein phosphorylation, vascular endothelial growth factor-induced endothelial cell proliferation, and retinal neovascularization. Proc Natl Acad Sci U S A 2002;99:721–726.
95. Chakravarthy U, Hayes RG, Stitt AW, McAuley E, Archer DB. Constitutive nitric oxide synthase expression in retinal vascular endothelial cells is suppressed by high glucose and advanced glycation end products. Diabetes 1998;47:945–952.
96. Cameron NE, Cotter MA, Jack AM, Basso MD, Hohman TC. Protein kinase C effects on nerve function, perfusion, Na(+), K(+)-ATPase activity and glutathione content in diabetic rats. Diabetologia 1999;42:1120–1130.
97. Danis RP, Bingaman DP, Jirousek M, Yang Y. Inhibition of intraocular neovascularization caused by retinal ischemia in pigs by PKCbeta inhibition with LY333531. Invest Ophthalmol Vis Sci 1998; 39:171–179.
98. Cotter MA, Jack AM, Cameron NE. Effects of the protein kinase C beta inhibitor LY333531 on neural and vascular function in rats with streptozotocin-induced diabetes. Clin Sci (Lond) 2002;103:311–321.
99. The PKC-DRS Study Group. The effect of ruboxistaurin on visual loss in patients with moderately severe to very severe nonproliferative diabetic retinopathy: initial results of the Protein Kinase C beta Inhibitor Diabetic Retinopathy Study (PKC-DRS) multicenter randomized clinical trial. Diabetes 2005;54:2188–2197.
100. Strom C, Sander B, Klemp K, Aiello LP, Lund-Andersen H, Larsen M. Effect of ruboxistaurin on blood-retinal barrier permeability in relation to severity of leakage in diabetic macular edema. Invest Ophthalmol Vis Sci 2005;46:3855–3858.
101. Aiello LP, Clermont A, Arora V, Davis MD, Sheetz MJ, Bursell SE. Inhibition of PKC beta by oral administration of ruboxistaurin is well tolerated and ameliorates diabetes-induced retinal hemodynamic abnormalities in patients. Invest Ophthalmol Vis Sci 2006;47:86–92.
102. Aiello LP, Davis MD, Girach A, et al. Effect of ruboxistaurin on visual loss in patients with diabetic retinopathy. Ophthalmology 2006;113:2221–2230.
103. Vinik AI, Bril V, Kempler P, et al. Treatment of symptomatic diabetic peripheral neuropathy with the protein kinase C beta-inhibitor ruboxistaurin mesylate during a 1-year, randomized, placebo-controlled, double-blind clinical trial. Clin Ther 2005;27:1164–1180.
104. Tuttle KR, Bakris GL, Toto RD, McGill JB, Hu K, Anderson PW. The effect of ruboxistaurin on nephropathy in type 2 diabetes. Diabetes Care 2005;28:2686–2690.
105. Beckman JA, Goldfine AB, Gordon MB, Garrett LA, Creager MA. Inhibition of protein kinase Cbeta prevents impaired endothelium-dependent vasodilation caused by hyperglycemia in humans. Circ Res 2002;90:107–111.
106. McGill JB, King GL, Berg PH, et al. Clinical safety of the selective PKC-beta inhibitor, ruboxistaurin. Expert Opin Drug Saf 2006;5:835–845.

21
Diabetic Foot Ulcers

Andrew Boulton and Frank Bowling

Introduction

The Wagner system describes the diabetic foot ulcer as a full thickness wound extending to tendons or deeper subcutaneous tissue but without bony involvement or osteomyelitis [1]. The university of Texas system refers to levels of ischemia [2] and infection while the SAD system [3] attends to size, area, depth, arteriopathy and any neuropathic involvement. The breadth of classification system in use reflects the complexity and range of signs/symptoms associated with diabetic foot ulceration, with a lower limb lost to amputation every 30 seconds [4]. Recent research has estimated that more than 50% of diabetic foot ulcers will recur within 3 years suggesting that the professionals involved in treatment are fighting a difficult battle especially when it is considered that the lifetime risk for developing such an ulcer is calculated to be in the region of 15–25% [5].

The cost implications of treatment products, amputation, rehabilitation and long-term care are colossal with US healthcare subscribers spending US$10.9 billion dollars in 2006 [6]. A UK estimate using the same calculations estimated a figure of £252 million [7]. While the cost to healthcare providers is seen as paramount, the price paid by the patient is a heavy psychological burden, which in itself may have a significant impact on healing [8].

In view of these statistics, it is fair to assume that prevention should be the focus of intervention and there is evidence to suggest that up to 50% of amputations and foot ulcers could be prevented by early identification and education of patients [9]. A diabetic foot ulcer does not appear spontaneously; there are multiple contributory factors and if these can be managed the incidence may be reduced. Unfortunately, the reality often demands the selection of treatments from an ever increasing source, with the choice dependent on the specifics of the presenting ulcer and the provision of optimum conditions for wound healing. Factors to be considered include aetiopathogenesis, size, and depth of the ulcer together with bacterial involvement.

In this chapter we will focus on a modern treatment approach to diabetic foot problems with special emphasis on pharmacological therapies.

Debridement

The key treatment for diabetic foot wounds is often debridement in its many guises. Despite the plethora of treatment available their success can be limited if the wound is not sufficiently prepared. The process of debridement removes non-viable tissue and the products remaining from an abnormal, sustained inflammatory response. Increased protease levels and an imbalance of matrix metalloproteinases and their tissue inhibitors [10] maintain the chronic wound state and their removal with associated hyperaemia will encourage an influx of the biological components of healing. The level of debridement used will depend on the aetiopathogenesis and the morphology of the ulcer.

The method of debridement selected will depend on the individual characteristics of the wound. Surgical and autolytic regimes are underpinned by encouraging the body's own healing response and mechanical techniques such as the Versa Jet (Smith & Nephew) work on a similar principle. Enzymatic debridement products attempt to impersonate natural biology but their efficacy is yet to be established.

The oldest form of debridement is by larval therapy with the earliest reference dating back to 1579. Throughout history there are references to the ability of larvae to debride wounds and secrete a healing substance [11]. The technique has seen a revival in modern medicine and there is growing evidence to support its use in the treatment of a range of wounds including diabetic foot ulcers. It also appears that not only do larvae selectively remove necrotic tissue but there is emerging data suggesting that their secretions and/or excretions have antibacterial properties, even towards Methicillin-Resistant Staphylococcus Aureus (MRSA), with a recent study reporting a 92% of MRSA from colonised diabetic foot wounds [12].

Antibiotics

An infected foot ulcer precedes approximately 60% of lower limb amputations in the diabetic population [13], thus the rapid and appropriate treatment of soft tissue infection is paramount. There is substantial evidence suggesting that people with diabetes are more susceptible to infection due to altered immune-response [14]. Polymorphonuclear neutrophil oxidative burst activity is thought to be reduced in addition to decreased bacterial killing [15]. Neutrophil and macrophage activity are thought to be prolonged [16].

The first step in treating an infected diabetic foot ulcer is to recognise infection, which must be defined clinically and is typically manifested by signs or symptoms of inflammation. This is sometimes difficult due to only one of the classical signs of infection being present. The clinical presentation will vary according to the extent and depth of the invading bacterial organisms [17]. It is worth noting at this point that colonisation is not infection and microflora on the base of the wound can be picked up by wound swabs and cultured for sensitivity. These microorganisms are usually part of the resident flora and do not present clinically as infection. Routine swab cultures of an ulcerative lesion are often difficult to interpret due to the number of pathogens found on the wound surfaces. Colonisation not only delays wound healing but is a source of cross contamination [18] and can reside on the wound for long periods of time.

A recent systematic review examined diagnostic methods used in suspected diabetic foot infections, but from a total of 2,762 references dating up to 2002 only 3 met the criteria for review [19] due to the evidence base being heavily weighted towards acute wounds. However, studies of acute post surgery and burns patients found quantities of bacteria at greater than ten colony forming units of bacteria/gram of tissue to be sufficient to impair healing and/or initiate a systematic response. Quantitative diagnostic tests to define infection may not be applicable to the heterogeneous group of diabetic foot ulcers and whilst an identified amount of bacteria may lead to infection in one patient it may have no impact on another [21]. The International Working Group on the Diabetic Foot suggested that diagnosis must be based upon clinical presentation. They developed a classification system [22], which may be more valuable in clinical practice with the laboratory to be used for the identification of specific pathogens present and their resistance profiles. This will enable the selection of appropriate antibiotic treatment. Superficial swabs can be unreliable as they may exclude anaerobic Gram-negative bacteria residing deep within the wound and so the group recommend curettage at the base of the ulcer.

In the current climate of ever-increasing strains of antibiotic-resistant pathogens, careful consideration of antibiotic selection is necessary.

Studies have shown that the pathogens responsible for diabetic foot infections are Staphylococcus aureus and beta haemolytic streptococci which respond to narrow spectrum antibiotics such as Flucloxacillin and cefalexin. However, progression in severity of infection will result in the emergence of bacteria such as Enterobacterium, Pseudomonas and obligate anaerobes, requiring a broader therapeutic target range.

The IWGDF propose that first-line treatment should be a broad spectrum antibiotic while culture results are awaited and when specific pathogens have been identified, targeted therapy can be administered. However, if a wound is clearly responding well to an empirical drug there may be little reason to narrow down the spectrum [20] simple, superficial infections can respond to topical or oral preparations with activity against Staphylococci and Streptococci. Clinically non-infected neuropathic ulcers do just as well without antibiotics [23]. Cephalosporins, penicillin and beta lactamase inhibitors, fluoroquinolones and clindamycin have all been shown to be effective treatments for diabetic foot infections [24]. Severity of infection will be a major consideration in patients with systemic involvement and broad-spectrum treatments are required to ensure maximum impact. Severe infections will often need to be treated with intravenous preparations, which can only be provided on an in-patient basis, for example, linezolid and vancomycin treatments for severe MRSA infections [24].

Diagnosis and treatment of osteomyelitis are fraught with controversy due to a limited evidence base but the point of diagnosis should begin with a clinical judgement regarding ulcer depth and chronicity in the presence of an appropriate but unsuccessful treatment episode. The IWGDF suggest the Probe to bone test (where the bone can be probed by a sterile instrument) to provide additional information during clinical examination but radiological procedures including simple x-ray and magnetic resonance imaging (MRI) would supply more information to contribute to an accurate diagnosis.

The treatment options for osteomyelitis are antibiotics for the infection and surgical resection or debridement. Some studies [25] have reported successful treatment with antibiotics alone but the best approach may be a combination of the two; clearly further research is needed [26]. The international guidelines advise that mild infections should be treated for approximately 1–2 weeks (with a single repeat of a treatment course before a radical review of the underlying aetiology).

Dressings

Wound healing is significantly impaired among the diabetic population and further complicated by neuropathy and/or ischaemia. The use of specialist dressings can provide favourable conditions for healing to occur by providing a moist protective environment. The range of dressings available is vast despite a questionable evidence base with products flooding the market claiming to fulfil all the requirements of the "ideal" dressing. Despite the development of complex preparations, the majority of foot ulcers will need a product that absorbs exudate, provides thermal insulation, is gas permeable but impermeable to microorganisms and will not adhere to the wound itself [27]. Health professionals require the dressing to allow wound monitoring and minimal changes while being easy to remove, as well as very cost-effective and easy to use.

Choosing the correct dressing will depend upon the condition and wound stage. The principle stages of healing are: cleansing, removal of debris, granulation, vascularisation and epithelisation. As the wound progresses through different stages of healing, it may be necessary to use a variety of different dressings to meet the wound criteria. Products available can be divided into broad categories of those with debriding properties, antiseptic-based dressings, moisture providing and those that influence the healing process itself.

Which type of dressing to choose is difficult due to the shear volume of dressing available. The field of wound care contains an enormous amount of literature regarding dressings but good quality, randomised controlled trials are not forthcoming and choice is often based on clinical experience rather than evidence. A thorough knowledge of the products available and their theoretical attributes is necessary for selection of the best dressing for the job. Table 1 summarises some of the dressings available and their application.

Cullum et al., in a comprehensive review of dressing trials of diabetic foot ulcers, found that the sample sizes of the studies they looked at were small with insufficient evidence of effect [28]. Clinicians should therefore question the validity of end point studies in wound healing experiments. A lot of the available information on wound healing refers to acute and experimental ulcers and therefore may not be relevant.

There is a wealth of evidence to show that dressings should never be used as a monotherapy. If the ulcer is not adequately offloaded, which occurs all too often in the diabetic foot, the wound will show no physical signs of improvement [29].

TABLE 1. Wound management products.

Dressing	Description	Contraindications	Example
Hydrocolloid	Facilitate rehydration and autolytic debridement.	Infected wounds.	Aquacel (Conva Tec)
	Dry, sloughy, necrotic wounds. Promote granulation.	Twice-weekly change.	Comfeel (Coloplast)
Hydrogels	Donates liquid to dry wounds and absorbs exudates.	Hydrogel sheets avoided in infected wounds.	Intrasite gel (S&N Hlth)
	Dry, sloughy wounds. Autyolitic debridement		Iodosorb (S&N Hlth)
Silver	Antimicrobial. Colonisation	Sensitivity to silver	Acticoat (S&N)
Vapour-permeable	Provide a moist healing environment. Mild exude.	Heavily exudating wound.	Tegaderm (3M)
Foam dressing	Primary or secondary cover. Light and Heavy exudates.	Remove if strike through occurs.	Allevyn (S&N Hlth) lyofoam (Medlock)
Odour absorbent	Absorbs odour. Malodorous.	Silver (sensitivity.)	Actisorb (J&J)
Larval Therapy	Debridement, promote granulation. Heavily sloughy necrotic wounds.	Increase in pain.	Maggots (Zoobiotic)
Alginate	Haemostat. Heavy exudates.	Blockage. Loose fibres.	Kaltostate (Conva Tec)
Skin substitutes	Living skin. Obstinate wounds.	Colonised. Infected wound.	Dermagraft (S&N Hlth)
Iodine	Antibacterial. Exudating wounds.	Iodine (sensitivity) Renal/ Thyroid conditions.	Iodosorb (S&N Hlth)
Honey	Antimicrobial. Sloughy necrotic wounds. Autyolitic debridement.	Medical grade only.	Mesitran (Medlock Medical)

Tobramycin Impregnated Calcium Sulphate Pellets

The diabetic population has been shown to have different patterns of absorption of medications particularly when the host is compromised and local delivery of antibiotics can have little impact on severe infections [30]. However, evidence is emerging to suggest that local treatment when combined with systemic therapies can increase treatment response. Local antibiotic therapy delivered in pellet form was first advocated by orthopaedic surgeons with the use of non-absorbent polymethylmethacrylate beads with antibiotic embedded in the wounds of patients with osteomyelitis. However, preparation and insertion was complex in addition to requiring a further episode of surgery for removal. More recently, Calcium sulphate has been demonstrated as having bone filling properties in clinical trials [31]. Although studies have been limited to orthopaedic patients with osteomyelitis, the attributes of the pellets are transferable to the diabetic population as a vehicle for delivery of antibiotics.

Calcium sulphate pellets impregnated with tobramycin are now available in a ready prepared pack and can be used with deep, severely infected ulcers in combination with systemic antibiotic treatment. The Osteoset T (Wright Medical) is a prefabricated plaster of paris pellet impregnated with tobramycin and the Bone Void Filler is available as a mixing kit allowing fabrication of pellets of various sizes and strengths. Following application the pellets remain in place and are reabsorbed over a 2–3-month period.

The efficacy of Osteoset as a bone graft substitute has been questioned [32] and the evidence base for use in treating diabetic ulcer infections is sparse but anecdotally UK and USA centres are reporting positive results. This is clearly an area for further research.

Offloading

Adequate offloading of an ulcer is a necessary adjunct to pharmacological-based treatments [33]. Therapies are likely to be limited in their success if the foot continues to be exposed to the stress and shear forces that contributed to the ulcer formation [34]. The principal behind offloading involves the redistribution of pressure over a wide area of the plantar aspect of the foot. The types of device available include removable or fixed casts, orthotic devices and custom made shoes. Studies have shown the gold standard to be total contact casts (TCC) [35] with healing times greatly reduced in comparison with other offloading devices [36]. It has been hypothesised that its great success lies with the fact that it is non-removable, thereby ensuring patient compliance. A study examining the activity patterns of patients with removable casts illustrated limited compliance with subjects only wearing the casts for a minority of steps per day [37]. This would appear to go some way towards explaining the longer healing times associated with removable offloading devices. However, not all patients are suitable for a TCC as there are limits to its use with contraindications for soft tissue infections and osteomyelitis.

Biogun

It has long been accepted that colonisation of wounds with MRSA delays healing and increases the risk of infection [37] and as such a reduction is desirable but in the current environment of increasing bacterial resistance to antibiotics the treatment sources are expanding and novel new treatments are emerging.

Another non-pharmological treatment is the Biogun (Dentron Limited), which is based on the ability of negative ions to exert a significant bactericidal effect [38]. It involves the ionisation of molecular oxygen thereby generating superoxide radical anions (O^{2-}), which Dentists have used to great effect in the treatment of dental caries. On a theoretical level the Biogun should be applicable to a range of pathologies but research is limited. Podiatrists have investigated its application to fungal and verrucae treatments with positive effects [39] and studies are now emerging with specific reference to diabetic foot ulcers. Negative ions have demonstrated activity against microorgansims at an in vitro level and more recently at soft tissue level, its ability to reduce MRSA colonisation in non-infected diabetic foot wounds. More research is necessary but the Biogun may become an adjunct to other more traditional treatments. Recently published data showed a 60% eradication of MRSA in diabetic foot ulcers [40].

Vacuum Assisted Closure Pump

The process of treating a diabetic foot ulcer begins with debridement and resolution of any infection and progresses towards dressing and offloading. However, the vacuum assisted closure (VAC) pump (KCI Medical) is emerging as an interim treatment to assist closure. The formation of a vacuum creates negative pressure, which when applied to a wound removes exudate and may stimulate the formation of granulation tissue by creating and maintaining a moist wound environment [41].

There are few studies available but the most extensive appears to be an RCT comparing the use of negative pressure via the VAC versus standard treatment for wounds post-partial amputation. The results show a significantly greater percentage of wounds achieved closure during VAC therapy and the rate of closure and formulation of granulation tissue was faster. A guideline published in 2004 recommended that this treatment be reserved for complex, deep extensive wounds including post-surgery [41].

Bisphosphonates in the Treatment of Charcot Foot

Charcot neuroarthropathy (CN) is a progressive condition that affects the bones and joints of the foot. It is characterised by joint dislocation, subluxation and pathological fractures of the foot in neuropathic patients resulting in debilitating deformity [42]. The incidence of CN is reported to be around 0.1–0.5. Although diabetes is the most common cause in the Western World CN can occur in other diseases associated with peripheral neuropathy. There is no sex predilection and it can occur at any age but is more commonly seen in the fourth or fifth decades of life and in patients with a long duration of diabetes [42].

Acute CN can be misdiagnosed as cellulitis, osteomyelitis or inflammatory arthropathy. A high level of suspicion is necessary to ensure that appropriate treatment is established immediately in order to prevent development of severe deformities. On examination the foot is generally warm and may be inflamed and swollen, temperature of >2°C from opposing limb. Once the acute phase has past there should be no temperature difference, just severe alteration in foot architecture. Most cases can be diagnosed by plain x-ray, but specialised investigations may be necessary. Three–phase ^{99m}Tc bisphosphonate bone scans demonstrate an early increase in bone uptake, which is due to increased blood flow through the bone that accompanies the active Charcot process. If the foot is ulcerated it may be difficult to rule out osteomyelitis In-labelled leukocyte scans and MRI may be required.

A multi-centre study [43] carried out a randomised double-blind placebo controlled trial. Patients received a single infusion of 90 mg of pamidronate or placebo (saline); foot temperatures, symptoms and markers of bone turnover (bone-specific alkaline phosphates and deoxypyridinoline cross links) were measured over the 12 months, in ten visits. There results were extremely promising showing bisphosphonate, pamidronate, given as a single dose leads to a reduction in bone turnover. A recent RCT carried out in 2005 [44] concluded that alendronate taken orally 70 mg once weekly over a 6-month period showed a significant reduction of ICTP and hydroxyprolin markers indicative of bone reabsorption. The test group showed an increase in bone density compared with the control group. Both groups received long-term immobilisation in an adequate offloading device. Offloading reduces inflammation and may help to prevent gross structural deformity.

References

1. Wagner FW. The dysvascular foot: A system for diagnosis and treatment. *Foot Ankle* 1981;2:64–122.
2. Armstrong DG, Lavery LA, Harkless LB. Validation of a diabetic foot wound classification system: contribution of depth infection and vascular disease to the risk of amputation. *Diabetes Care* 1998;21:855–859.
3. Treece KA, MacFarlane RM, Pound P, Game FL, Jeffcoate WJ. Validation of a system of foot ulcer classification in Diabetes Mellitus. *Diabet. Med.* 2004;21:987–991.
4. International Diabetes Federation time to act: Diabetes and foot care. Brussels: International Diabetes Federation, 2005.
5. Singh N, Armstrong DG, Lipsky BA. Preventing foot ulcers in patients with diabetes. *JAMA* 2005;293:217–228.
6. Gordois A, Scuffham P, Shearer A, Oglesby A, Tobian JA. The health care costs of Diabetic Peripheral Neuropathy, in the US. *Diabetes Care* 2003;26:1790–1795.
7. Gordois A, Scuffham P, Shearer A, Oglesby A. The healthcare costs of Diabetic Peripheral Neuropathy, in the UK. *Diabet. Foot* 2003;6:62–73.
8. Vileikyte L. Stress on wound healing. Clinics in Dermatology 2007;25:49–55.
9. Boulton AJM. The Diabetic Foot. *Diabet. Med.* 2006;34:87–90.
10. Lobmann R, Ambrosch A,, Waldmann K, Schultz G, Lehnert H, Schiweck S. Expression Matrix-metalloproteinases and inhibitors in the wounds of diabetic and non-diabetic patients. *Diabetologia* 2002;45:1011–1016.
11. Thomas S. Sterile maggots and the preparation of the wound bed. In: Cherry GW, Harding KG, Ryan TJ (eds). *Wound bed preparation. Proceedings of a symposium sponsored by the European Tissue Repair Society*, 2000 Nov 24–25; Oxford UK. International Congress and Symposium Series 250. Royal Society of Medicine Press Limited, 2001:59–66.
12. Bowling FL, Salgami E, Boulton AJM. Larval therapy a novel treatment in eliminating MRSA from diabetic foot wounds. *Diabetes Care* 2007;30:370–371.
13. Pecoraro RE, Reiber GE, Burgess EM. Pathways to diabetic limb amputation. Basis for prevention. *Diabetes Care* 1990;3:513–521.
14. Mc Manon MM, Bistrian BR. Host defences and susceptibility to infection in patients with diabetes mellitus. *Infect. Dis. Clin. North Am.* 1995;9:1–10.
15. Marhoffer W, Stein M, Schleinkofer L, Federlin K. Evidence of ex vivo and in vitro impaired neutrophil oxidative burst and phagocytic capacity in type 1 diabetes mellitus. *Diabet. Res. Clin. Pract.* 1993;193:183–188.
16. Wetzler C, Kampfer H, Stallmeyer B, Pfeilschifter J, Frank S. Large and sustained induction of chemokines during impaired wound healing in the genetically diabetic mouse: prolonged persistence of neutrophilils and macrophages during the late phase of repair. *J. Invest. Dermatol.* 2006;11520:245–253.
17. Bridges RM, Deitch EA. Diabetic foot infections. Pathophysiology and treatment. *Surg. Clin. North Am.* 1994;74:537–545.
18. Roghmann MC, Siddiqui A, Plaisance K, Standiford H. MRSA colonization and the risk of bacteraemia in hospitalized patients with chronic ulcers. *J. Hosp. Infect.* 2001;47:98–103.
19. O'Meara S, Nelson EA, Golder S, Dalton JE, Craig D, Iglesias C. Systematic review of methods to diagnose infection in foot ulcers in diabetes. *Diabet. Med.* 2006;23(4):341–347.

20. Lipsky BA. A report from the international consensus on diagnosing and treatment the diabetic foot. *Diabet./Metab. Res. Rev.* 2004;20(Suppl. 7):586–577.
21. McMahaon MM, Bistrian BR. Host defences and susceptibility to infection in patients with diabetes mellitus. *Infect. Dis. Clin. North Am.* 1995;9:1–10.
22. International Working Group on the Diabetic Foot. International consensus on the diabetic foot. European Association for the Study of Diabetes. CD ROM 2003, May.
23. Chantelau E, Tanudjaja T, Altenhofer F, Ersanli Z, Lacigova S, Metzeger C. Antibiotic treatment for uncomplicated neuropathic forefoot ulcers in diabetes. *Diabet. Med.* 1996;13:156–159.
24. Cunha BA. Antibiotic selection for diabetic foot infections: a review. *J. Foot Ankle Surg.* 2000;39:253–257.
25. Venkatesan P, Lawn S, Macfarlane R, Fletcher EM, Finch RG, Jeffcoate WJ. Conservative management of osteomyelitis in the feet of diabetic patients. *Diabet. Med.* 1997;14:487–490.
26. Jeffcoate W, Lipsky B. Controversies in diagnosing and managing osteomyelitis of the foot in diabetes. *Clin. Infect. Dis.* 2004;39:S115–S122.
27. Bradley M, Cullum N, Nelson EA, Petticrew M, Sheldon T, Torgeson D. Systematic reviews of wound care management. *Health Technol. Assess.* 1999;3:1–35.
28. Cullum C, Majid M, O'Meara S, Shelocn T. Use of dressings: is there an evidence base? In: Boulton AJM, Connor H, Cavanagh PR (eds). *The foot in diabetes*, 3rd edn, Chichester: Wiley; 2000:153–163.
29. Armstrong DG, Lavery LA, Wu S, Boulton AJM. Evaluation of removable and irremovable cast walkers in the healing of diabetic foot wounds: a randomized controlled trial. *Diabetes Care.* 2005;28(3):551–554.
30. Armstrong DG, Findlow AH, Cybil SC, Boulton AJM. Absorbable antibiotic-impregnated calcium sulphate pellets in the management of diabetic foot infections. *Diabet. Med.* 2001;18:937–948.
31. Kelly CM, Wilkins RM, Gitelis S, Hartjen C, Watson JT, Kim PT. The use of a surgical grade calcium sulfate as a bone graft substitute: results of a multicentre trial. *Clin. Orthop. Relat.* 2001;382:42–50.
32. Petruskeukius J, Nielsen S, Faalunis S, Fnudsen PR, Cvergaards NC. Effects of osteoset, a bone craft substitute on bone healing in humans. *Acta Orthop. Scand.* 2002;5:575.
33. Armstrong DG, Lavery LA, Nixon BP, Boulton AJM. It is not what you put on, but what you take off: techniques for debriding and offloading the diabetic foot wound. *Clin. Infect. Dis.* 2004;39:S92–S99.
34. Brand PW. The diabetic foot. In: Ellenberg M, Rifkin H (eds), *Diabetes mellitus, theory and practice*, 3rd edn., Medical examination publishing: New York; 1983:803–828.
35. Mueller MJ, Diamond JM, Sinacore DR. Total contact casting in treatment of diabetic planter ulcers. Controlled clinical trial. *Diabetes Care* 1989;12:384–388.
36. Armstrong DG, Lavery LA, Kinbriel HR, Nixon BP, Boulton AJM. Activity patterns of patients with diabetic foot ulceration. Diabetic foot ulceration. *Diabetes Care* 2003;26:1–4.
37. Tentolouris N, Jude EB, Smirnoff I, Knowles EA, Boulton AJM, Methicillin Resistant Staphylococcus aureus: an increasing problem in the diabetic foot clinic. *Diabet. Med.* 1999;16:767–771.
38. Kellogg EW III, Yost MG, Barthakurn, Kreveger AP. Superoxide involvement in the bacteriocidal effects of negative air ions on staphylococcus albus. *Nature* 1979;4:281–400.
39. Vernon CJ. Long term experience of the Dentron Biogun in verruca pedis, mosaic verruca and hand warts. *J. Pod. Med.* 2000;65:4–8.
40. Dang CN, Anwar R, Thomas G, Prasad YDM, Boulton AJM, Malik R. The Biogun: A novel way of eradicating MRSA colonization in diabetic foot ulcers. *Diabetes Care* 2006;29:1176–1177.
41. Armstrong DG, Attinger CE, Boulton AJM, Frykberg RG. Guidlines regarding negative wound therapy (NWPT) in the diabetic foot. *Ostomy. Wound Manage.* 2004;50(4b Suppl.):35–27s.
42. International Diabetes Federation. Working Group on The Diabetic Foot. Diabetes Monitor 2007 volume 19:21–27.
43. Jude EB, Selby PL, Burgess J, Lilleystone P, Mawer EB, Page Sridcnohce M, Foster AV, Edmonds ME, Bolton AJM. Bisphosphonates in the treatment of Charcot neuroarthropathy. *Diabetologia* 2001;44(11):2032.
44. Pitocco D, Rudtolov V, Caputos, Mancin L, Collina MC, Manto A, Caradonna P, Chirlanda G. Six-month treatment with alendronate in acute Charcot neuroarthropathy. *Diabetes Care* 2005;5:1214–1215.

22 Pharmacotherapy in Diabetic Neuropathy

Anders Dejgaard and Jannik Hilsted

Introduction

Diabetic neuropathy was defined at the San Antonio Consensus Conference as "a descriptive term meaning a demonstrable nerve disorder, either clinically evident or subclinical, that occurs in the setting of diabetes mellitus without other causes for peripheral neuropathy. The neuropathic disorder includes manifestations in the somatic or autonomic parts of the peripheral nervous system" [1]. Diabetic neuropathy is a chronic condition caused by hyperglycaemia, characterized by progressive morphological destruction of the peripheral nervous system, accompanied by loss of peripheral nerve function. Clinically, loss of function is defined by distal loss of sensibility, muscular strength and loss of deep tendon reflexes as well as by autonomic dysfunction of viscera and blood vessels.

Peripheral neuropathy is the complication with the highest impact on Quality of life (QOL) and the major cause of morbidity in diabetic patients. Diabetic neuropathy is one of the most common neuropathies globally. Diabetic neuropathy develops in parallel with the other long-term diabetic complications. Presence of diabetic neuropathy increases the risk of foot ulcer development and subsequent amputation, and diabetic neuropathy carries an increased mortality.

Over the years a number of pharmacological treatment modalities for the prevention and treatment of diabetic neuropathy have been proposed. This chapter attempts to give an overview of studies and trials carried out in the past decades in this area.

Pathogenesis and Pathophysiology

Hyperglycaemia is the central aetiological factor for the development of diabetic neuropathy. Studies of large cohorts of patients, followed for up to 25 years have shown that poor glycaemic control and diabetic neuropathy are interrelated [2]. In the DCCT study (Diabetes Control and Complications Trial) [3] type 1 diabetic patients with high glucose concentrations receiving conventional insulin treatment more frequently developed neuropathy than the patients treated with multiple daily insulin injections or continuous insulin infusion by a portable insulin pump, resulting in lower blood glucose concentrations. Similar results have been obtained in Type 2 diabetic patients as in the UKPDS (UK Prospective Diabetes Study) [4].

Increased blood glucose concentrations induce a number of biochemical changes where each may be involved in the processes that result in destruction of nerve cells and myelin sheaths. The most significant hypotheses include the polyol pathway, oxidative stress, non-enzymatic glycation, changes in growth factors and gene expression, and microvascular abnormalities [5]. These changes may alone or in concert be involved not only in the pathogenesis of peripheral nerve dysfunction but also in the development of microangiopathy. Since peripheral nerve function is dependent on vascular supply of oxygen, the vascular (microangiopathic) hypothesis is also relevant.

Polyol accumulation is directly dependent on blood glucose concentrations. Sorbitol and fructose are polyols derived from glucose by an enzymatic process facilitated by the enzyme Aldose

Reductase. The polyols are accumulated in nervous tissue (the nerve cell membrane is not permeable for polyols) causing osmotic damage to the nerve cell with reduction in myo-inositol and Na+/K+-ATPase activity and increased oxidative stress. A number of Aldose Reductase inhibitors have been developed, and several of these have been tested in diabetic patients [6].

Oxidative stress causes increased formation of free radicals that potentially may cause destruction of nerve tissue. Diabetes is characterized by increased amounts of free radicals, and accordingly a number of antioxidants have been tested in diabetic neuropathy.

Non-enzymatic glycosylation of slow turnover proteins may be involved in the development of long-term diabetic complications [7]. One example of non-enzymatic glycosylation is glycosylation of the axonal structural proteins actin and tubulin, a process which is capable of changing their function in axonal transport.

Growth factors and gene expression. Nerve Growth Factor (NGF) and a number of growth factors such as BDNF, NT3, NT4, NT5 and NT6 with their specific receptor systems may influence survival and growth of nerve cells. Mitogen-Activated-Protein-kinases (MAP-kinases) may be the link between the biochemical changes caused by hyperglycaemia, and the structural changes in the nerve tissue characteristic of the neuropathic process.

Microvascular abnormalities. Neurons depend on capillaries for nutrition and there is a strict correlation between microangiopathia, haemodynamic changes, neuronal ischaemia, oxidative stress and clinical neuropathy.

These theories are by no means mutually exclusive, and there is experimental evidence for interrelationships as depicted in Fig. 1.

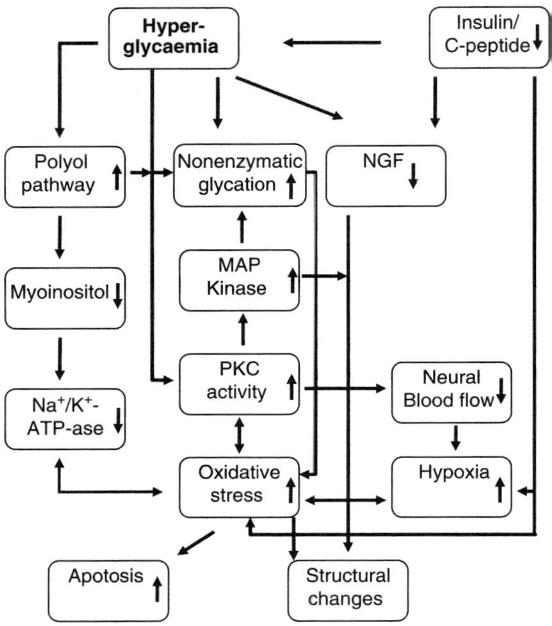

FIG. 1. Aetiological factors in the development of diabetic neuropathy.

Histopathology

Morphological abnormalities in diabetic neuropathy include changes in the axon as well as in the myelin sheath. The early stages of the disease are characterized by changes in axonal calibre and myelin sheath disintegration, whereas axonal degeneration and subsequent atrophy are the dominating features at a later stage [8]. Essentially, these changes are found throughout the nervous system, albeit the morphological changes are most obvious in the distal regions of the somatic nerves. Accordingly, diabetic neuropathy is encountered in the somatic nervous system, the autonomic nervous system and the central nervous system (CNS) – symptoms and clinical findings being much more prominent in the two former than in the latter system, the existence of CNS neuropathy being a matter of debate until quite recently [9].

Diagnostic Criteria

Whereas diagnostic criteria for other long-term diabetic complications such as nephropathy and retinopathy have been well established for a number of years, a number of different tests have been introduced for the diagnosis of diabetic neuropathy. This is explained by the fact that diabetic neuropathy may be encountered in all regions of the peripheral nervous system with an inherent opportunity to investigate these different regions. Furthermore, several different methodologies may be applied (e.g. nerve conduction velocity, neurological examination and autonomic function tests). Taken together, it is not surprising that many different diagnostic criteria have been applied over the years.

The DCCT trial was conducted with diagnostic criteria subsequently used in other investigations, that is, the coexistence of clinical signs and symptoms characteristic of neuropathy and decreased nerve conduction velocity in at least two different somatic nerves and/or abnormal autonomic nerve function tests. Standardized scoring systems are used for the characterization of clinical signs and symptoms, increasing reproducibility and allowing to some extent monitoring of the progression of clinical neuropathy.

Measurements of nerve conduction velocities and autonomic nerve function tests require considerable efforts in terms of standardization in order to reduce intra- and interobserver variation. In the DCCT study the use of core-labs was introduced to reduce variation in these parameters between centres, and subsequent metacentre studies have used similar approaches. Evidently, clinical routine practise requires a more simplistic and flexible approach.

Neuropathy assessment in outpatient settings. Daily routine practise requires methods that are robust, reliable and simple. Easy outpatient clinic tests includes knee and ankle tendon reflexes, pin prick pain test, light touch (Cotton wisp), vibration sense using a 128 Hz tuning fork, pressure perception using a 10-g monofilament. Regarding the somatic nerve system, the most commonly used test is the determination of threshold for sense of vibration by a Biothesiometer. The vibration perception threshold has been found to correlate with a number of other measures of somatic and autonomic function tests and is therefore considered a good all-round marker of the functional state of the peripheral nervous system in diabetic patients [10]. The method has been shown to give more detailed and reliable information than qualitative methods for the determination of sensory nerve loss (like the 128-Hz tuning fork and the 10-g "monofilament" technique).

Autonomic nerve function tests basically consist in measurements in integrated cardiovascular reflex arches, the heart most often being the effector organ. Different physiological stimuli are applied, and changes in heart rate and heart rate variation are used as markers of cardiac vagal function. The most commonly used tests are heart rate variability during deep respiration, standing or Valsalva's manoeuvre. Tests for the sympathetic nerves system involve blood pressure response to standing and the Quantitative sudomotor axon reflex test (QSART) [11]. Abnormal test results are associated with premature cardiovascular disease and death in diabetic patients.

Experimental settings require a more detailed description of the functional state of the peripheral nervous system. As regards the somatic nervous system, determination of sensory and motor nerve conduction velocity and amplitude by neurophysiological techniques are applied, along with quantitative estimation of thresholds for various sensory functions (Quantitative Sensory Assessment, QSA), including tests for proprioception, temperature, vibratory sense, tactile sensation and pain. Characterization of the motor unit (one motor neuron and the muscle cells innervated by the neuron) requires electromyography with registration of denervation potentials. Quantitative dynamographic analysis is used for quantitative biomechanical estimation of striated muscle power and dynamics.

The San Antonio conference recommended that at least one parameter from the following five categories is measured to classify diabetic neuropathy: (i) symptom profile, (ii) neurological examination, (iii) QSA, (iv) nerve conduction study, and (v) autonomic functioning testing. Several questionnaires have been developed to quantify signs and symptoms of diabetic neuropathy like the McGill pain questionnaire, Dycks neuropathic staging and the Michigan Neuropathy Screening Instrument. Visual analogue scales seem preferable to follow responses on treatment.

As regards the autonomic nervous system a description of parasympathetic and sympathetic function is generally applied. Heart rate variation as a marker of cardiac parasympathetic activity is widely used; the investigation may be expanded for longer periods of time by means of Holter monitoring. There are no methods for estimation of integrated (global) parasympathetic activity or methods for the determination of extracardiac parasympathetic activity. The functional state of the sympathetic nervous system is mirrored by plasma concentrations of norepinephrine (derived mainly from sympathetic nerve endings) and epinephrine (from the adrenal medulla). Unlike parasympathetic techniques plasma concentrations of catecholamines do provide a global estimate of sympathetic activity. Regional estimation of sympathetic activity may be performed by microneurography (electrophysiological estimation of impulse frequency in sympathetic nerves from skin and muscle).

Epidemiology

The incidence and prevalence of diabetic neuropathy in the literature varies more than similar estimates of diabetic nephropathy and retinopathy, due to the diagnostic complexity and lack of a mutually agreed definition as described above. Furthermore, different methods have been applied and to some extent also different normal intervals for these methods are described and many studies have included a mixture of type 1 and type 2 diabetic patients. Furthermore, diabetic neuropathy is more frequent in male gender, smokers and elderly, which makes the population tested a potentially important bias. Finally, a distinction between the symptomatic state and measurable non-symptomatic abnormalities has often not been made.

With these reservations in mind, the frequency of symptomatic neuropathy seems to be 15–20% in unselected diabetes patient populations, whereas the frequency of more or less pronounced abnormalities in the peripheral nervous system varies between 20% and 50%, depending on the methodology applied. The prevalence in type 2 diabetes seems to be higher than in type 1 diabetic patients although data are somewhat contradictory [11]. At the onset of diabetes the frequency of nervous system abnormalities is 5–10%, increasing linearly as a function of duration of diabetes and amounts to 50% of the population after 25 years duration of diabetes. Ten to twenty per cent of patients with peripheral diabetic neuropathy will have painful diabetic neuropathy that requires treatment.

Signs and Symptoms

Diabetic neuropathy is characterized by a spectrum of clinical neuropathic syndromes, which includes dysfunction of almost every segment of the somatic peripheral and autonomic nervous system. Diabetic neuropathy is classified as either mononeuropathy or polyneuropathy. Focal and multifocal mononeuropathies involve both mononeuropathies and entrapment syndromes. Mononeuropathies occurs most often in the elderly and in contrast to entrapment syndromes they are characterized by sudden onset, not progressive, resolves spontaneously and needs only symptomatic treatment. They are caused by endoneurial ischaemic lesions leading to nerve infarctions. Entrapment syndromes most often affect the peroneal, median, ulnar, medial and lateral plantar nerves. The typical symptoms are loss of function and pain.

Multifocal proximal motor neuropathy was for many years considered a component of diabetic neuropathy. Although more frequent in patients affected by diabetes mellitus this syndrome is now known to be secondary to other causes than diabetes [12].

Distal symmetric sensorimotor polyneuropathy is the most common form of diabetic neuropathy. Small fibre neuropathies involving unmyelinated C and Aδ fibres are involved in symptoms like pain, which is burning and superficial and associated with allodynia, hypoalgesia and defective warm thermal sensation. Patients can experience dys-, para, hypo- or hyperaesthesia, tingling, pins and needles or electric-shock-like sensations.

Autonomic neuropathy is also a small fibre neuropathy leading to symptoms like resting tachycardia, orthostatic hypotension, gustatory sweating, delayed gastric emptying, diarrhoea/constipation, erectile dysfunction, urinary retention/incontinence and exercise maladaptation. Cardiac symptoms like dysrhytmias and even sudden cardiac death are linked to autonomic neuropathy. When larger myelinated Aα or Aα/β fibres get affected more deep pain and muscle weakness, atrophy and cramps appear.

The large-fibre neuropathy may involve both sensory and motor nerves. Large fibres facilitate motor function, vibration sense, position sense and cold thermal perception. Most patients with a distal symmetric polyneuropathy have a mixed variety of neuropathy with involvement of both large and small-fibre damages. Above symptoms are characterized by having a "glove and stocking" distribution.

Persistent pain due to neuropathy is experienced by approximately 10% of diabetic patients. Acute pain includes the insulin neuritis syndrome, which occurs in the beginning of insulin therapy for diabetes and is self-limiting. Chronic pain with duration of more than 6 months can be constant, intermittent or hyperalgesic, that is, increased response to a painful stimulation. The presentation and character of pain in diabetic neuropathy can be highly diverse and typically worsens at night. The pain is usually divided into a cutaneous dysaesthetic pain and a deeper nerve trunk pain, the first being characterized by burning and tingling, whereas the last is more aching and knife like.

The mechanism behind pain in diabetic neuropathy is not fully understood but various mechanisms have been proposed, such as hyperglycaemia lowering the threshold for pain, increased firing of abnormally excitable nociceptive fibres, and/or ectopic impulse generation with erratic transmission, which relates to electrical cross talk between damaged nociceptive afferents and perhaps sympathetic nerves. Central changes can follow peripheral nerve damage as dorsal root ganglion can spontaneously generate impulses when peripheral nerves are damaged. Arteriovenous shunting that occurs in small nerve fibre disease involving the autonomic nerve system may also be a source of pain.

Therapeutic Approaches

Numerous investigational studies have been undertaken to test for various pharmaceuticals for prevention and intervention of diabetic neuropathy. Most studies have been disappointing partly due to poor study designs involving patients with advanced disease with loss of a majority of nerve fibres, where improvements cannot be expected. Many have involved too few subjects in too short an observation period to get any meaningful results. Another obstacle is the fact that diabetic neuropathy is a multifactorial dynamic and progressing disease, which make a simple approach unlikely to succeed. Finally, reproducibility of clinical measurements and definition of clinical meaningful end points have been an additional problem.

In the following a thorough review is given as regards studies directed towards various pathogenetic factors.

Hyperglycaemia

Several studies have shown a relationship between hyperglycaemia and the development and severity of diabetic neuropathy. Pirart et al. [2] showed by following more than 4,000 diabetic patients over 25 years that the prevalence of diabetic neuropathy increased over time from 12% at diagnosis to 50% after 25 years of duration. Those patients with the poorest metabolic control had the highest prevalence. In the DCCT study a primary intervention sub-study in 726 patients showed that intensified glycaemic control reduced the risk of developing neuropathy by 69% compared with conventional therapy. It is noteworthy that despite near-normal blood glucose control over 5 years 8% still developed abnormal clinical signs and 18% developed abnormal nerve conduction tests. In the secondary intervention cohort of DCCT a 57% reduction in prevalence of diabetic neuropathy was seen in the intensified treatment group. In the Epidemiology of Diabetes Intervention and Complication (EDIC) study, which is a follow-up stud on the DCCT study, showed that the beneficial effect persisted at least 8 years after the end of DCCT, in spite of no difference in glycaemic control between the arms in EDIC advocating for a "glycaemic memory" as regards effect [13].

The major role of hyperglycaemia in the development of diabetic neuropathy is furthermore seen in other interventions trials with pancreatic transplantation where a normalization in blood glucose has resulted in improvement in nerve conduction velocity and symptomatology [14]. Accordingly, strict metabolic control needs to be applied in patients with diabetes in order to reduce the risk of developing or worsening diabetic neuropathy. However, it has to be recalled that insulin levels is increased in all the above interventions and aside its metabolic effects insulin does have specific neurotrophic properties that might play a role in the above outcomes separate from the metabolic effects. Insulin stimulates neurite outgrowth, is required for the survival of sensory and sympathetic neurons, and stabilizes neurofilaments and tubulins in a dose-dependent manner. Furthermore, insulin is required for an optimal interaction between NGF and its receptors. These effects are not investigated separately in clinical studies in man. Interestingly, there are recent data from animal and early data from human beings including patients with diabetic neuropathy indicating that C-peptide might play a role in the treatment of diabetic neuropathy [15]. In vivo studies have shown that C-peptide corrects the Na+/K+-ATPase and endothelial NO synthase, and expression of neurotrophic factors. In studies in type 1 diabetic patients C-peptide has shown significant improvements in sural nerve conduction velocity, vibration and thermal perception [16].

Polyol Pathway

Aldose Reductase (AR) is the rate limiting enzyme of the polyol pathway, which converts glucose to sorbitol in the presence of NADPH as cofactor. The pathway is completed by the second enzyme, sorbitol dehydrogenase, which converts sorbitol to fructose with NAD^+ as cofactor. In the hyperglycaemic state there is accordingly an accumulation of sorbitol in the cell leading to a cascade of metabolic abnormalities causing hypoxia and tissue ischaemia. Aldose reductase hyperactivity increases the oxidative stress in the cell through a number of mechanisms. AR-mediated oxidative stress leads to such detrimental consequences as MAPK activation and PARP activation [17]. Both MAPKs and PARP control numerous transcription factors leading to downstream up-regulation of inflammatory genes that may increase free radical generation.

Aldose reductase inhibitors (ARI) reduce the flux of glucose through the polyol pathway thereby inhibiting the accumulation of sorbitol and fructose and preventing NADPH consumption and oxidative stress. Numerous studies of ARI in animal models of diabetic complications have demonstrated the potential of ARI against diabetic neuropathy. However, animal models of neuropathy do not predict outcome in human beings well.

A number of ARIs have reached phase II or III clinical trials but only three are presently in clinical development (Fidorestat, Lidorestat and Ranirestat). In general most studies have been disappointing either due to lack of efficacy or evolvement of severe side effects. Some studies including recent long-term studies have shown effect with moderate to minor improvements in electrophysiological (i.e. 1 m/s in NCV) and symptomatic end points [18,19]. However, ARI's are not presently established as a treatment modality for diabetic neuropathy, and critical factors for success of ARI's in the future will depend on development of non-toxic compounds with sufficient nerve tissue selectivity and affinity to ensure tissue penetration to normalize sorbitol generation in the nerve.

Oxidative Stress

Increased oxidative stress, which according to accumulating data, contributes to the pathogenesis of diabetic neuropathy, which is the consequence of either enhanced ROS production or attenuated ROS scavenging capacity, resulting in tissue damage [20]. α-lipoic acid is a derivative of octanic acid and a potent antioxidant that scavenges hydroxyl, superoxide and peroxyl radicals and regenerates glutathione and has been investigated in various recent trials. The ALADIN II and III and the SYDNEY study have demonstrated a significant improvement in neuropathy score, neuropathy impairment score, sensory and motor NCV, and sensory nerve action potential [21]. Furthermore, α-lipoic acid has been shown to have beneficial effects on autonomic neuropathies and mononeuropathies in diabetes as well [22]. Results from ongoing large-scale trials (NATHAN I and II) are awaited to determine the therapeutic potential of this compound.

Glycosylation

Hyperglycaemia results via the Maillard reaction in the formation of advanced glycation end products (AGE), which in turn binds on specific receptors (RAGE), inducing monocytes and endothelial cells to increase the production of cytokines and adhesion molecules [23] The formation of AGE will furthermore increase the formation of reactive oxygen species. Aminoguanidine is a hydrazine compound that prevents AGE formation and has shown promising results in animal studies but controlled clinical trials testing in diabetic patients of aminoguanidine have been discontinued due to severe adverse effects [24]. However, modified successors are being tested for this approach presently.

Vascular Factors

Endoneurial ischaemia is considered to play a major role in the pathogenesis of diabetic neuropathy [25]. Improvements of tissue blood flow by revascularization have been shown to improve status of diabetic neuropathy with improvements in NCV, which is one prominent proof of an ischaemic element in diabetic neuropathy. γ-linolenic is an important constituent of neuronal membrane phospholipids and also serves as a substrate for prostaglandin E formation, seemingly important for preservation of blood flow. In diabetes, conversion of linoleic acid to gamma linolenic acid and subsequent metabolites is impaired, possibly contributing to the pathogenesis of diabetic neuropathy. A 1-year multi-centre placebo-controlled randomized trial of gamma linolenic acid showed improvement in clinical and neurophysiologic measures [26]. Later trials have been less promising and more data are needed to finally settle its role in the treatment of diabetic neuropathy. Angiotensin – converting enzyme (ACE) inhibitors mediate increased flow-dependent release of endothelium derived relaxing factors (EDRF) and endothelium-dependent vessel relaxation. ACE has been tested in patients with diabetic neuropathy and has shown beneficial effects on neurophysiological tests such as NCV. However, the recent Appropriate Blood pressure Control in Diabetes (ABCD) trial did not show any effect, and further studies are needed before ACE can be recommended in the treatment of diabetic neuropathy.

Other vasodilating agents such as prostacyclin analogues have been tested in small-term trials and shown effect on neurophysiologic end points and clinical end points like pain. However, again more long-term trials are needed.

Diabetes and hyperglycaemia induce an increase in the synthesis of diacylglycerol resulting in the activation of Protein Kinase C (PKC). The activation of vascular PKC is considered to lead to impairment in vasodilatation and an increase in vasoconstriction, which can occur in the endoneurial microvessels and cause a decrease in neural blood flow, resulting in neural dysfunction in diabetes. PKC inhibition has shown beneficial effects in animal studies and preliminary studies in diabetic patients. However, disappointing results in recent phase 2 studies have led to the discontinuation of the development of this compound for the diabetic neuropathy indication.

Neurotrophic Factors

NGFs play an important trophic role in the maintenance of the peripheral nervous system and are deficient in diabetic neuropathy. Several trials have been undertaken to test for an effect of recombinant NGF supplementation in diabetic neuropathy. Although some of these trials have been positive with an improvement in nerve fibre function and neuropathic symptoms later large-scale phase 3 trials in patient with sensory polyneuropathy were unable to demonstrate any significant effect compared with placebo [27]. Accordingly, this treatment is not pursued further presently. Studies are presently ongoing to test if Vascular Endothelial Growth Factor (VEGF) can improve sensory neuropathy in diabetic patients.

Symptomatic Treatment of Pain

Neurogenic pain is seen in approximately 10% of all diabetic patients, and is associated with substantial impairment in QOL. Except for optimization of metabolic control and α-linoic acid none of the above pathogenetically directed treatments have shown long-term clinical effect. Accordingly, various symptomatic treatments have been tested. These are all without any effect on the underlying disease process.

Antidepressants

A. *Tricyclic antidepressants* are among the widest studied drugs for treatment of painful diabetic neuropathy. It has a documented effect in these patients and meta-analysis has shown a 50% reduction in pain intensity in 30% of patients with diabetic neuropathic pain [28]. Effects are probably due to an inhibition of both 5 HT, norepinephrine and serotonin presynaptic reuptake. Sodium and calcium channel blockade and *N*-methyl-D-aspartate receptor antagonism are other potential mechanisms. Imipramine, Desipramine, Amitriptyline, Clomipramine and Nortriptyline are the most tested and used. Based on their effect ratio of norephinephrine and serotonin reuptake, effects may differ within patients. Side effects include dry mouth, weight gain, drowsiness, and orthostatic hypotension. The secondary amines nortriptyline and desipramine have less cholinergic side effects but may show to be less efficacious as well. Starting dose should be 25 mg given at bedtime with increases of 25 mg every week until effect or adverse effects appear, which includes cholinergic effects such as dry mouth, sweating, sedation and dizziness. Maximal doses are 150 mg/day, and tricyclic antidepressants are contraindicated in patients with coronary heart disease.

B. *Selective serotonin reuptake inhibitors.* Studies have shown that citalopram and serotonin in doses of 20–40 mg/day are effective in the treatment of painful diabetic neuropathy but not as efficacious as tricyclic antidepressants [29]. However, they do have less adverse effects, and accordingly they are recommended to be given to patients that do not tolerate tricyclic antidepressants. Upper gastric bleeding is a reported adverse effects and concomitant use of NSAID increases this risk.
C. *Selective norepinephrine reuptake inhibitors.* Few studies have been done with selective norephinephrine inhibitors. Bupropion have shown effect but the adverse event profile does not place these compounds as a first line treatment option.
D. *Selective norepinephrine and serotonin reuptake inhibitors.* Both Venlafaxine and Duloxetine have shown significant higher effect than placebo in the treatment of pain in diabetic patients and both compounds are being used with increasing frequency in these patients. Duloxetine is a more potent inhibitor than Venlafaxine and seems from clinical studies to be more efficacious. Doses tested in trials are 60 and 120 mg/day and side effects include nausea, somnolence, dizziness, dry mouth and decreased appetite.

Anticonvulsants

Carbamazepine and Phenytoin are first generation anticonvulsants that have been used in for many years in the treatment of diabetic painful neuropathy. However, although Carbamazepine has shown effect in controlled clinical trials high rates of adverse events like somnolence, dizziness and allergy have placed these compounds late in the armentarium against painful diabetic neuropathy [30].

Second generation anticonvulsants with a demonstrated effect against pain in diabetic neuropathy includes gabapentin, pregabalin and oxcarbazepine. These anticonvulsants act by binding to the alpha-2-delta subunit of the calcium channel reducing neurotransmitter release. Gabapentin is an anticonvulsant with a structure related to GABA, which is a neurotransmitter that plays a role in the transmission and modulation of pain. In controlled clinical trials gabapentin (900–3600 mg/day) has shown to be as efficacious as amitriptyline with improvements in symptom score and QOL [31]. Due to its rather low adverse effect profile and lack of cardiac adverse effects this compound is one of the most prescribed for the treatment of painful diabetic neuropathy.

Pregabalin is another second-generation anticonvulsant that has recently obtained FDA approval for treatment of neurogenic pain, and several randomized placebo controlled studies have shown that this compound is efficacious in the treatment of painful diabetic neuropathy [32]. Doses between 300 and 600 mg/day have shown effect already apparent after 1 week of treatment. There are few clinically important drug interactions as there is no interference with the cytochrome 450 system. This compound requires minimal dose titration and seems easy to use. Side effects to gabapentin and pregabalin include drowsiness, dizziness and peripheral edema.

Oxcarbazepine is another second-generation anticonvulsant structurally related to carbamazepine. Oxcarbazepine have been tested in clinical trials for its effect against painful diabetic neuropathy and in a recently published study no effect was seen on VAS score between oxcarbazepine and placebo [33].

Antiarrhytmic Agents

Single 30-min intravenous infusions of Lidocaine (5 mg/kg BW) has shown to be effective in relieving painful diabetic neuropathy with a duration of the effects up to 21 days [34]. The oral analogue Mexilitin has been tested in several studies and has shown effect in doses below the doses required for antiarrythmic effect [35]. The effect was especially seen for burning and stabbing effect. This compound should due to its relatively weak efficacy and need for ECG monitoring be reserved for those patients failing on above therapies.

Opiates

Long-term use of opioids in diabetic patients remains controversial and many find the neurogenic pain to be insensitive to opioids and not be used due to the risk of abuse. Tramadol is a weak opioid with inhibitory effects on reuptake of serotonin and norepinephrine as well. Tramadol has been shown to be effective in the treatment of painful diabetic neuropathy. Sindrup showed that slow release tablets (doses between 200 and 400 mg/day) effectively relieved pain [36]. Side effects are nausea, dizziness and constipation.

Topical agents

Various topical agents have been tested. Capsaicin is an alkaloid and a main ingredient in chilli peppers, and is available in a cream for topical use. This neurotoxin depletes substance P from the terminals of unmyelinated C-fibres. Substance P is considered the primary neurotransmitter of pain from the periphery to the CNS. Data suggest that Capsacain application produces degeneration followed by reinnervation of epidermal nerve fibres. This in combination with inconsistent results from clinical trials as regards its efficacy for treatment of painful diabetic neuropathy has resulted in limitation of its use [37].

Topical lidocaine 5% is approved by FDA for use in postherpetic neuralgia. Studies have shown it to be effective in relieving pain due to diabetic neuropathy as well.

Non-Pharmacologic Treatment

Non-pharmacologic treatment like acupuncture, transcutaneous electric nerve stimulation, electrical spinal cord stimulation, physical approaches and psychological support is not addressed in this chapter.

Symptomatic Treatment of Autonomic Failure

Autonomic neuropathy is rather common in patients with diabetic neuropathy especially the sensory polyneuropathy type. Treatment of symptoms due to autonomic failure in patients with diabetic neuropathy is rather complex and directed towards the physiologic changes that are consequences of the non-functioning autonomic nervous system. It is for these patients critical that detailed explorations of differential diagnosis are performed before a symptomatic treatment is instituted. In this section we mention the most used and documented pharmacological intervention directed to specific symptoms of the autonomic diabetic neuropathy. Non-pharmacological interventions are not addressed.

A. *Orthostatic hypotension.* The most important is to limit use of vasoactive substances. If non-pharmacologic measures are not enough then fludrocortisone should be tried starting with a dose of 0.1 mg at bedtime and increased to 0.4 mg/day [38]. Side effects are oedema and recumbent hypertension. Other compounds that have been tested with positive results include Erythropoietin, Octreotide, desmopressin and midodrine.
B. *Gastroparesis.* Drugs like cisapride, domperidone, metoclopramide and erythromycin have in clinical trials shown effects on symptoms and QOL.
C. *Diarrhoea.* Diarrhoea is a common symptom in diabetic autonomic neuropathy. First line treatment includes a short course of antibiotics such as tetracycline or erythromycin. Opiate-like anti diarrhoeal agents like loperamide and codeine sulphate represents other first line treatments. Cholestyramine given with loperamide might be beneficial, and octreotide have shown to be effective as well.
D. *Constipation.* For this syndrome osmotic laxatives seems efficient and erythromycin might be effective as well in some patients.
E. *Erectile dysfunction.* For this condition sildenafil, tadalafil and vardenafil have all shown effect in improving erectile dysfunction allowing intercourse.

Clinical Recommendation

In practical daily life it is important to establish near normoglycaemic control in the all patients with diabetes mellitus, which means a HbA1c of <6.5% to reduce the risk for patients being affected by late diabetic micro- and macro-vascular complications. This will in most patient mean a rather intensive treatment and at least more intensive than present where average HbA1c are far above in most regions of the world.

It is furthermore important to evaluate the status of the peripheral and autonomic nervous system by routine measurements as described on a regular basis, that is, at least once a year. If signs of neuropathy appear it is important to rule out other causes of neuropathy that might be treatable. Furthermore precautional instructions must be given to the patient. Treatment with α-lipoic acid can be evaluated at this stage. When and if the patient experience painful diabetic neuropathy, treatment is often a matter of trial and error and treatment needs often to be changed either due to lack of effect or appearance of side effects. There is unfortunately very limited data on combination of various therapeutic modalities. We recommend the following treatment guideline based on present literature on effect and adverse events experience. Furthermore, this algorithm is in line with recent ADA guidelines.

1. Start with a tricyclic antidepressant (Amitriptyline, nortriptyline, desipramine, imipramine or clomipramine).

If inefficient or too many adverse effects:

2. Treat with serotonin and norepinephrine reuptake inhibitor (duloxetine, venlafaxine) or alternatively with serotonin reuptake inhibitors, (citalopram, paraoxetine).

If inefficient or too many adverse effects:

3. Start treatment with second-generation anticonvulsants like gabapentin or pregabalin.

If inefficient or too many adverse effects:

4. Start treatment with tramadol.

If inefficient or too many adverse effects:

5. Try mexilitine

If inefficient or too many adverse effects:

6. Consider short-term topical treatment especially if the patient is affected by superficial discomfort and pain (burning, tingling, etc.)

If symptoms of autonomic failure appear, each symptom must be addressed based on a clinical evaluation.

Summary and Future Directions

Pharmacological treatment to prevent and intervene with established diabetic neuropathy has so far been disappointing. A number of compounds have been tested, yet none of these have been implemented in daily clinical practice. A major reason seems that many biochemical mechanisms seem to be in play, and most intervention has so far been directed towards single individual abnormalities. Increasing knowledge and understanding of the interplay between these mechanisms establishing oxidative stress with mitochondrial overproduction of ROS as a central pathogenetical defect holds promise for new mechanistically directed interventions [39,40]. Several compounds have shown effect in symptomatic relief of painful diabetic neuropathy. However, most drugs show only a number needed to treat 3–4 to relieve pain more than 50%, and more effective compounds are still warranted.

Intensified insulin treatment remains a documented and effective way of reducing the rate of progression of established neuropathy and is also essential in the primary prevention of diabetic neuropathy.

For a number of years, it has been hoped that a pharmacological principle would evolve that would significantly reduce the burden of diabetic neuropathy in combination with intensified insulin treatment. The efforts to identify such compounds is ongoing and the possibility of linking the various known etiologies into one holds promise for more successful interventions in the future.

References

1. Consensus statement. Report and recommendation of the San Antonio Conference on diabetic neuropathy. American Diabetes Association American Academy of Neurology. Diabetes Care 1988;11:592–597.
2. Pirart J. Diabetes mellitus and its generative complications: A prospective study of 4400 patients observed. Diabetes Care 1978;1:168–188.
3. DCCT research group. The effect of intensive treatment of diabetes on the development and progression of long-term complications in insulin-dependent diabetes mellitus. N Engl J Med 1993;329:977–986
4. UK Prospective Diabetes Study group. Intensive blood glucose control with sulphonylureas or insulin compared with conventional treatment and risk of complications in patients with Type 2 diabetes. Lancet 1998;352:837–853.
5. Duby JJ, Campbell RK, Setter SM et al. Diabetic neuropathy: An intensive review. Am J Health Syst Pharm 2004;61:160–173.
6. Sima AAF, Pierson CR. Pathogenesis and Pathology of diabetic neuropathy. In: Gries FA, editor. Textbook of diabetic neuropathy, Stuttgart. New York: Georg Thieme verlag, 2003, 83–169.
7. Boel E, Selmer J, Flodgaard HJ et al. Diabetic late complications: Will aldose reductase inhibitors or inhibitors of advanced glycosylation endproducts formation hold promise? J Diab Compl 1995;9:104–129.
8. Dyck P. Pathology and pathophysiology- Human and experimental. In Dyck PJ, editor. Diabetic neuropathy. London: WB Saunders Company, 1987, 223–237.
9. Dejgaard A, Gade A, Larsson H et al. Evidence of diabetic encephalopathy. Diabet Med 1991;8:162–167.

10. Garrow AP, Boulton AJM. Vibration perception threshold- a valuable assessment of neural dysfunction in people with diabetes. Diabet Metab Res Rev 2006;22:411–441.
11. Dejgaard A. Pathophysiology and treatment of diabetic neuropathy. Diabet Med 1988;15:97–112.
12. Jensen TS, Backonja M, Jimenez SH et al. New perspectives on the management of diabetic peripheral neuropathic pain. Diabet Vasc Dis Res 2006;3(2):108–119.
13. Martin CL, Albers J, Herman WH et al. Neuropathy among the diabetes control and complications trial cohort 8 years after trial completion. Diabetes Care 2006;29:340–304.
14. Allen RDM, Al-Habri IS, Morris JGL et al. Diabetic neuropathy after pancreas transplantation: determinants on recovery. Transplantation 1997;63:830–838.
15. Sima AAF. Pathological mechanisms involved in diabetic neuropathy: Can we slow the process? Curr Opin Investig Drugs 2006;7(4):324–337.
16. Ekberg K, Brismar T, Johansson BL et al. Amelioration of sensory nerve dysfunction by C-peptide in patients with Type 1 Diabetes. 2003;52:536–541.
17. Obrosova IG, Pacher P, Szab C et al. Aldose reductase inhibition counteracts oxidative-nitrosative stress and poly(ADP-ribose) polymerase activation in tissue sites for diabetic complications. Diabetes Nutr Metab. 2005;54:234–242.
18. Hotta N, Akanuma Y, Kawamori R et al. Long-term clinical effects of Epalrestat, an aldose reductase inhibitor, on diabetic peripheral neuropathy. Diabetes Care 2006;29(7):1538–1544.
19. Bril V, Buchanan RA, Ranistat study group. Long term effects of ranirestat on peripheral nerve function in patients with diabetic sensimotor polyneuropathy. Diabetes Care 2006;29(1):68–72.
20. Vincent MV, Feldman EL. New insights into the mechanism of diabetic neuropathy. Rev Endocr Metab Disord 2004;5(3):227–236.
21. The SYDNEY trial. The sensory symptoms of diabetic polyneuropathy are improved with alfa-lipoic acid. Diabetes Care. 2003;26:770–776.
22. Tankova T, Chernikova S, Koev D. Treatment for diabetic mononeuropathy with alfa-lipoic acid. Int J Clin Pract 2005;59(6):645–650.
23. Peyroux J, Sternberg M. Advanced glycation endproducts (AGEs): pharmacological inhibition in diabetes. Pathologie Biologie 2006;54:405–419.
24. Goldin A, Beckman JA, Schmidt AM et al. Advanced glycation end products- sparking the development of diabetic vascular injury. Circulation 2006;114:597–605.
25. Cameron NE, Eaton SEM, Cotter MA et al. Vascular factors and metabolic interactions in the pathogenesis of diabetic neuropathy. Diabetologia 2001; 44:1973–1988.
26. Keen H, Payan J, Allawi J. et al. Treatment of diabetic neuropathy with gamma-linolenic acid. Diabetes Care 1993;16:8–15.
27. Apfel SC, Schwartz S, Adornato BT et al. Efficacy and safety of recombinant human nerve growth factor in patients with diabetic polyneuropathy: A randomized controlled trial. rhNGF Clinical Investigator Group. JAMA 2000;284(17):2215–21.
28. Argoff C, Backonia MM, Belgrade MJ et al. Consensus guidelines: Treatment planning and options. Mayo Clin Proc. 2006;81:s12–s25.
29. Boulton AJM. Management of diabetic peripheral neuropathy. Clin Diab. 2005;23(1):9–15.
30. Vinik A. Clinical review: Use of antiepileptic drugs in the treatment of chronic painful diabetic neuropathy. J Clin Endocrinol Metab 2005;90:4936–4945.
31. Morello CM, Leckband SG, Stoner CP et al. Randomized double-blind study comparing the efficacy of gabapentin with amitriptyline on diabetic peripheral neuropathy pain. ArchIntern Med 1999;159:1931–1937.
32. Griesing T, Freeman R Rosenstock et al. Efficacy, safety and tolerability og pregabalin treatment for diabetic peripheral neuropathy: findings from 6 randomized controlled trials. Diabetologia 2005;48 (suppl 1):A351.
33. Grosskopf J, Mazzola J, Wan J et al. A randomized, placebo controlled study of oxcarbazepine in painful diabetic neuropathy. Acta Neurol Scand 2006;114:177–180.
34. Kastrup J, Petersen P, Dejgaard et al. Treatment of chronic diabetic neuropathy with intravenouis lidocaine infusion. Br Med J 1986;292:173–174.
35. Dejgaard A, Petersen P, Kastrup J. Mexilitine for treatment of chronic diabetic neuropathy. Lancet 1988;29:9–11.
36. Sindrup SH, Andersen G, Madsen C et al. Tramadol relieves pain and allodynia in polyneuropathy: a randomised double blind, controlled trial. Pain 1999;83:85–90.
37. Jensen PG, Larson R. Management of painful diabetic neuropathy. Drugs and aging. 2001;18(10):737–749.
38. Vinik AI. Diabetic neuropathies. Med Clin N Am 2004;88:947–999.
39. Boulton AJM, Vinik AI, Arezo JC et al. Diabetic neuropathies. Diabetes Care 2005;28(4):956–962.
40. Brownlee M. The pathobiology of diabetic complications – a unifying mechanism. Diabetes 2005;54: 1615–1625.

23
Pregnancy – Pharmacological Problems

Elisabeth R. Mathiesen and Peter Damm

This chapter covers the use of insulin, insulin analogues, and oral hypoglycemics, as well as other drugs relevant for use before or during pregnancy and lactation in women with diabetes.

Insulin Analogues

The most physiological way to correct hyperglycemia apart from diet and exercise is insulin supplementation. Insulin molecules do due to their size generally not cross the placental barrier, but a transfer of the insulin–insulin antibody complex is possible [1]. Although transplacental crossing of the insulin antibody complex has repeatedly been described, the amount of insulin crossing this way is probably not of clinical significance. There is no evidence of any relationship between insulin antibodies in maternal serum and fetal outcome [1]. Treatment with human insulin has during the last 10 years been the golden standard of insulin treatment during pregnancy.

The aim of insulin replacement is to mimic the physiological pattern of insulin secretion. Conventional insulin preparations have in this respect some major pharmacodynamic pitfalls. The action of rapidly acting preparations is slower and of longer duration than the physiological meal time-stimulated insulin secretion. Preparations for basal use have peak action 5–8 h after a subcutaneous application. In addition, the absorption of intermediate-acting insulin varies a lot.

In order to obtain a more useful pharmacodynamic profile, insulin analogues have been developed [2]. All analogues show a more physiological time–action profile with either a shorter onset and shorter duration of action (insulin lispro and aspart) or a more constant effect lasting up to 24 h (insulin glargine and levemir). Currently, the rapid-acting insulin analogues such as lispro, aspart, and glulisin as well as the long-acting analogues glargin and detemir are commercially available.

Lispro has been tested in a randomized study of pregnant women ($n = 33$) with type 1 diabetes and found comparable with human insulin [3]. Data of more than 500 pregnancies with insulin lispro is now published without any excess malformation or other bad outcomes observed [4]. Initially case reports suggested an accelerated progression of retinopathy [5] but studies specifically designed to investigate this issue did not find an accelerated progression of diabetic retinopathy using insulin lispro in pregnancy [6]. Insulin lispro does not induce excess amount of insulin antibodies when used in pregnancy, and lispro has not been observed in the fetal circulation in women using insulin lispro during pregnancy [7].

In a randomized, controlled, multicenter trial treatment with insulin aspart and human insulin were compared in 332 pregnant women with type 1 diabetes [8]. The incidence of severe hypoglycemia tended to be lower in the insulin aspart group, especially at night, and pregnancy outcome was comparable in the two groups with a trend toward less fetal losses and preterm deliveries using insulin aspart. Diabetic retinopathy was stable during pregnancy using insulin aspart. Stimulation of insulin antibodies in women using insulin aspart during pregnancy did not occur, and insulin aspart was not observed in the fetal circulation [9]. Data regarding Glulisin in pregnancy are at present not available.

In vitro studies have shown a correlation of metabolic effects to insulin receptor affinity and mitogenic effects with IGF-1 receptor affinity [10]. Both short-acting insulin analogues and insulin detemir have a comparable affinity with these receptors as human insulin [10].

The long-acting analogue glargine has a somewhat higher affinity to IGF 1 in the cell line tested [10]. However, preclinical and clinical studies with glargine did not show relevance of that in a clinical setting. Until now, the limited existing reports of the use of glargine during pregnancy have not revealed any concerns [11]. A documentation of maternal and perinatal outcome in a large sample of pregnant women using insulin glargine is awaited before a general recommendation for its use in pregnancy can be given.

Insulin detemir has been on the market for a short period, and no concerns are registered in the few pregnancies using detemir observed. A large randomized study investigating the efficacy and safety of using insulin detemir are initiated in spring 2007, and the data are expected to be available in 2010.

Based on this evidence, the use of short-acting analogues in pregnancy is considered safe and insulin aspart is labeled for use in pregnancy in Europe and USA. However, a documentation of outcome in a large sample of pregnant women using the long-acting insulin analogues insulin glargine or detemir in pregnancy is awaited before a general recommendation for its use in pregnancy can be given.

Oral Hypoglycemics

Sulfonylureas are the oldest and most widely used oral hypoglycemic agents. Data on older preparations show transplacental crossing of these compounds. Prolonged neonatal hypoglycemia was more frequently described in infants exposed to sulfonylureas during pregnancy [12].

A second generation of sulfonylureas has been developed, and glibencamide (glyburide) has been found not to cross the placenta in significant amounts [13]. To date, no randomized study addressing the use of oral hypoglycemic agents during organogenesis has been performed, but the use of glyburide in women with GDM has been compared with insulin treatment [14]. The mean blood glucose values obtained were comparable in the glyburide and insulin group, and a similar low incidence of macrosomia (7% vs. 4%) and poor neonatal outcomes was registered. These results are promising but the use of sulfonylureas is still rare in USA and Europe.

Metformin does cross the placenta in significant amounts [15]. Metformin is often used as adjuvant treatment in polycystic ovary syndrome [16] and might improve the pregnancy rate [17]. It has been tested in diabetic pregnancy [18] but there are reports from cohort studies of the serious adverse effects of metformin in pregnancy. A significantly higher incidence of preeclampsia was found in 50 women treated with metformin when compared with 68 women treated with sulfonylurea and 42 women treated with insulin [19]. In the same study, perinatal mortality was significantly higher in those treated with metformin in the last trimester. Until the results of large randomized trials using metformin are present the use of metformin in pregnancy cannot be recommended.

Regarding postnatal use, metformin seems to be safe in lactating mothers since it appears in milk in insignificant amounts and is not detectable in the circulation of breastfed infants [20]. There are virtually no data on the use of other classes of oral hypoglycemic agents in pregnancy.

Antihypertensive Drugs

Angiotensin-converting enzyme inhibitors (ACE-I) and angiotensin II receptor blockers (AIIRB) are both frequently used for treatment of hypertension and microalbuminuria in young diabetic women. For both drugs, teratogenicity and fetotoxicity have been reported [21–23]. The relative risk of congenital malformations in offspring of 209 women taking ACE-I during organogenesis was 2.7 times compared with those not taking antihypertensive drugs [23]. The relative risk of malformations in 202 women taking other types of antihypertensive was 0.66. The most common malformations were in the cardiovascular or central nervous system [23]. In addition to congenital malformations, fetal and neonatal renal failure and oligohydramnios have been observed [21,22]. A change from ACE-I or AIIRB to other types of antihypertensive prior to a planned pregnancy is therefore recommended. However, in women suffering from diabetic nephropathy, an individual judgment must be offered. A weighing of the benefit of using drugs to inhibit the renin angiotensin system while waiting to become pregnant and then stopping this treatment as soon the pregnancy is diagnosed [24] or to have a period without inhibition of the renin angiotensin system might lead to the progression of the disease prior to pregnancy. This period may be of long duration if the women do not easily become pregnant.

Beneficial effect of treating women with type 1 diabetes and established microalbuminuria with methyldopa with addition of other antihypertensive drugs if blood pressure or urinary albumin excretion increase during pregnancy has been suggested [25]. Using this strategy, a reduction of preterm delivery before week 34 has been demonstrated [25]. In the same way, women with diabetic nephropathy probably benefit from early and aggressive antihypertensive treatment in pregnancy.

Antihypertensive drugs such as methyldopa, the alfa-betablocker labetalol, and nifedipine are widely used and regarded safe to use in pregnancy and during lactation [26], and other types of calciumblockers such as diltiazem have also been used in pregnant women with proteinuria [27].

Regarding postnatal use, ACE-I captopril and enelapril are regarded compatible with breast feeding since the amount occurring in the milk is 0.002% [28] of the maternal dose for captopril and 0.01% for enalapril [29]. No information regarding AIIRB occurring in breast milk is available at present. Thus, so far, the use of AIIRB cannot be recommended for use during lactation.

Statins

Cholesterol-lowering drugs known as statins modulate the lipid synthesis and are regarded contraindicated during pregnancy [30].

Aspirin

Aspirin are widely used in patients with diabetes to reduce the incidence of cardiovascular events. In addition, aspirin from gestational week 12 might reduce the prevalence of preeclampsia in high-risk women [31]. Whether aspirin is associated with a slightly increased risk of malformations is a matter of debate [32]. Use of aspirin during organogenesis is therefore not routine and should be based on an individual risk/benefit assessment, but after gestational week 12 it might be useful in high-risk pregnancy.

Steroids and Other Drugs Used in Women with Imminent Preterm Labor

Corticosteroids for lung maturation, if preterm delivery before week 34 is threatening, are widely used. Steroids lead to severe insulin resistance and often result in increased blood glucose values from 4 h after the first injection and up to 5 days later. If insulin dose is not adjusted accordingly, diabetic ketoacidosis might evolve. The need for increase in insulin dose is very individual but on average 50%. An early rise in insulin dose at initiation of the steroid treatment, prior to the first elevated blood glucose, is of uppermost importance in keeping the blood glucose values near normal, and an algorithm has been described [33].

Betasymptomemitics used as tocolytic agents to inhibit contractions result in severe insulin resistance with a very high risk of ketoacidosis. A need of intravenous infusion of more than 10 IU per h of fast-acting insulin during treatment with betasymptomemitica has been reported The oxytosin inhibitor atosiban does not seem to have a significant influence on the glucose metabolism [34]. We therefore recommend that atosiban is used as the primary tocolytic agent in women with diabetes and that betasymptomemetics are used only with extreme caution.

Folic Acid Supplementation

The general risks of congenital malformations are 2–4 times higher in women with diabetes, and the risk of having a fetus with an open neural tube defect is 2.5 times higher [35]. Folic acid supplementation induces diminished diabetes-induced dysmorphogenesis in rat embryos [36]. Pre-pregnancy supplementation of folic acid extended through the first 12 weeks of pregnancy in diabetic women is therefore extra important as it is in women suffering from epilepsy. At present, there is no consensus whether a daily dose of 400 μg or 5 mg should be recommended to women with diabetes.

Contraception in Diabetic Women

Pregnancy in women with diabetes mellitus is associated with an increased risk for the mother and her infant. It is well described that pregnancy in women with type 1 diabetes is associated with significantly increased risks for preterm delivery, preeclampsia, polyhydramnios, operative delivery, major congenital malformations, birth trauma, and various neonatal complications. Planned pregnancy is therefore mandatory in women with diabetes, and their need for contraception is essential. Basically, the same methods can be used as in women without diabetes, but a number of specific conditions have to be considered in the guidance of women with diabetes. Unfortunately, the field is limited in studies in certain areas, especially considering contraception for women with type 1 diabetes and late diabetic complications and women with type 2 diabetes. These women also have the greatest risk for complications due to an unplanned pregnancy. Thus, in the real clinical world, the choice of contraceptive method often will be a kind of compromise balancing the pros and cons for the different available methods.

Thus, contraceptive counseling should be an integrated part of the preconceptional care for all women with diabetes and is described in detail in two recent reviews [37,38]. In essence, barrier methods are well suited for the well-motivated couple, but when an increased risk of user's failure can be predicted, intrauterine devices or combined oral contraceptives may be the only acceptable reversible alternative. Intrauterine devices are very efficient and without metabolic side effects and can be used on the same indications and with the same reservations as in nondiabetic women. Intrauterine devices are therefore well suited for women with diabetes, especially parous women.

Combined oral contraceptives are widely used in the general population and short-term studies support low dose combined oral contraceptives prescription in type 1 diabetic women. These studies indicate that the changes in insulin sensitivity, glucose tolerance, lipid metabolism, and the coagulation/thrombotic system are very similar to the findings in healthy women and do not appear to be of clinical significance [37]. Whether prescription of combined oral contraceptives influence the risk of microvascular complications is only sparsely investigated [38].

Due to a possible increased risk of vascular disease, combined oral contraceptives should be restricted to women below 35 years without evidence of vascular complications who have no other risk factors. Progestin-only pills can in most cases be used as in women without diabetes and will therefore often be a good choice for women with contraindications for combined oral contraceptives.

Theoretically, there is no difference in the methods available to diabetic and nondiabetic women, but the state of disease alters the risk–benefit ratio that is normally taken into consideration when contraceptive advice is given [37–39]. It is therefore important that the woman/couple have a thorough discussion with their physician about the pros and cons of the different methods, as individual considerations should be balanced with the general recommendations in each particular case.

References

1. Weiss PA, Kainer F, Purstner P, Zehetleitner G, Huttner U, Haas J. Anti-insulin antibodies and birthweight in pregnancies complicated by diabetes. Early Hum Dev 1998;53:145–154.
2. Heise T, Heinemann L: Rapid and long-acting analogues as an approach to improve insulin therapy: An evidence-based medicine assessment. Curr Pharm Des 2001;7:1303–1325.
3. Persson B, Swahn ML, Hjertberg R, Hanson U, Nord E, Nordlander E, Hansson LO: Insulin lispro therapy in pregnancies complicated by type 1 diabetes mellitus. Diabetes Res Clin Pract 2002;58:115–121.
4. Wyatt JW, Frias JL, Hoyme HE, Jovanovic L, Kaaja R, Brown F, Garg S, Lee-Parritz A, Seely EW, Kerr L, Mattoo V, Tan M, IONS study group. Congenital anomaly rate in offspring of mothers with diabetes treated with insulin lispro during pregnancy. Diabet Med. 2005;22(6):803–807.
5. Kitzmiller JL, Main E, Ward B, Theiss T, Petereson DL: Insulin lispro and the development of proliferative diabetic retinopathy during pregnancy (Letter). Diabetes Care 1999;22:874–876.
6. Looukovaara S, Immonen I, Teramo KA, Kaaja R. Progression of retinopathy during pregnancy in type 1 diabetic women treated with insulin lispro. Diabetes Care 2003;26:1193–1198.

7. Jovanovic L, Ilic S, Petitt DJ, Hugo K, Gutierrez M, Browsher RR, Bastyr EJ: Metabolic and immunologic effects of insulin lispro in gestational diabetes. Diabetes Care 1999;22:1422–1427.
8. Elisabeth R. Mathiesen, Brendan Kinsley, Stephanie A. Amiel, Simon Heller, David McCance, Santiago Duran, Shannon Bellaire, Anne Raben on behalf of the Insulin Aspart Pregnancy Study Group: Maternal Glycemic Control and Hypoglycemia in Type 1 Diabetic Pregnancy: A randomized trial of insulin aspart versus human insulin in 322 pregnant women. Diabetes Care 30:771–776.
9. David McCance D, Damm P, Mathiesen ER, Kaaja K, Dunne F, Hod M, Jensen LE, Mersebach H. No increase in insulin antibodies and no clear evidence of transfer of insulin aspart across the placenta in pregnant women with type 1 diabetes. Abstrakt ADA 2007.
10. Kurtzhals P, Schaffer L, Sorensen A, Kristensen C, Jonassen I, Schmid C, Trub T: Correlations of receptor binding and metabolic and mitogenic potencies of insulin analogs designed for clinical use. Diabetes 2000;49:999–1005.
11. Woolderink JM, van Loon AJ, Storms F, de Heide L, Hoogenberg K. Use of insulin glargine during pregnancy in seven type 1 diabetic women. Diabetes Care 2006;29:471–472.
12. Slocum JM, Soso MEB: Use of antidiabetic agents in pregnancy: Current practise and controversy. J Perinat Neonatal Nurs 2002:16:40–53.
13. Elliot B, Langer O, Schenker S, Johnson RF. Insignificant transfer of glyburide occurs across the human placenta. Am J Obest Gynecol 1991;165:807–812.
14. Langer O, Conway DL, Berkus M, Xenakis EMJ, Gonsales O. A comparison of glyburide and insulin in women with gestationel diabetes mellitus. et al. NEJM 2000;343:1135–1138.
15. Vanky E et al. Placental passage of metformin in women with polycystic ovary syndrome. Fertil Steril. 2005;83:1575–1578.
16. Vandermolen DT, Ratts VS, Evans WS, Stovall DW, Kauma SW, Nestler JE. Metformin increases the ovulatory rate and pregnancy rate from clomiphene citrate in patients with polycystic ovary syndrome who are resistant to clomiphene citrate alone. Fertil Steril 2001;75:310–315.
17. Lilja AE, Mathiesen ER. Polycystic ovary syndrome and metformin in pregnancy. Acta Obstetrica et Gynaecologica. 2006;85:861–868.
18. Coetzee EJ, Jackson WPU. Metformin in management of pregnant insulin dependent diabetics. Diabetologia 1979;16:241–245.
19. Hellmuth E, Damm P, Molsted-Pedersen L. Oral hypoglycemic agents in 118 diabetic pregnancies. Diabetic Medicine 2000;17:507–511.
20. Hale TW, Kristensen JH, Hackett LP, Kohan R, Ilett KF: Transfer of metformin into human milk. Diabetologia 2002:45:1504–1514.
21. Shotan A, Widerhorn J, Hurst A, Elkayam U. Risks of angiotensin-converting enzyme inhibition during pregnancy: experimental and clinical evidence, potential mechanisms, and recommendations for use. Am J Med 1994;96:451–456.
22. Alwan S, Polifka JE, Friedman JM: Angiotensin II receptor antagonist treatment during pregnancy. Birth Defects Res A Clin Mol Teratol. 2005;73:123–130.
23. Cooper WO, Hernandez-Diaz S, Arbogast PG, Dudley JA, Dyer S, Gideon PS, Hall K, Ray WA: Major congenital malformations after first-trimester exposure to ACE inhibitors. N Engl J Med 2006; 354:2443–2451.
24. Hod M, van Dijk DJ, Karp M, Weintraub N, Rabinerson D, Bar J, Peled Y, Erman A, Boner G, Ovadia J. Diabetic nephropathy and pregnancy: the effect of ACE inhibitors prior to pregnancy on fetomaternal outcome. Nephrol Dial Transplant 1995;10:2328–2333.
25. Nielsen LR, Muller C, Damm P, Mathiesen ER. Reduced prevalence of preterm delivery in women with diabetes type 1 and microalbuminuria – possible effect of early antihypertensive treatment during pregnancy. Diabetic Medicine 2006;23:426–431.
26. National High Blood Pressure Education Program. National Institutes of Health Publication No. 00–3029. Revised 2000.
27. Khandelwai M, Kumanova M, Gaughan JP, Reece EA: Role of diltiazem in pregnant women with chronic renal disease. J Matern Fetal Neonatal Med 2002;12:408–412.
28. Devlin RG, Fleiss PM. Captopril in human blood and breastmilk. J Clin Pharmacol 1981;21:110–113.
29. Rush JE, Snyder DL, Barrish A, Hichens M: Comment on Huttunen K, Gronhagen-Riska C and Fyhrquist F, 1989. Enalapril treatment of a nursing mother with slightly impaired renal function. Clin Nephrol 31: 278. Clin Nephrol 1991;35:234.
30. Statins: beware during pregnancy. Prescrire Int. 2006;15:18–19.
31. Ruano R, Fontes RS, Zugiab M: Prevention of preeclampsia with low-dose aspirin – a systematic review and meta-analysis of the main randomized controlled trials. Clinics. 2005;60:407–414.
32. Norgard B, Puho E, Czeizel AE, Skriver MV, Sorensen HT. Aspirin use during early pregnancy and the risk of congenital abnormalities: a population-based case-control study: Am J Obstet Gynecol 2005;192:922–923.
33. Mathiesen ER, Christensen AB, Hellmuth E, Horness P, Stage E, Damm P. Insulin dose during glucocorticoid treatment for foetal lung maturation in diabetic pregnancy - test of an algorithm. Acta Obstet Gynecol Scand 2002;81:835–839.

34. Worldwide Atosiban versus Beta-agonists Study Group. Effectiveness and safety of the oxytocin antagonist atosiban versus beta-adrenergic agonists in the treatment of preterm labour. The Worldwide Atosiban versus Beta-agonists Study Group. BJOG 2001;108:133–142.
35. Ray JG, Vermeulen MJ, Meier C, Wyatt PR: Risk of congenital anomalies detected during antenatal serum screening in women with pregestational diabetes. QJM 2004;97:651–653.
36. Wentzel P, Gareskog M, Eriksson UJ: Folic acid supplementation diminishes diabetes- and glucose-induced dysmorphogenesis in rat embryos in vivo and in vitro. Diabetes 2005;54:546–553.
37. Damm P, Mathiesen E, Clausen TD, Pedersen KR. Contraception for women with diabetes mellitus. Metabolic Syndrome and Related Disorders 2005;3: 244–249.
38. Damm P, Mathiesen ER, Petersen KR, Kjos S. Contraception after GDM. Diabetes Care in press 2007.
39. World Health Organisation. Medical eligibility criteria for contraceptive use. 3rd Edition WHO, Geneva, Switzerland 2004.

24
Pharmacotherapy of Diabetic Retinopathy

Toke Bek

Keywords: Ocular pharmacotherapy, aldose reductase inhibitors, PKC inhibitors, VEGF inhibitors, ACE inhibitors, somatostatin analogues, intravitreal steroids.

Introduction

Retinal photocoagulation is the current standard for the treatment of diabetic retinopathy. The treatment destroys the diseased retina in the extrafoveal areas with the purpose of preventing the disease from reaching the visual axis and reduce central vision. However, the destruction of the retina in extrafoveal areas imposes adverse effects such as blurring of vision, constriction of the visual field, and impaired dark adaptation. Consequently, during the past years, considerable efforts have been invested in developing treatment modalities with less or no adverse effects based on pharmacological intervention.

Generally, pharmacological treatment of diseases in the eye is limited by special pharmacokinetic properties inherent in the anatomy of the eye. Diseases in the anterior segment of the eye are predominantly treated by local application of the active compound in the conjunctiva. These drugs will diffuse into the eye to affect the vitreous body and the retina, but for practical purposes this mode of administration is less suitable for diseases in the posterior segment of the eye. The vitreous body is avascular, which implies that the treatment of diseases in and around this structure depends on intravitreal injection of the active compound. On the contrary, the retina is richly vascularized, but the access to this structure of drugs administered through the systemic circulation is limited by a tight barrier system. In cases where the drug cannot pass this barrier system or when the active compound undergoes degradation in the systemic circulation, it is possible to obtain a pharmacological effect from the anterior aspect of the retina by diffusion from the vitreous body after intravitreal injection of the compound. Therefore, the preferred route of administration for drugs to treat diabetic retinopathy will depend on the bioavailability of the drug and its profile of systemic adverse effects.

Basic Pathophysiology

Pharmacological intervention on diabetic retinopathy is aimed at blocking specific stages of the disease development. These stages can be appropriately described on the basis of a modification of Michaelson's hypothesis [1] for the pathophysiology of diabetic retinopathy (Fig. 1). According to this working hypothesis, the metabolic dysregulation in diabetic retinopathy induces disturbances in retinal perfusion. These disturbances result in ischemia in the retinal periphery and hyperperfusion in the central retina. The peripheral ischemia will initiate the release of growth factors that diffuse to the nearest venule with an angiogenic potential. This initiates the proliferation of new vessels that will later result in vitreous hemorrhage or retinal detachment. The central hyperperfusion leads to retinal edema with a direct destructive effect on the retinal neurons and a consequent loss of central vision. In this chapter, this hypothesis will be used as frame of reference

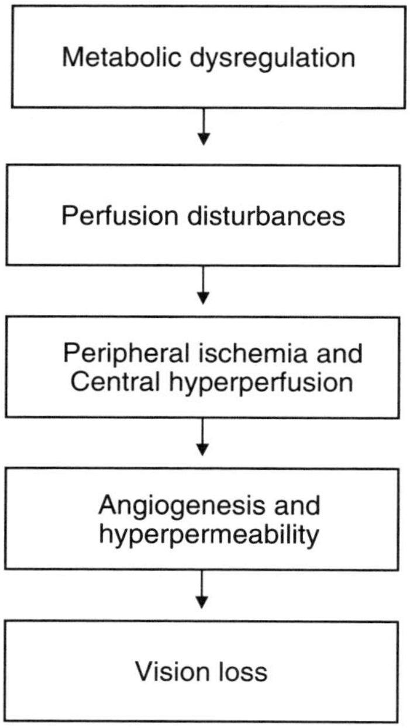

FIG. 1. A modified scheme of Michaelson's hypothesis for the development of vision loss secondary to diabetic retinopathy.

to structure the account of finished and ongoing trials of pharmacological intervention to treat diabetic retinopathy.

Therapeutic Approaches

Intervention on Metabolic Dysregulation

A number of hypotheses have been proposed to explain how metabolic dysregulation in diabetic patients may lead to the development of diabetic retinopathy. Several of these hypotheses have been tested in pharmacological intervention studies.

Aldose Reductase Inhibition

It has been suggested that the key element in the development of diabetic retinopathy is metabolism of glucose by other pathways than the normal route through glycolysis. This might include an involvement of aldose reductase with a consequent accumulation of sorbitol to be deposited in the intercellular matrix of the tissues. The significance of this pathway is supported by the fact that activation of aldose reductase in experimental animals fed on a diet enriched with galactose leads to retinal changes that resemble the changes observed in clinical diabetic retinopathy. Additionally, the aldose reductase enzyme is present in high concentrations in the retinal vascular pericytes, which are one of the first cell types lost in diabetic retinopathy. A number of studies on animal models and smaller clinical intervention studies have supported the assumption that the aldose reductase inhibitor sorbinil was able to halt the development of diabetic retinopathy. On the basis of this preliminary data, a larger prospective randomized study was carried out, but this study was unable to show an effect of 2 years treatment with this drug [2]. Therefore, the interest for further investigation of this treatment modality has tapered considerably.

Protein Kinase C Inhibitors

A number of intracellular messenger molecules, including protein kinase C (PKC), are involved in the general cellular metabolism. PKC constitutes a group of enzymes with a number of subtypes, including PKCβ1 and PKCβ2 that are specific for Langerhans' cells in the pancreas and cells in the nervous system including the retina. PKCβ is activated by hyperglycemia with a consequent destructive effect on the retinal blood vessels [3]. This activation involves several pathways, including the binding of diacyl glycerol, activation of intracellular calcium, excessive production of superoxide, and production of advanced glycosylated end products. The resulting increase in the activity of PKCβ leads to changes in muscle contractility, thickening of the vascular basement membranes, and retinal neovascularization [4]. Since these changes are also central pathophysiological manifestations of diabetic retinopathy, the increased activity of PKCβ secondary to hyperglycemia has been linked to the development of diabetic retinopathy.

Ruboxistaurin (LY333531) mesylate is a synthetic compound with a specific inhibitory effect on the PKCβ isoforms 1 and 2 in the pancreas and the retina. In animal studies, the compound has been shown to have a stabilizing effect on retinal perfusion, to reduce the permeability of retinal vessels, and to block the neovascular response in retinal vessels during retinal ischemia [5]. Ruboxistaurin is a pro-drug which is administered as tablets and is metabolized to the active compound in the liver. The compound has not been shown to have any appreciable adverse effects, but simultaneous use of the antifungal compound ketokonazol is contraindicated since this compound inhibits the formation of the active metabolite with a consequent systemic accumulation of ruboxistaurin.

At present three larger prospective randomized clinical trials of the effect of ruboxistaurin on diabetic retinopathy have been carried out. The first study, PKC-DMES (PKC-Diabetic Macular Edema Study), carried out on patients with mild to moderate diabetic retinopathy with diabetic macular edema showed no significant effect of the drug on visual acuity or on progression of the macular edema over 2½ years [6]. A subsequent study, PKC-DRS (PKC-Diabetic Retinopathy Study), performed on patients with moderately severe and very severe retinopathy showed a similar negative effect on the development of diabetic maculopathy and treatment requiring changes over a period of 3 years, but the study showed a significant delay in the development of visual loss [7]. In these studies, the effects of different arms administering respectively 4, 8, 16, and 32 mg per day indicated a dose-dependent effect, and suggested the initiation of a larger study using the highest of the tested doses. Consequently, in a third study, PKC-DRS2 patients were randomized to 32 mg Ruboxistaurin orally once daily for 36 months. This study showed significantly fewer cases developing visual loss in the treatment group (5.5%) as compared with the placebo group (9.1%), and the difference was significant after 12 months. In addition to this, significantly fewer patients in the treatment group than in the placebo group experienced that the macular edema approached the fovea or developed into laser requiring retinopathy [8]. These findings have prompted the initiation of other intervention studies focusing on the effect of ruboxistaurin on diabetic retinal edema. The results of these studies are awaited with interest, and altogether there is promising evidence that ruboxistaurin may become a central drug for the treatment of diabetic retinopathy in the future.

Perfusion Disturbances

ACE Inhibitors

Several studies have demonstrated a relation between increased blood pressure and the development of diabetic retinopathy [9,10]. This relation is assumed to be a consequence of impaired autoregulation of the retinal blood vessels so that increases in the systemic blood pressure are transmitted to the capillary network to exert damage there. Conversely, a reduction of the blood pressure will reduce the hydrostatic pressure in the capillaries and prevent the development of retinopathy lesions. Evidence suggests that especially the use of ACE inhibitors has a positive effect on the barrier function in the retinal capillaries and reduces diabetic retinopathy in a more pronounced manner than can be explained from the blood pressure lowering effect alone [11]. The background for this additional effect of ACE inhibitors is at present unknown, but may be linked to an observed activity of the renin–angiotensin system in the retina.

Peripheral Ischemia and Central Hyperperfusion

Inhibitors of the Thrombocyte Aggregation

One of the hypotheses for the development of vascular occlusion that precedes proliferative diabetic retinopathy is that disturbances in the thrombocyte aggregation lead to leukostasis and formation of microthrombosis in the retinal capillaries. Consequently, attention has been focused at treating diabetic retinopathy with inhibitors of thrombocyte aggregation. However, a prospective study has shown that acetyl salicylic acid does not reduce the development of diabetic retinopathy. Additionally, this treatment does not increase the risk of developing complications such as vitreous hemorrhage. This is important evidence since inhibitors of thrombocyte aggregation are often used to reduce the risk of the development of the macrovascular complications of the disease [12].

Angiogenesis and the Formation of Central Edema

Somatostatin Analogues

More than 50 years ago, a patient was observed with severe proliferative diabetic retinopathy that regressed totally after infarction of the hypophysis while giving birth [13]. This stimulated the hypothesis that there might be a relation between the hormone production in the pituitary gland notably growth hormone, and the development of diabetic retinopathy. The hypothesis was tested in clinical trials using hypophysectomy to treat diabetic retinopathy, but the trials were discontinued because of the severe systemic adverse effects. Subsequently, the working hypothesis has been tested by pharmacological inhibition of the effect of growth hormone. In the retina, this effect is mediated through growth factors such as IGF-I, which has been shown to be present in increased concentrations in the retina and the vitreous body of diabetic patients. Consequently, clinical trials have been carried out with the aim of elucidating the significance of both growth hormone and various growth factors for the development of diabetic retinopathy.

The most prominent clinical trials have tested the growth hormone inhibitor octreotide, which is a ligand to the somatostatin receptor. As a precondition for its use in clinical practise, this synthetic compound has been designed to have a half-life that is much longer than that of native somatostatin. Octreotide has the significant disadvantage of requiring intramuscular administration. Additionally, many patients experience gastrointestinal adverse effects such as diarrhea, and the treatment needs to be administered under surveillance of endocrinological expertise since the insulin requirement may change. Octreotide inhibits the proliferation of vascular endothelial cells stimulated by the growth factors VEGF, IGF, and bFGF during hypoxia in vitro [14]. In smaller intervention series in the earlier stages of diabetic retinopathy, no effect of the drug has been found on the development of diabetic retinopathy, whereas other clinical observations indicate that treatment with octreotide to patients with advanced diabetic retinopathy may reduce the development of diabetic retinopathy, the number of late complications, and may improve visual acuity [15,16]. In a recent unpublished prospective randomized intervention study on patients with moderate to advanced nonproliferative diabetic retinopathy, the effect of the drug was not found to be sufficiently convincing to justify further development at the moment.

Angiostatins

VEGF is a growth factor that increases the permeability of retinal vessels and stimulates the proliferation of vascular endothelial cells in proliferative diabetic retinopathy. VEGF is synthesized as several isoforms with different molecular lengths. This synthesis is stimulated by IGF-I [17] and by retinal ischemia, and the intraocular concentration of VEGF has been found to be increased in proliferative diabetic retinopathy.

During the recent years, several new compounds have been developed that inhibit the effect of VEGF in the eye. The compound pegaptanib (Macugen) is a nucleotide (aptamer) that binds specifically to the VEGF-165 isoform, whereas ranibizumab (Lucentis) consists of FAB fragments of immunoglobulin molecules with binding affinity against all VEGF isotypes. Additionally, the VEGF inhibitor bevacizumab (Avastin) registered for the treatment of gastrointestinal cancers has been used casuistically. The ocular use of these VEGF inhibitors has been initiated for the treatment of subretinal neovascularizations in exudative age-related macular degeneration, but clinical studies in both diabetic maculopathy and proliferative diabetic retinopathy are ongoing [18–20].

VEGF inhibitors are easily degraded in the systemic circulation. Consequently, direct injection of the compound into the vitreous body is required in order to achieve an effect on the retina. The pharmacokinetic properties of currently available VEGF inhibitors necessitate repetition of the treatment with 4–6-week intervals, but work is ongoing to achieve longer administration intervals or to develop alternative routes of administration in order to increase the interval between individual treatments. Intravitreal injections are accompanied with risks of provoking an acute increase in the intraocular pressure, risks of intraocular infection, and in the long run an increased risk of developing cataract. However, cataract operation is performed in advance in most type 2 diabetic patients since this condition is age related and is accelerated in patients with diabetes mellitus. Therefore, in spite of its novelty and potential complications, intravitreal injection of VEGF inhibitors appears to have a promising potential for the treatment of diabetic retinopathy in the future.

Intravitreal Steroids

Intravitreously administered steroids have been used for decades for treating intraocular inflammation and retinal edema. However, during the recent years, increased attention has also been focused on the potential of this treatment to reduce diabetic macular edema. The effect is assumed to be due to a direct or an indirect restoration of the blood retina barrier to reduce the increased permeability observed in the retinal capillaries in diabetic retinopathy. The positive effect of the treatment requires that the drug is applied locally to allow it to diffuse to the retina in a high concentration, an effect that can be achieved both by intravitreal and peribulbar injection. Several steroid drugs have been used [21]. The initial treatments were carried out using dexamethason, but during the recent years intravitreal injection of triamcinolone has received increased focus. The positive effect of the treatment has been shown in a number of case series, but the effect has also been documented in prospective randomized studies with a follow-up time of up to 1 year. Administration of 4 mg triamcinolone is effective in reducing the diabetic macular edema for approximately 6 months, but thereafter the macular edema often recurs. A major drawback of the treatment is that the effect is reduced when the injections are repeated. Since the treatment is not curative and the adverse effects accumulate for each treatment session, the treatment should be restricted to transient edema or be used as a supplement to other treatment modalities. Thus, it has been suggested to restrict the use intravitreal injection of steroids to cases of diffuse diabetic macular edema that respond poorly to retinal laser photocoagulation.

Summary

A number of new pharmacological treatment options for diabetic retinopathy are presently under investigation to replace the currently used retinal photocoagulation. These new treatments differ from the existing by interfering with specific and well-described steps in the pathophysiology of the disease. The major challenge for the future is to improve visual prognosis by achieving at least the same positive effect as can be achieved with retinal photocoagulation, but at the same time avoid the adverse effects of this treatment. These goals may potentially be reached with new treatment modalities based on peroral intake of drugs with no systemic adverse effects. The drugs that depend on, for example, intravitreous injection should have additional effects that balance the risks of this invasive route of administration. The treatment of diabetic retinopathy is a dynamic field undergoing immense development. The current evidence points at several promising pharmacological treatments for future improvement of the visual prognosis for patients with diabetic retinopathy.

References

1. Michaelson JC. Retinal circulation in man and animals (Thomas, Springfield, Illinois, 1954) 1–146.
2. Sorbinil Retinopathy Trial Research Group. A randomozed trial of sorbinil, an aldose reductase inhibitor, in diabetic retinopathy. Arch Ophthalmol 1990;108(9):1234–1244.
3. Tomlinson DR. Mitogen-activated protein kinases as glycose transducers for diabetic complications. Diabetologia 1999;42:1271–1281.
4. Koya D and King GL. Protein Kinase C Activation and the development of diabetic complications. Diabetes 1998;47:859–866.
5. Danis RP, Bingaman DP, Jirousek M et al. Inhibition of intraocular neovascularisation caused by retinal ischemia in pigs by af PKC β inhibition with LY333531. Invest Ophthalmol Vis Sci 1998;39:171–179.
6. Aiello LP. Medical and pharmacologic treatment of diabetic macular oedema. AAO Subspecialty Day, Anaheim CA, November 15, —vol. 18, 2003.
7. The PKC-DRS study group. The effect of ruboxistaurin on visual loss in patients with moderately severe to very severe nonproliferative diabetic retinopathy: initial results of the protein kinase C beta inhibitor diabetic retinopathy study (PKC-DRS) multicenter randomized clinical trial. Diabetes 2005;54:2188–2197.
8. PKC-DRS2 Group. Effect of Ruboxistaurin on visual loss in patients with diabetic retinopathy. Ophthalmology 2006;113:2221–2230.
9. Diabetes Control and Complications Trial Research Group. Progression of retinopathy with intensive versus conventional treatment in the Diabetes Control and Complications Trial. Ophthalmology 1995;102(4):647–661.
10. UKPD Study Group 38. Tight blood pressure control and risk of macrovascular and microvascular complications in type 2 diabetes. Brit M J 1998;317(7160):703–712.
11. Wilkinson-Berka JL. Diabetes and retinal vascular disorders: role of the rennin angiotensin system. Expert Rev Mol Med 2004;6:1–18.
12. ETDRS Research Group. Effects of aspirin treatment on diabetic retinopathy. ETDRS Report No 8. Ophthalmology 1991;98(5):757–765.
13. Poulsen J. The Houssay phenomenon in man: recovery from retinopathy in a case of diabetes with Simmond's disease. Diabetes 1953;2:7–1284,722–733.
14. Baldysiak-Figiel A, Lang GK, Kampmeier J et al. Octreotide prevents growth factor-induced proliferation

of bovine retinal endothelial cells under hypoxia. J Endocrin. 2004;180:417–424.
15. Boehm BO, Lang GK, Jehle PM et al. Octreotide reduces vitreous hemorrhage and loss of visual acuity risk in patients with high-risk proliferative diabetic retinopathy. Horm Met Res. 2001;33: 300–306.
16. Grant MB, Mames RN, Fitzgerald C et al. The efficacy of octreotide in the therapy of severe nonproliferative diabetic and early proliferative diabetic retinopathy. Diabetes Care 2000;23:504–509.
17. Poulaki V, Joussen AM, Mitsiades N et al. Insulin-like growth factor-I plays a pathogenic role in diabetic retinopathy. Am J Pathol 2004;165:457–469.
18. Cunningham ET Jr, Adamis AO, Altaweel M et al. Macugen Diabetic Retinopathy Study Group. A phase II randomized double-masked trial of pegaptanib, an anti-vascular endothelial growth factor aptamer for diabetic macular edema. Ophthalmology 2005;112(10):1747–1757.
19. Chun DW, Heier JS, Topping TM et al. A pilot study of multiple intravitreal injections of ranibizumab in patients with center-involving clinically significant macular edema. Ophthalmology 2006;113(10):1706–1712.
20. Avery RL, Pearlman J, Pieramici DJ et al. Intravitreal bevacizumab (Avastin) in the treatment of proliferative diabetic retinopathy. Ophthalmology 2006;113(10):1695–1705.e6.
21. Sivaprasad S, McCluskey P, Lightman S. Intravitreal steroids in the management of macular oedema. Acta Ophthalmol Scand 2006;84(6):722–733.

25
Pharmacotherapy in Diabetic Sexual Dysfunction

Niels Ejskjaer

Introduction

Since the dawn of times the sexual act has been paramount to mankind. First of all, obviously to secure the propagation of generations and secondly as a remedy for physical and psychological well-being. Everybody, women and men, have the right to a well-functioning sexual life according to a WHO (World Health Organisation) resolution from 1995. However, quite naturally, expectations vary from one person to the next and throughout the course of a lifetime. The feeling of sexual inadequacy may be a reason for problems individually and in relationships. As many as 10–15% of all patients attending general practice suffer sexual dysfunction to such a degree that qualified advice and treatment are needed. It is often very difficult for patients to "bring up the topic", and perhaps more worryingly, equally so for the clinician. Therefore, many suffer in silence and remain untreated resulting in reduced quality of life and negative impact on relationships.

People with diabetes, type 1 and 2, are at higher risk than others of developing sexual problems. This is true for both women and men. Not many decades ago it was generally assumed that erectile dysfunction in men was of a psychogenic nature in perhaps 90% of all cases and organic in 10%. After the appearance of efficient pharmacotherapy for this condition it has become obvious that quite the opposite is true. There is no efficient pharmacotherapy available for women with diabetes and it is generally acknowledged that about 90% of all cases are of a psychogenic nature. This statement may be challenged over the coming years.

A number of studies report prevalence figures of erectile dysfunction of 50% or more in type 2 diabetic men above 50 years of age. Probably comparable figures may be true for women with diabetes. Diabetes, type 1 and 2, remains the most common cause of sexual dysfunction and it is generally acknowledged that these problems are two or three times as common as in the background population.

Sexual problems among diabetic patients are considerably better described for men than women. Over the last 35 years hundreds of publications on male sexual problems have become available, whereas relatively few studies have been published on female sexual dysfunction. Much along the same line most therapeutic possibilities have been directed towards diabetic men with erectile dysfunction, whereas only very few or practically no therapies have been developed for diabetic women with sexual problems. Over the last years more focus has been placed on female sexual problems and research efforts in developing efficient drugs have been intensified, undoubtedly driven by considerable commercial interests, but also as recognition of the importance of a well-functioning sexual life in both men and women with diabetes.

Background

Public interest in male erectile dysfunction was briskly awakened in 1998 with the media coverage of the release of *sildenafil citrate* (Viagra) for the treatment of male erectile dysfunction. Following the development of *sildenafil citrate* two drugs with the same therapeutic indication were developed, *tadalafil* (Cialis) and *vardenafil* (Levitra). Thus there are currently three drugs on the market for the treatment of male erectile dysfunction. All in all it has been a positive effect that more interest is directed towards this often forgotten, but very common late complication of diabetes, and more men are now aware of their condition and seek treatment. All this attention to male problems has resulted in increased awareness to female problems. Physiology in men and women is very similar and so are anatomic structures, although different in proportions. This has led to the assumption that the above-mentioned drugs might be efficient in women also. *Sildenafil* and *tadalafil* have been shown to increase genital blood flow, lubrication and sensitivity in diabetic women. On the other hand libido, mental arousal and sexual satisfaction are unchanged and further development for female use is not ongoing. However, it is likely that particularly diabetic women with considerable microangiopathy and neuropathy may benefit. Some case reports support this view. Currently there is no efficient pharmacotherapy available for diabetic women with sexual problems.

As mentioned physiology and anatomy may be similar in men and women, whereas pathophysiology and mechanisms necessary for achieving sexual satisfaction are not.

Diabetes may result in a number of sexual problems in men: reduced libido, premature ejaculation and erectile dysfunction. Diabetes may result in a number of sexual problems in women: reduced or absent libido, problems with arousal, absence of orgasms and genital pain. Generally, diabetic sexual problems in women are of a more complex and multifactorial nature than that of men and is not well described and understood.

Definitions and Physiology

Erectile dysfunction in men is defined as the inability over a minimum of 3 months to achieve and maintain an erection sufficient for sexual intercourse. The mechanism resulting in an erection is complex and depends on a number of factors. By sexual stimulation (smells, sounds, visual inputs, tactile sensations or sexual thoughts) the brain generates signals, primarily from the hypothalamus via the medulla and nerve tracts to the penis resulting in increased blood flow and relaxation of smooth muscle cells in the penis. The latter obstructs venous return of blood resulting in the erection. The most important signal molecule is nitrogen oxide (NO), which is released from nerve endings in the penis and endothelial cells in the cavernous tissue. The erection mechanism is thus dependent upon a well-functioning blood flow and nervous system.

Female sexual dysfunction is defined as "a sexual problem", where the woman is bothered by her condition. This diagnose differs much from the above, which is very clear and objective, whereas this is subjective and may vary greatly from one woman to the other. It is a composite definition consisting of problems regarding libido, sexual aversion, arousal, orgasm and pain. Anyone of these may lead to the diagnosis of female sexual dysfunction. Equally to men, women depend on vasculature and nervous tissue for physiological function.

Pathogenesis

The debut of sexual dysfunction in diabetes occurs after many years of diabetes. This is highlighted by the striking finding that erectile dysfunction may lead to the diagnosis of type 2 diabetes. Autonomic neuropathy and microangiopathy are both important, but their relative relationship is not known. Metabolic factors such as glycaemic control and lipid metabolism contribute as well as cardiovascular disease, hypertension and obesity. A common denominator is *endothelial dysfunction*, which is a common condition in diabetes and forms the basis for pharmacological treatment. Prophylactic and therapeutic pharmacotherapy is mandatory for most diabetics, but unfortunately sometimes may provoke sexual dysfunction, perhaps particularly so in predisposed individuals. It is obvious that organically based sexual dysfunction may result in psychogenic disturbances further complicating the condition. Purely psychogenic cases tend to evolve and resolve promptly, whereas organic conditions are of more slow onset and remains a chronic condition. A number of other causes could be mentioned. Low testosterone levels in men, oestrogen deficiency in women, stress, alcohol and drug abuse, surgery, endocrine and systemic diseases and cancer are among these.

Epidemiology and Examination

Sexual dysfunction increases in the background population with increasing age. Studies have shown that in men below 40 years of age the prevalence is 1–9%, in 40–59 year olds 20–30% and for the 60–69 year olds 40–50% with a steep increase in the above 70-year olds up to 75%. A number of studies have shown that diabetes significantly increases the risk of sexual dysfunction and generally any person with diabetes has a risk of 35–75% of developing sexual dysfunction. This condition arises earlier in the diabetic person than in the non-diabetic and is most often promoted by the co-existence of late complications of diabetes. There is a very close association to cardiovascular disease and type 2 diabetic patients are therefore at high risk. Sexual problems may even lead to the diagnosis of cardiovascular disease and type 2 diabetes. The above is probably true for women with diabetes as also. In a Swedish survey 47% of women between 18 and 74 years of age had one or several sexual problems and between 60% and 80% were not satisfied with their sex life. There is not much evidence on the impact of diabetes on female sexual function, but it is safe to say that women with diabetes more commonly suffer sexual problems than women without diabetes.

It is important to exclude other reasons for sexual dysfunction than diabetes. Taking a thorough patient history is most important and it is always helpful to include the partner. Addressing sexual issues specifically helps identifying the nature of the problem and thereby aids one in performing a full clinical examination. A full assessment of late complications is a natural part, as is a neurological examination. Pelvic and genital examinations should always be performed. Other endocrine diseases, anaemia and organ-specific conditions can be excluded by a full biochemical screening.

Therapeutic Approaches and Pharmacotherapy

Treatment of diabetic sexual problems is to a large extent the same for women and men and for most clinicians follow a logics strategy. Applying lifestyle measures (physical activity, weight loss, diet, reducing alcohol consumption and cessation of tobacco smoking) in parallel to optimising glycaemic control, cholesterol levels and lipid profiles is often the first step. Possible side effects of often extensive medication of a number of diabetes-related conditions are evaluated and suspected drugs should be exchanged for others or stopped if possible. Antihypertensive drugs are believed to be particularly harmful. These measures are often not sufficient and pharmacotherapy is introduced. A vacuum apparatus is used by a few couples. It evokes erection during vacuum applied to the penis and a rubber ring is put on the root of the penis to maintain the erection. It may be used by men where all other treatment has failed and surgery is not indicated. Only rarely is surgical correction of anatomical abnormalities indicated, but conditions in men such as penile deviation, Peyronie's disease and venous leakage may need intervention. Surgery in women is not indicated apart perhaps from correction of post-surgical conditions. Implantation of penile prostheses is a highly specialised procedure and should only be used as an ultimatively last resort, when the patient suffers irrevocable damage to vasculature and nervous tissue and when other treatments have been without success. Any surgical treatment in diabetic patients bear an increased risk of infection, which always must be taken into consideration. Psychosocial therapy is sometimes needed and it is helpful to include the partner.

For thousands of years pharmacotherapy has been the mainstay in treating sexual problems in men with little or no attention pointed towards the problems of women. Ironically enough, the first efficient tablet treatment was developed only some years ago in 1998.

Topical treatment applied as an injection into the penis of vasoactive substances, such as prostaglandin E (*alprostadil*) has been available for years and is still used by a few patients. It was only a few years ago the only very efficient treatment. The injection results in an erection independent of sexual stimulation and libido. The treatment is efficient in up to 70% of patients and can be applied as a test of ability, psychogenic factors not influencing the outcome. Pain as a result of the injection is common, priapismus (prolonged erection) occurs, fibrous degeneration at injection sites may develop after repetitive injections.

However efficient the treatment is, patients find it difficult to accept due to the form of administration. If oral treatment fails this may be a possibility to some patients. Prostaglandin E (*alprostadil*) may also be administered by application in the urethra of men in the form of a pellet that resolves and the active compound diffuses to the cavernosae. This treatment is less efficient and side effects are dominated by pain in the urethra.

Apomorphine is administered sublingually and affects cerebral dopaminerge areas. This aids sexual stimulation and erection. Side effects comprise nausea, yawning and tiredness. The product has not found extensive use and efficiency parameters are a matter of discussion. *Yohimbin* is taken over 2–3 months and effect evolves after 2–3 weeks of treatment. This drug is a vasodilator with general effects and drops in blood pressure is the predominant side effect. These two drugs are not widely used after the appearance of efficient oral treatment with little or no side effects.

Sildenafil (Viagra), *Tadalafil* (Cialis) and *Vardenafil* (Levitra) have revolutionised treatment of male erectile dysfunction and failed to do so in female sexual dysfunction, where it is only extremely rarely efficient. The drug is efficient in about 50% of treated diabetic men. The mode of action is near the physiological, as effect depends on libido and some erectile function, which is supported by diminishing degradation of *nitrogen oxide* (NO). Side effects are scarce in most patients and varies between the different tablets (headache, flushing, dyspepsia, muscle pain). There is a clear contraindication for administering this drug to patients taking *nitrates* to control angina pectoris. This may lead to life threatening drops in blood pressure. The most substantial difference in mode of action is *Tadalafil* (Cialis), which is active for about 24 hours, whereas the others duration of action is about 5–6 hours. All three set on 25–45 min after ingestion, good clinical practice recommends minimal dosing to achieve treatment goals and thereby also minimizing side effects. Side effects are all self-limiting, but common, and varies from one drug to the next.

Efficient drugs as the above are not available for diabetic women with sexual problems. However, there are a number of symptom alleviating drugs, which may be useful in some cases. In postmenopausal women topical or systemic administration of *oestrogen* may resolve lubrication problems and in some cases have a positive effect on libido. Long-term side effects on cardiovasculature and cancer must be considered. *Testosterone* (DHEA) is being administered in some countries to treat women with reduced libido and a *testosterone-gel* has been approved in Europe for treatment of women prematurely postmenopausal due to surgical removal of their ovaries. The drug has not been studied in women with diabetes, but has been investigated in premenopausal women with normal levels of *oestrogen,* where testosterone is administered until high in the reference interval for *free testosterone*. About 60% of women experience increased libido. There are a number of possible side effects not tolerable to women. The development of efficient pharmacological treatment for sexual problems in diabetic women is still pending.

Summary and Perspectives

Everybody has the right to a well-functioning sexual life according to the WHO (World Health Organisation, 1995), but unfortunately treatment options are limited, in spite of the introduction of efficient oral treatment for erectile dysfunction. Efficient treatment for women with diabetes does not exist and only inefficient symptom-relieving treatment can be offered the unfortunate.

Diabetes is rapidly increasing in prevalence, especially type 2 diabetes, and great efforts are needed to prevent the development of late complications including sexual dysfunction. Sexual dysfunction severely impacts quality of life in the affected, who are becoming younger and younger as the average age at time of diagnosis of type 2 diabetes is steadily lowered. This problem now affects a number of people in their fertile years, which certainly underlines the graveness and magnitude of this issue.

References

Fisher WA, Rosen RC, Eardley I, Niederberger C, Nadel A, Kaufman J, Sand M. The Multinational Men's Attitudes to Life Events and Sexuality (MALES) Study Phase II: understanding PDE5 inhibitor treatment seeking patterns, among men with erectile dysfunction. J Sex Med. 2004;1(2):150–160.

Kostis JB, Jackson G, Rosen R, Barrett-Connor E, Billups K, Burnett AL, Carson C 3rd, Cheitlin M, Debusk R, Fonseca V, Ganz P, Goldstein I, Guay A, Hatzichristou D, Hollander JE, Hutter A, Katz S, Kloner RA, Mittleman M, Montorsi F, Montorsi P, Nehra A, Sadovsky R, Shabsigh R. Sexual dysfunction and cardiac risk (the Second Princeton Consensus Conference). Am J Cardiol. 2005;96(12B):85M–93M.

McMahon CG, Abdo C, Incrocci L, Perelman M, Rowland D, Waldinger M, Xin ZC. Disorders of orgasm and ejaculation in men. J Sex Med. 2004;1(1):58–65.

Boulton AJ, Selam JL, Sweeney M, Ziegler D. Sildenafil Citrate for the treatment of erectile dysfunction in men with Type II diabetes mellitus. Diabetologia 2001;44(10):1296–1301.

Masters WH, and Johnson VE. Human sexual response. Boston, MA: Little; Brown; 1966.

Kaplan HS. The new sex therapy. New York: Brunner Mazel; 1974.

Goldstein I, Giraldi A, Kodigliu A, van Lunsen RH, Marson L, Nappi RE. Pfaus J, Salonia A, Traish A, Vardi Y. Physiology of female sexual function and pathophysiology of female sexual dysfunction. Lue T F, Basson R, Rosen R, Giuliano F, Khoury S, and Montorsi F. Sexual Medicine. Sexual dysfunctions in men and women. 2nd International Consultation on Sexual Dysfunctions. 2 ed. Paris: Health Publications; 2004, pp. 683–748.

Basson R, Weijmar Schultz WCM, Binik YM, Brotto L A, Eschenbach DA, Laan E, Utian WH, Wesselmann U, Lankveld Van J, Wyatt G, Leiblum S, Althof SE, Redmond G, Woman's sexual desire and arousal disorders and sexual pain. Lue TF, Basson R, Rosen R, Giuliano F, Khoury S, and Montorsi F. Sexual Medicine. Sexual dysfunctions in men and women. 2nd ed. Paris: Health Publications; 2004, pp. 851–990.

Basson R, Althof SE, Davis SR, Fugl-Meyer K, Goldstein I, Heiman J, Leiblum S, Meston C, Rosen R, Wagner G, Weijmar Schultz WCM, Summary of the Recommendations on Women's sexual Dysfunctions. Lue TF, Basson R, Rosen R, Giuliano F, Khoury S, and Montorsi F, Sexual Medicine. Sexual Dysfunctions in men and women. 2 ed. Paris: Health Publications; 2004, pp. 975–990.

Fugl-Meyer AR, and Fugl-Meyer KS, Sexual Disabilities, Problems and Satisfaction in 18–74 Year Old Swedes. Scand J Sexol 1999;2(2):79–97.

Enzlin P, Mathieu C, Van Den Bruel A, Vanderschueren D, and Demyttenaere K, Prevalence and Predictors of Sexual Dysfunction in Patients with Type 1 Diabetes. Diabetes Care 2003;26(2):409–414.

26
A Bone Perspective

Lars Rejnmark

Glitazones improve insulin sensitivity through the activation of the nuclear receptor, peroxisome proliferator-activated receptor-γ (PPAR-γ). In addition to sensitizing cells to insulin, the PPAR-γ may affect bone. Thus, an increasing body of evidence suggests that genetic mutations in the PPAR-γ as well as treatment with glitazones affect skeletal tissue.

Mechanisms

Although the exact mechanism by which glitazones may affect bone needs further clarification, in vitro studies have indicated that treatment may inhibit osteoblastogenesis. Osteoblasts and bone marrow adipocytes are derived from common mesenchymal progenitor stem cells [1], and treatment with glitazones may increase adipogenesis on the expense of osteoblasts, leading to bone loss [2,3]. In a recent study it was shown that this effect may be due to decreased circulating IGF-I concentrations [4].

Clinical and Biochemical Findings

These findings are in line with the results of studies in PPAR γ heterozygous-deficient mice, showing a higher trabecular bone volume, a notable absence of marrow fat, and protection against age-related bone loss [5,6]. This hypothesis is further supported by the findings from animal experimental studies showing a decreased osteoblast differentiation in rodents treated with rosiglitazone. Thus, the number of marrow adipocytes increased in response to treatment, whereas the ratio of osteoblasts to osteoclasts decreased causing bone loss [3]. Similarly, treatment with rosiglitazone has been shown to decrease bone mineral density (BMD) in mice [7,8]. Concomitantly with decreased BMD, treatment may change bone morphology, as a decreased trabecular number and an increase in trabecular spacing has been reported [8].

There are only few studies on the effects of glitazones on human bone. Most recently, the results of a 14-week randomized, double-blind, placebo-controlled trial was published [9]. The study included 50 healthy postmenopausal women in whom treatment with rosiglitazone 8 mg/day caused a 1.7% (95% CI 0.6–2.7 $p < 0.01$) decrease in BMD at the total hip compared with placebo. BMD at the lumbar spine also decreased, but did not differ significantly between groups (1.0%, 95% CI –0.2–2.3, $p = 0.13$) at the end of treatment. However, compared with placebo, treatment caused an approximately 10% ($p < 0.05$) decrease in levels of biochemical markers of bone formation (osteocalcin and procollagen type I N-terminal propeptide), whereas markers of bone resorption did not change in response to treatment [9]. The findings from the randomized controlled trial are in line with the results from a previous cohort study showing that treatment with glitazones is associated with an approximately 50% increased annualized rate of bone loss in elderly diabetic women, but not in men [10]. The reason for a potential differential effect of glitazones in women and men is not clear. It may be due to the fact that women compared with men have an increased bone turnover, and therefore the consequence of a reduced osteoblastic activity is more pronounced. In addition, glitazones may affect the synthesis of sex steroids, as they have been shown to inhibit the aromatase pathway, which is the main source for oestrogen in postmenopausal women [11]. Moreover, in women with polycystic ovary syndrome glitazones decrease testosterone levels, whereas the effect on testosterone levels in men is largely unknown [12].

Most importantly, treatment with glitazones seems to increase risk of fracture. Thus, in the ADOPT study, 4 years of treatment with rosiglitazone caused an increased risk of fractures in women, but not in men, in the foot and at the upper limb, involving the humerus and hand [13]. The risk of fracture was approximately doubled compared with treatment with either metformin or glyburide [13]. Moreover, in a subsequent interim analysis of fractures in a large, ongoing, controlled clinical trial, preliminary analysis are reported as being consistent with the results from the ADOPT-study (http://www.fda.gov/MEDWATCH/SAFETY/2007/Avandia_GSK_Ltr.pdf).

Conclusion

An increasing body of evidence suggests that therapy with glitazones exerts detrimental skeletal effects, by inhibiting bone formation. This may worsen bone loss and increase fracture risk. Importantly, most antiosteoporotic treatments act by inhibiting osteoclast activity (so called antiresorptive therapies). Therefore, conventional treatment against osteoporosis may not compensate for an impaired osteoblast function induced by treatment with a glitazone. Taking into account the widespread use of glitazones, there is an urgent need for further studies on skeletal effects, and whether current anti-fracture treatment regimes are able to reduce fracture risk in patients on treatment with glitazones.

References

1. Nuttall ME, Patton AJ, Olivera DL, Nadeau DP, Gowen M. Human trabecular bone cells are able to express both osteoblastic and adipocytic phenotype: implications for osteopenic disorders. J Bone Miner Res 1998;13:371–382.
2. Lecka-Czernik B, Moerman EJ, Grant DF, Lehmann JM, Manolagas SC, Jilka RL. Divergent effects of selective peroxisome proliferator-activated receptor-{gamma}2 ligands on adipocyte versus osteoblast differentiation. Endocrinology 2002;143:2376–2384.
3. Ali AA, Weinstein RS, Stewart SA, Parfitt AM, Manolagas SC, Jilka RL. Rosiglitazone causes bone loss in mice by suppressing osteoblast differentiation and bone formation. Endocrinology 2005;146:1226–1235.
4. Lecka-Czernik B, Ackert-Bicknell C, Adamo ML, Marmolejos V, Churchill GA, Shockley KR, Reid IR, Grey A, Rosen CJ. Activation of peroxisome proliferator-activated receptor {gamma} (ppar{gamma}) by rosiglitazone suppresses components of the insulin-like growth factor regulatory system in vitro and in vivo. Endocrinology 2007;148:903–911.
5. Akune T, Ohba S, Kamekura S, Yamaguchi M, Chung Ui, Kubota N, Terauchi Y, Harada Y, Azuma Y, Nakamura K, Kadowaki T, Kawaguchi H. PPAR {gamma} insufficiency enhances osteogenesis through osteoblast formation from bone marrow progenitors. J Clin Investig 2004;113:846–855.
6. Bennett CN, Longo KA, Wright WS, Suva LJ, Lane TF, Hankenson KD, MacDougald OA. Regulation of osteoblastogenesis and bone mass by Wnt10b. Proc Natl Acad Sci USA 2005;102: 3324–3329.
7. Soroceanu MA, Miao D, Bai XY, Su H, Goltzman D, Karaplis AC. Rosiglitazone impacts negatively on bone by promoting osteoblast/osteocyte apoptosis. J Endocrinol 2004;183:203–216.
8. Rzonca SO, Suva LJ, Gaddy D, Montague DC, Lecka-Czernik B. Bone is a target for the antidiabetic compound rosiglitazone. Endocrinology 2004;145: 401–406.
9. Grey A, Bolland M, Gamble G, Wattie D, Horne A, Davidson J, Reid IR. The peroxisome-proliferator-activated receptor-gamma agonist rosiglitazone decreases bone formation and bone mineral density in healthy postmenopausal women: a randomized, controlled trial. J. Clin Endocrinol Metab 2007;92: 1305–1310.
10. Schwartz AV, Sellmeyer DE, Vittinghoff E, Palermo L, Lecka-Czernik B, Feingold KR, Strotmeyer ES, Resnick HE, Carbone L, Beamer BA, Park SW, Lane NE, Harris TB, Cummings SR, for the Health AaBCHAS. Thiazolidinedione use and bone loss in older diabetic adults. J Clin Endocrinol Metab 2006;91:3349–3354.
11. Rubin GL, Zhao Y, Kalus AM, Simpson ER. Peroxisome proliferator-activated receptor {{gamma}} ligands inhibit estrogen biosynthesis in human breast adipose tissue: possible implications for breast cancer therapy. Cancer Res 2000;60:1604–1608.
12. Azziz R, Ehrmann D, Legro RS, Whitcomb RW, Hanley R, Fereshetian AG, O'Keefe M, Ghazzi MN. troglitazone improves ovulation and hirsutism in the

polycystic ovary syndrome: a multicenter, double blind, placebo-controlled trial. J Clin Endocrinol Metab 2001;86:1626–1632.
13. Kahn SE, Haffner SM, Heise MA, Herman WH, Holman RR, Jones NP, Kravitz BG, Lachin JM, O'Neill MC, Zinman B, Viberti G, the ADOPT Study Group. Glycemic durability of rosiglitazone, metformin, or glyburide monotherapy. N Engl J Med 2006;355:2427–2443.

Section: Notes from Major Pharmaceutical Companies (all major companies asked to participate)

27
Achieving Guideline Control with New Pharmacotherapies: Albumin-Binding by Acylation of Insulin and GLP-1

Mads Krogsgaard Thomsen

The Need for Control

Over the last 15 years, it has become apparent that substantial reduction in the risk of micro- and macro-vascular complications follows from intensified treatment regimens in type 1 and 2 diabetes [1–3]. In simple terms, reducing HbA1c from 9% to 7% in patients with type 1 diabetes leads to an approximate halving of the risk of angiopathy-related diabetic complications [1,2].

Unfortunately, the flipside of the coin is the high risk of hypoglycaemia and weight gain associated with bringing HbA1c below the target of 7%, which is now recommended [1,2,4]. Since it is well-established that glycaemic control deteriorates during oral anti-diabetic drug therapy [5], recent research at Novo Nordisk has focused heavily on improving the pharmacodynamic profile of insulin and GLP-1, two human hormones that are known to provide superior blood glucose control over extended treatment periods [4,6]. Specifically, research has aimed at discovering predictable, long-acting compounds while minimizing the risk of hypoglycaemia and weight increase that together represent the treatment-related complications that are the most feared by patients [7].

Discovery of Insulin Detemir and Liraglutide by Fatty Acid Derivatization

None of the classical approaches (precipitation of acidic analogues and polymer-based protraction) fulfilled the full list of selection criteria that was

1. Efficacy based on ability to bring patients to target HbA1c
2. Predictability of response as assessed by FPG variability
3. Durability as assessed by glucose control after one daily injection
4. Low or no rate of hypoglycaemia in spite of target achievement
5. Body weight maintenance or reduction during therapy
6. Good local tolerability as assessed by low risk of injection site reactions and antibody formation
7. Convenient administration as estimated by lack of need for re- suspension/reconstitution, and injection *via* >30 G needle.

Albumin-binding represents a classical mechanism of protraction of small molecule drugs [8] and furthermore, peptide hormones are known to circulate in the human body bound to albumin due to endogenous acylation with a fatty acid [9]. Based on this, it was tempting to follow a drug discovery strategy of protracting and smoothening the profile of insulin and GLP-1 by attaching a tailor-made fatty acid to the protein backbone. It was early on realized that the fatty acid charge, lipophilicity and distance from the protein backbone were among the factors crucial for achieving the desired predictable, long-acting anti-hyperglycaemic profile [10,11].

The benefit of a long and predictable half-life is related to the buffering capacity of albumin [12], and the associated favourable safety profile is related to a large excess of fatty acid binding sites on albumin at therapeutic levels of insulin/GLP-1, leading to a minimal risk of drug displacement interactions [10,12].

During the drug discovery process, the insulin/GLP-1 selection criteria were not fulfilled until numerous fatty acid chain lengths and structures had been tested in a multi-year process. The discovery of insulin detemir (Levemir) was accomplished by adding the C14 length myristic acid to Lysine at position B29 in des-B30 human insulin [10], whereas liraglutide was created as a human GLP-1 analogue by selectively adding a C16 fatty acid to GLP-1 at position 26 [11]. For use in type 2 diabetes, both compounds are characterized as being neutral and soluble, and both having a predictable 24-h action profile with good local tolerability and lack of neutralizing antibodies [6,12].

Clinical Profile of Insulin Detemir

The day-to-day variability in the glucose-lowering effect of basal insulins is a major problem in the management of diabetes [13]. To assess differences between marketed basal insulin products, a euglycaemic clamp study was performed in type 1 diabetic subjects [14]. When compared with insulin glargine and NPH insulin, insulin detemir was found to exhibit significantly less within-subject variability as regards both pharmacokinetic and dynamic parameters [14]. For insulin detemir, the approximate 50% reduction in the coefficient of variation has been observed to correlate with a reduction in the occurrence of nocturnal hypoglycaemia of about 50%, both in type 1 [15] and type 2 [16] diabetes, as shown in Fig. 1. In the presence of identical glucose control, overall hypoglycaemia was reduced by 25–45% in the insulin detemir arm of the two analogue versus human insulin comparator trials [15,16].

Obesity represents a global epidemic that drives the type 2 diabetes problem of today and historically, insulin therapy has – due to its adipogenic effect and reduced glucosuria – been considered to be associated with aggravation of the problem [17]. A body weight difference in favour of insulin detemir has been a finding of statistical significance in every insulin detemir trial conducted [12]. Furthermore, it appears that the weight benefit of insulin detemir increases with increasing BMI, albeit the underlying mechanism remains a matter for further investigation:

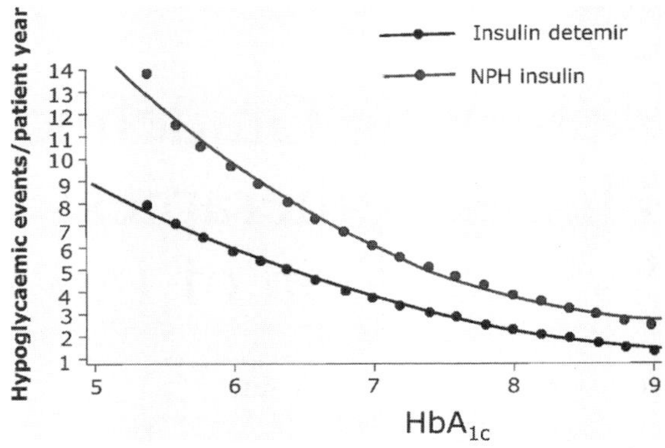

FIG. 1. Relationship between incidence of hypoglycaemia (Confirmed minor and major events, excluding "symptoms only") in the previous 12 weeks of the study and A1C at end point, as modelled using negative-binomial distribution with a log-link function. (copyright © 2006 American Diabetes Association from Diabetes Care®, Vol. 29, 2006; 1269–1274. Reprinted with permission from The American Diabetes Association).

- CNS-mediated satiety response related to insulin detemir crossing the blood-brain barrier
- Hepato-selectivity related to preferential distribution of the albumin-bound insulin detemir to the liver
- Reduced snacking due to predictable 24-h plasma profile of insulin detemir, with reduced hypoglycaemia risk.

The above-mentioned phase 1–3 findings related to glucose control, predictability and lack of weight gain have recently been confirmed in a major observational study of 30,000 type 1 and 2 diabetes patients.

Clinical Profile of liraglutide

Prolongation of the 2-min half-life of native human GLP-1 was achieved through a rational analysis of the structure–activity relationship of numerous fatty acid-derivatized human GLP-1 analogues that showed resistance to DPPIV-mediated inactivation and avoided renal clearance through binding to albumin that exceeds the molecular threshold for glomerular filtration [11].

Based on the above, as well as the observation of pronounced weight reduction in obese rats [18], liraglutide was selected for further development. Early clinical studies subsequently revealed

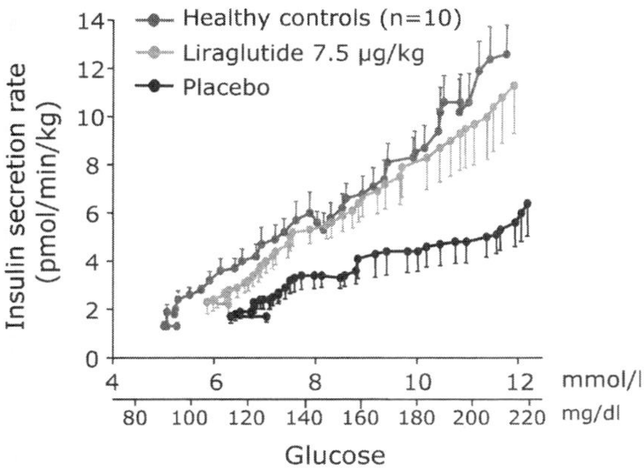

FIG. 2. Type 2 diabetes patients ($n = 10$) received a single injection of liraglutide or placebo (crossover trial) 9 h before a 3-h graded glucose infusion. β-cell sensitivity, as assessed by insulin secretion, was measured during graded glucose infusion. Liraglutide restored β-cell responsiveness, only when glucose was elevated. (copyright © 2003 American Diabetes Association from Diabetes®, Vol. 52, 2003; 1786–1791. Reprinted with permission from The American Diabetes Association).

that liraglutide acts to reduce both fasting and postprandial glucose in type 2 diabetic subjects in a glucose-dependent manner [19]. Figure 2 shows a clamp study assessing the insulin secretory rate that was profoundly reduced in patients with type 2 diabetes. Intriguingly, liraglutide improved insulin secretion to the level of healthy controls, with insulin secretion approaching zero as glucose was lowered to the normal level.

Recently, results from a 14-week study, with HbA1c at baseline of approximately 8.5%, have demonstrated an HbA1c reduction of 1.75% in the absence of any cases of minor or major hypoglycaemia [6]. Treatment success rate, defined as the proportion of patients achieving HbA1c of 7% or less in the absence of hypoglycaemia during the preceding 12 weeks, was 50% and thus exceeds that reported for other diabetes drug classes at this baseline HbA1c.

Weight reduction of around 3 kg bodyweight following treatment with liraglutide for 12 weeks has been observed, thus being consistent with the preclinical findings [18] that are assumed to relate primarily to the specific satiety-promoting effect of liraglutide at the hypothalamic level [6].

The placebo-corrected level of gastrointestinal side effects was below 10% and consistently with previous studies, no antibody formation was observed [20].

In conclusion, the technology of attaching tailor-made fatty acids through site-selective acylation of insulin and GLP-1 has proven to provide new and long-acting pharmacotherapies with superior properties.

References

1. The Diabetes Control and Complications Trial Research Group. The effect of intensive treatment of diabetes on the development and progression of long-term complications in insulin-dependent diabetes mellitus. N Engl J Med 1993;329:977–986.
2. The Diabetes Control and Complications Trial/Epidemiology of Diabetes Interventions and complications (DCCT/EDIC) Study Research Group. Intensive diabetes treatment and cardiovascular disease in patients with type 1 diabetes. N Engl J Med 2005;353:2643–2653.
3. UK prospective Diabetes Study (UKPDS) Group. Intensive blood-glucose with sulphonylureas or insulin compared with conventional treatment and risk of complications in patients with type 2 diabetes (UKPDS 33). Lancet 1998;352:837–853.
4. Nathan DM, Buse JB, Davidson MB, Heine RJ, Holman RR, Sherwin R, Zinman B. Management of hyperglycaemia in type 2 diabetes: a consensus algorithm for the initiation and adjustment of therapy. Diabetologia 2006;49:1711–1721.
5. Cook MN, Girman CJ, Stein PP, Alexander CM, Holman RR. Glycemic control continues to deteriorate after sulfonylureas are added to metformin among patients with type 2 diabetes. Diabetes Care 2005;28:995–1000.
6. Drucker DJ, Nauck MA. The incretin system: glucagon-like peptide-1 receptor agonists and dipeptidyl peptidase-4 inhibitors in type 2 diabetes. Lancet 2006;368:1696–1705.
7. Gonder-Frederick LA et al. Predictors of fear of hypoglycemia in adolescents with type 1 diabetes and their parents. Pediatric Diabetes 2006;7:215–222.
8. Ghuman J, Zunszain PA, Petitpas I, Bhattacharya AA, Otagiri M, Curry S. Structural basis of the drug-binding specificity of human serum albumin. J Mol Biol 2005;353:38–52.
9. Kojima M, Hosoda H, Date Y, Nakazato M, Matsuo H, Kangawa K. Ghrelin is a growth-hormone-releasing acylated peptide from stomach. Nature 1999;404:656–660.
10. Kurtzhals P, Havelund S, Jonassen I, Kiehr B, Larsen UD, Ribel U, Markussen J. Albumin binding of

insulins acylated with fatty acids: characterization of the ligand-protein interaction and correlation between binding affinity and timing of the insulin effect *in vivo*. Biochem J 1995;312:725–731.

11. Knudsen LB, Nielsen PF, Huusfeldt PO, Johansen NL, Madsen K, Pedersen FZ, Thøgersen H, Wilken M, Agersø H. Potent derivatives of glucagon-like peptide-1 with pharmacokinetic properties suitable for once daily administration. J Med Chem 2000;43:1664–1669.
12. Home P, Kurtzhals P. Insulin detemir: from concept to clinical experience. Expert Opin Pharmacother 2006;7:325–343.
13. Galloway JA, Spradlin CT, Howey DC, Dupre J. Intrasubject differences in pharmacokinetic and pharmacodynamic responses: the immutable problem of present-day treatment. In Diabetes 1985, Serrano-Rios M, Lefebvre PJ, Eds. New York, Excerpta Medica, 1986:877–886.
14. Heise T, Nosek L, Rønn BB, Endahl L, Heinemann L, Kapitza C, Draeger E. Lower within-subject variability of insulin detemir in comparison to NPH insulin and insulin glargine in people with type 1 diabetes. Diabetes 2004;53:1614–1620.
15. Hermansen K, Fontaine P, Kukolja KK, Peterkova V, Leth G, Gall M-A. Insulin analogues (insulin detemir and insulin aspart) versus traditional human insulins (NPH insulin and regular human insulin) in basal-bolus therapy for patients with Type 1 diabetes. Diabetologia 2004;47:622–629.
16. Hermansen K, Davies M, Derezinski T, Martinez G, Clauson P, Home PA. 26-week, randomized, parallel, treat-to-target trial comparing insulin detemir with NPH insulin as add-on therapy to oral glucose-lowering drugs in insulin-naïve people with type 2 diabetes. Diabetes Care 2006;29: 1269–1274.
17. Finkelstein EA, Ruhm CJ, Kosa KM. Economic causes and consequences of obesity. Annu Rev Public Health 2005;26:239–257.
18. Larsen PJ, Fledelius C, Knudsen LB, Tang-Christensen M. Systemic Administration of the long-acting GLP-1 derivative NN2211 induces lasting and reversible weight loss in both normal and obese rats. Diabetes 2001;50:2530–2539.
19. Chang AM, Jakobsen G, Sturis J, Smith MJ, Bloem CJ, An B, Galecki A, Halter JB. The GLP-1 derivative NN2211 restores β-cell sensitivity to glucose in type 2 diabetic patients after single dose. Diabetes 2003;52:1786–1791.
20. Vilsboll T, Exp Opin Investig Drugs 2007;16:231–237.

28
Pharmacotherapy of Diabetes

Post Scriptum by the Editor

Notes on the Past, the Present, and the Future

Editorials in major journals may provide an important review of opinion regarding diabetes and pharmacotherapy of diabetes as well as the nature of treatment. Many years ago Siperstein argued against support of rigid glycemic control. According to Siperstein [1,2] most studies on better glycemic control were inconclusive. This left the clinicians with the impression that complications were related to genetic patterns and not to the phenotypic risk factors occurring with diabetes. Later he argued that the muscle capillary basement membrane could be influenced by the level of blood glucose, but whether this was related also to other organs such as the kidney and the retina was in doubt, thus arguing against results in the important work of Østerby. I believe that this really influenced the clinical practice in the USA for many years.

Thus, Siperstein was a challenge to the architects of the DCCT (Diabetes Control and Complication Trial) and the UKPDS (The United Kingdom Prospective Diabetes Study) study, which later firmly documented that glycemic control was important although also blood pressure was a clear factor involved at least in type 2 diabetes and certainly also according to other studies in type 1 diabetes, especially regarding renal function. Gerich [3] later discussed the role of growth hormone as a possible critical factor for the progression of diabetic retinopathy. We are still missing convincing evidence here, and so far, growth hormone inhibition has not really been documented as beneficial [3]. Immunotherapy has potentially played a role in possible prevention of type 1 diabetes in people at high risk, but so far it has not proven effective [4,5].

A major step forward was the publication of the landmark study, DCCT published in 1993 [6]. The conclusion was that effective treatment lowering blood glucose not merely relieves symptoms, but it is also beneficial in the long run to prevent complications, especially microvascular complications. It was also documented later that macrovascular complications can be reduced considerably by intensified insulin treatment either with pumps or multiple injections [7]. Later this was confirmed as far as type 2 diabetes is concerned in the UKPDS study [8], where they combined the effect of high blood pressure and glucose was documented as the so-called "double jeopardy." Indeed, blood pressure treatment in type 2 diabetes was more efficient than lowering blood glucose; it also came sooner and the relevant editorial also suggested that dyslipidemia was a bad companion. This was confirmed later by the Heart Protection Study from the UK. In 1993, another landmark study was published [9]. It was documented that treatment with Captopril and ACE-inhibitor was somewhat efficient in slowing the progression of diabetic nephropathy in type 1 diabetes. Earlier studies had indicated that blood pressure reduction in general was beneficial and in the author's opinion blood pressure reduction is a key element, but blocking the renin–angiotensin system is an efficient way to reduce the blood pressure in these patients. The effect of Captopril on microalbuminuric patients with type 1 diabetes was also documented [10]. And indeed, early treatment seems to be more effective than waiting to overt nephropathy – a strategy that has been prevailing for many years in Europe. As discussed by Parving, both initiation and progression of diabetic nephropathy are related to poor metabolic control and high blood pressure and there is no major difference between type 1 and type 2 diabetes in this respect. Early intervention is a key issue [11].

Turning to type 2 diabetes, traditional oral treatment and the use of Metformin have been common in Europe for many years, which later came to the USA, as discussed by Crofford [12]. American studies confirmed the beneficial effect, but obviously the contraindications of Metformin should be taken into consideration and regarding long-term complications, only post hoc analyses, as documented in the UKPDS, confirmed the beneficial effect of Metformin. Here again, strict glycemic control is the key issue, but side effects of any treatment should be taken into consideration.

A few years later, another class of antidiabetic drugs came into consideration, namely Troglitazone [13], and there were some reasons for hope but also concerns. This was obviously for Troglitazone (but it is also the case for the newer agents, Rosiglitazone and Proglitazone). A new concern is more fractures by the use of glitazones. Maybe well-known agents being used for many years should be the preference when we are confronted with a difficult situation in treating patients with type 2 diabetes where glycemic control is difficult, often ending up with HbAc1 values around 8% or even more.

A critical issue regarding treatment is pancreas transplantation and later also islet transplantation for diabetic complications [14,15]. There is only one study documenting that renal complications in diabetes as evaluated by biopsies could be reversed by the long-term effect of normalizing blood glucose by pancreas transplantation. However, no beneficial effect on renal function was documented, rather the opposite. Immunosuppressive treatment has side effects and isolated pancreas transplantation is, according to the author, not a real option considering that good metabolic control can be obtained by optimized insulin treatment. As mentioned earlier, a challenge in treatment is a key issue in preventing complications in both type 1 and type 2 diabetes, and therefore in patients at risk of diabetes, the treatment type for blood pressure should be taken into consideration (9,16–20). Turning to another strategy, more and more studies now support the use of agents that block the renin–angiotensin system as the prime agent, which also seems to have some effect on preventing diabetes. It is, however, a consideration that other agents like diuretics and beta-blockers may be involved in an increased risk for type 2 diabetes [16,18].

Prospective studies on the use of ACE and ARBs with beta-blockers or diuretics are of interest, and the ACCOMPLISH study [18] may find the solution for what is the best combination when blocking the renin–angiotensin system for preventing diabetes and associated side effects [19].

Regarding type 2 diabetes, the two studies, RENAAL and IDNT as well as IRMA using ARBs suggested the beneficial effect of these agents. A major issue regarding this study was that ARBs were not compared to ACE-inhibitors, and new studies therefore suggest that the effect is very similar [20]. Thus, the use ACE-I and ARBs was discussed by William E. Mitch [20]. Both seem to be effective and Barnett studied patients with microalbuminuria and found that ACE-I is just as effective as an ARB. In an interesting study from Bergamo it was shown that ACE-I is quite effective in preventing microalbuminuria in contrast to a CCB [20]. On the other hand, there are so far no such studies using ARBs.

Albuminuria as well as microalbuminuria and macroalbuminuria and indeed also normoalbuminuria in the upper normal range are documented to have a very strong predictive power in predicting vascular damage, not only renal damage but also cardiovascular damage as reviewed by Ritz [21]. The key issue in reducing cardiovascular risk in type 2 diabetes is, however, to use a multifactorial intensified intervention strategy, especially in microalbuminuric patients considering not only glycemic control, but also lipid control and blood pressure control, as suggested in the UKPDS study. The STENO II [22] study documented the beneficial effect on cardiovascular end point, but after 7.8 not on total mortality. However, this was found after 13 years of follow-up with a clear-cut effect on mortality in general. The STENO II is a paradigm shift study: it documented that the best way to reduce cardiovascular risks in type 2 diabetes was to use a multifactorial approach as long as we do not have any effective way to reduce diabetes itself [22].

In the last 2 years some long-term studies regarding the use of glitazones have been published, namely the PROactive study using Proglitazone as well as the ADOPT study using Rosiglitazones. The PROactive study was not really so convincingly positive regarding combined cardiovascular end points. The bad news were oedema and increase of body weight and that the long-term prognosis regarding heart failure is not known [23]. The newer ADOPT study [24] suggested that diabetes could be postponed in at risk patients, but the drug was not compared with the combination of Sulfonylurea and Metformin and obviously the cost of newer drugs is much higher than the well-examined drugs. David Nathan continues in a new editorial that the epidemic of type 2 diabetes is really alarming and we need much more effective treatment of type 2 diabetes with lifestyle measures. This author can only agree with Dr Nathan: "ensuring the effective and cost effective use of medications that have already been established by high quality clinical trial to control glycemia and to prevent diabetes should have a high priority than flowing the market with ever more medications" [25]. The same is the case regarding diabetic complications where already established drugs are effective. In the ADOPT study it was clear that both Metformin and Sulfonylurea were quite effective. Interestingly, Sulfonylurea was associated with fewer long-term diabetic complications [24], including coronary heart disease [26,27]. The effect of Rosiglitazone to delay progression to diabetes was not persistent when the drug was discontinued as shown in a follow-up of the DREAM study, which was reported at the IDF congress in Cape Town. Long-term preventive treatment with Rosiglitazone in pre-diabetes is, according to these authors, out of the question.

Indeed, the use of glitazones has been found to be associated with increased risk of fractures in women, both in the ADOPT study and in the PROactive study [28] as inferred by FDA (http://www.fda.gov/medwater). Effectiveness and the costs per life saved as well as unwanted effects are of importance. Indeed, Rosiglitazone may increase the risk of MI and death from CV-disease [29] as well as heart failure [30].

The following is a list summarizing some ongoing trials in diabetes.

Some ongoing trials in diabetes

Acronym	Head investigator	Sponsor	Purpose	Patients (n)	Trial ends
ACCOMPLISH	Kenneth A. Jameson	Novartis	Comparing first-line treatment (also to prevent DM)	Patients with hypertension and risk for CV disease (12,600)	2009
ACCORD (Action for Central CV-risk in Diabetes)	ACCORD investigators	NIH/NHLBI/ NIDDK	(a) Better Hba1c, and/or (b) better SBP, and/or (c) use of fenofibrate + statin vs. statin alone.	T2 DM patients (10,251)	2010
ADDITION	Torben LauritzenKnut Borch-Johnsen	Multiple sponsors	Multifactorial intervention	T2 DM patients (3,000)	2010
ADVANCE	John Chalmers Stephen MacMahon	Servier/NHMRC Australia	Factorial 2×2 design on BP and BG control	T2 DM patients (11,140)	2007 (BP) 2008 (BG)
ALTITUDE	Hans-Henrik Parving	Novartis	Effect on renin-inhibition on high -risk diabetic patients	T2 DM patients (8,600)	2008
AVOID	Hans-Henrik Parving	Novartis	Change in albuminuria with Aliskiren	T2 DM patients (600)	2007
BARI 2D	–	NIKKD & NHBLI	T2 DM sensitizer versus insulin secretagogues	(2800) T2 DM	2007

(*continued*)

Some ongoing trials in diabetes—*Continued*

Acronym	Head investigator	Sponsor	Purpose	Patients (*n*)	Trial ends
DIRECT	AK Sjølie	AstraZeneca	Candesartan effect on retinopathy	T2 DM (1,421)	2008
EDIT	–	–	Comparison of Met. and Acarbose	T2 DM (631)	–
HEART 2D	–	Lilly	Post MI Type of insulin	T2 DM (1,355)	2008
LEVEMIR in pregnancy	Elisabeth Mathiesen	Novo	Diabetic glycemic control in pregnancy	–	–
NANSY	–	–	Treatment with gliclazide	FPG - 5.6–6 (2000)	–
NAVIGATOR	Rury Holman et al.	Novartis	Valsartan and/or Nateglinide vs. placebo	IGT (9,578)	2007
ONTARGET	–	Boehringer Ingelheim	Comparison of Telmisartan vs. Ramipril vs. dual blockade	(also DM) (25,600)	2008–9
ORIGIN	ORIGIN investigators	Sanofi Aventis	Glargine vs. standard and Omega 3 PUFA vs. placebo	IGT or DM (12,612)	2010
PHIDIAS	Alberto Zanchetti	Ministry of Health, Italy	Prevention of diabetes by lifestyle + blocking RAS	At risk persons	2011
PLANET	Dick de Zeeuw	AstraZeneca	Comparison of Crestor and Lipitor on albuminuria	T1 + T2 + proteinuria	2008
RASS	Michael Mauer	NIH/Merck	Renal biopsy and retinopathy study ARB vs. ACEi	T1 DM with normoalb. (285)	2007
RECORD	Philip Home	GSK	Comparing Rosi/ SU/Met	T2DM (4500)	2009
SHARP	Rory Collins Collin Baigent (Oxford)	Merck/ Schering Plough	Statin on CV and renal progression ± Ezetimile	Not only diabetes	–
SMART	A. Kashiwagi Shiga University	None	Microalb. Reduction ARB/CCB	T2 DM (150)	2007
SUN – overt nephropathy Keryx 4001	Ed Lewis	Keryx	Time to doubling of S-creatinine on Sulodexide	T2 DM with proteinuria (2,240)	2012
SUN-micro Keryx 301	Ed lewis	Keryx	Change in microalb.	T2 DM (–)	2008
Transcend	–	Boehringer Ingelheim	Comparison of Telmisartan vs. placebo	(some diabetics) (5,304)	2008
TREAT	Marc Pfeffer	Amgen	Darbepoetin in diabetic nephropathy	T2 DM patients (4,000)	2010
VA DT	Carlos Abraira	VA	Better control and better HbA1c	T2 DM (1,800)	2009
VITAL	Dick de Zeeuw	Abbott	Albuminuria reduction with Paricalcitol	T2 DM (258)	–

The list cannot be completed, but it gives an overview of some ongoing trials. It is, however, unlikely they will provide a breakthrough in the treatment of diabetes. Progress is more likely to come from mechanistic studies in clinical and experimental medicine: Serendipity. Interestingly, the most recent interim request on the Record-study did not find increased mortality from Rosiglitazone [31].

References

1. Siperstein MD, Foster DW, Knowles HC *et al.* Control of blood glucose and diabetic vascular disease. *N Engl J Med* 1977;296(1):1060–1063.
2. Siperstein MD. Diabetic microangiopathy and the control of blood glucose. *N Engl J Med* 1983;309:1577–1579.
3. Gerich JF. Role of growth hormone in diabetes mellitus. *N Engl J Med* 1984;310(13):848–850.
4. Fathman CG, Myers BD. Cyclosporine therapy for autoimmune disease. *N Engl J Med* 1992; 327(4):271–273.
5. Gale EAM. Can we change the course of beta-cell destruction in type 1 diabetes? *N Engl J Med* 2002;346:1740–1741.
6. Lasker RD. The diabetes control and complications trial – implications for policy and practice. *New Engl J Med* 1993;329:1035–1036.
7. William T and Cefalu MD. Glycemic control and cardiovascular disease – should we reassess clinical goals? *New Engl J Med* 2005;353:2707–2709.
8. Mogensen CE. Combined high blood pressure and glucose in type 2 diabetes: double jeopardy. British trials show clear effects of treatment, especially blood pressure reduction. *Br Med J*; 1998; 317:693–694.
9. Remuzzi G. Slowing the progression of diabetic nephropathy. *N Engl J Med* 1993;329:1496–1497.
10. Viberti CG. A glycemic threshold for diabetic complications? *N Engl J Med* 1995;332:1293–1294.
11. Parving H-H. Initiation and progression of diabetic nephropathy. *N Engl J Med* 1996;335:1682–1683.
12. Crofford OB. Metformin. *N Engl J Med* 1995;333:588–589.
13. Imura H. A novel antidiabetic drug – troglitazone – reason for hope and concern. *N Engl J Med* 1998;338:908–909.
14. Luzi L. Pancreas Transplantation and diabetic complications. *N Engl J Med* 1998;339:115–117.
15. Robertson RP. Successful islet transplantation for patients with diabetes – fact or fantasy? *N Engl J Med* 2000;343:289–290.
16. Bakris GL. Antihypertensive therapy and the risk of type 2 diabetes mellitus. *N Engl J Med* 2000;342: 969–970.
17. Ingelfinger JR, Solomon CG. Angiotensin-converting-enzyme inhibitors for impaired glucose tolerance – is there still hope? *N Engl J Med* 355:1608–1610.
18. Jamerson KH, Bakris GL, Wun C-C *et al.* Rationale and design of the avoiding cardiovascular events through combination therapy in patients living with systolic hypertension (ACCOMPLISH) trial. *Am J Hypertens* 2004;17:793–801.
19. Hostetter TH. Prevention of end-stage renal disease due to type 2 diabetes. *N Engl J Med* 2001;345:910–911.
20. Mitch WE. Treating diabetic nephropathy is – are there only economic issues. *N Engl J Med* 2004;35: 348:1934–1936.
21. Ritz E. Albuminuria and vascular damage – the vicious twins. *N Engl J Med* 2003;348:2349–2351.
22. Solomon CG. Reducing cardiovascular risk in type 2 diabetes. *N Engl J Med* 2003;348:457–459.
23. Yki-Järvinen H. The PROactive study: some answers, many questions. *The Lancet* 2005;366:1241–1242.
24. Nathan DM. Thiazolidinediones for initial treatment of type 2 diabetes. *N Engl J Med* 2006;355:2477–2480.
25. Nathan DM. Finding new treatments for diabetes – how many, how fast . . . how good? *N Engl J Med* 356:437–440.
26. Berry C, Tardif J-C, Bourassa MG. Coronary heart disease in patients with diabetes. part 1: recent advances in prevention and noninvasive management. *J Am Coll Cardiol* 2007;49:631–642.
27. Berry C, Tardif J-C, Bourassa MG. Coronary heart disease in patients with diabetes. part ii: recent advances in coronary revascularization. *J Am Coll Cardiol* 2007;49:643–656.
28. Short R. Fracture risk is a class effect of glitazones. *Br Med J* 2007;334:551.
29. Nissen SE, Wolski K. Effect of rosiglitazone on the risk of myocardial infarction and death from cardiovascular causes. *N Engl J Med* 2007;356:xx–xx.
30. Singh S, Loke YK, Furberg CD. Thiazolidinediones and Heart Failure: A Teleo-Analysis. *Diabetes Care* 2007; DOI:10.2337/dc07–0141.
31. Home PD, Pocock SJ, Beck-Nielsen H, et al. Rosiglitazone evaluated for cardiovascular outcomes – an interim analysis. *N Engl J Med* 2007;DOI: 0.1056/NEJMoa073394.

Index

Printed in the United States of America.